AHA Hospital Statistics™

2014 Edition

AHA Institutional Members $196
Nonmembers $258
AHA Catalog NUMBER 082014
Telephone ORDERS 1-800-AHA-2626

ISSN 0090-6662
ISBN-13: 978-0-87258-922-3

Contents

Acknowledgements
& Advisements

Acknowledgments

The 2014 edition of AHA Hospital Statistics is published by Health Forum, an affiliate of the American Hospital Association, Richard J. Umbdenstock, President and CEO.

Advisements

The data published here should be used with the following advisements: The data are based on replies to an annual survey that seeks a variety of information, not all of which is published in this book. The information gathered by the survey includes specific services, but not all of each hospital's services. Therefore, the data do not reflect an exhaustive list of all services offered by all hospitals. For information on the availability of additional data, please contact Health Forum, (800) 821-2039.

Health Forum does not assume responsibility for the accuracy of information voluntarily reported by the individual institutions surveyed. The purpose of this publication is to provide basic data reflecting the delivery of health care in the United States and associated areas, and is not to serve an official and all-inclusive list of services offered by individual hospitals.

Beyond Health Care
The Economic Contribution of Hospitals

For most people, the hospital "H" connotes care and curing – the 133 million people served in emergency departments, the 34 million patients admitted, the 27 million surgeries performed, the nearly 4 million babies delivered, and the 542 million other outpatients treated.[1] Every year, hospitals provide vital health care services like these to millions of people in thousands of communities. However, many people don't realize that the importance of hospitals to their communities extends far beyond health care.

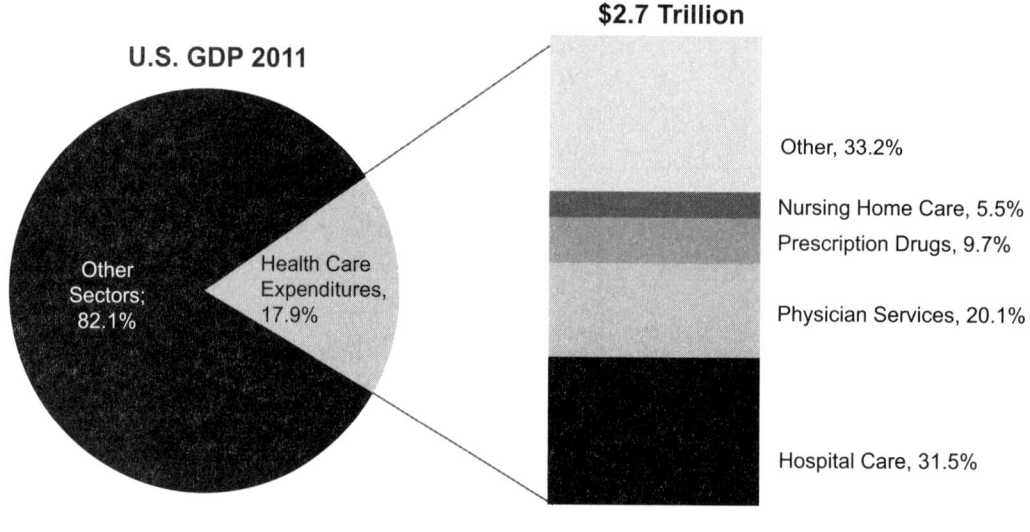

Chart 1: National Health Expenditures as a Percentage of Gross Domestic Product (GDP) and Breakdown of National Health Expenditures, 2011

U.S. GDP 2011

Other Sectors; 82.1%

Health Care Expenditures, 17.9%

$2.7 Trillion

Other, 33.2%

Nursing Home Care, 5.5%

Prescription Drugs, 9.7%

Physician Services, 20.1%

Hospital Care, 31.5%

Source: Centers for Medicare & Medicaid Services, Office of the Actuary. Data released Jan. 9, 2013.

Hospital care is the largest component of the health sector, which itself is a growing segment of the U.S. economy. In 2011, health care represented nearly 18 percent of the gross domestic product (GDP) – a measure of economic output – or approximately $2.7 trillion.[2] Hospitals accounted for $851 billion of that total (Chart 1).[3] The health sector is an economic mainstay providing stability and growth, even during the most recent recession.[4]

In 2012, community hospitals employed nearly 5.6 million people and spent about $380 billion on goods and services in their own and other communities in addition to employee compensation (Chart 2). These purchases and the purchases of hospital workers support other businesses. Nationally, each hospital job supports almost two additional jobs, and every dollar spent by a hospital supports more than $2 of additional business activity.[5] With these "ripple effects" included, hospitals support nearly $2.5 trillion of economic activity (Chart 3).

A strong health care network, in which hospitals play a key role, also adds to the attractiveness of a community as a place to settle, locate a business or retire.

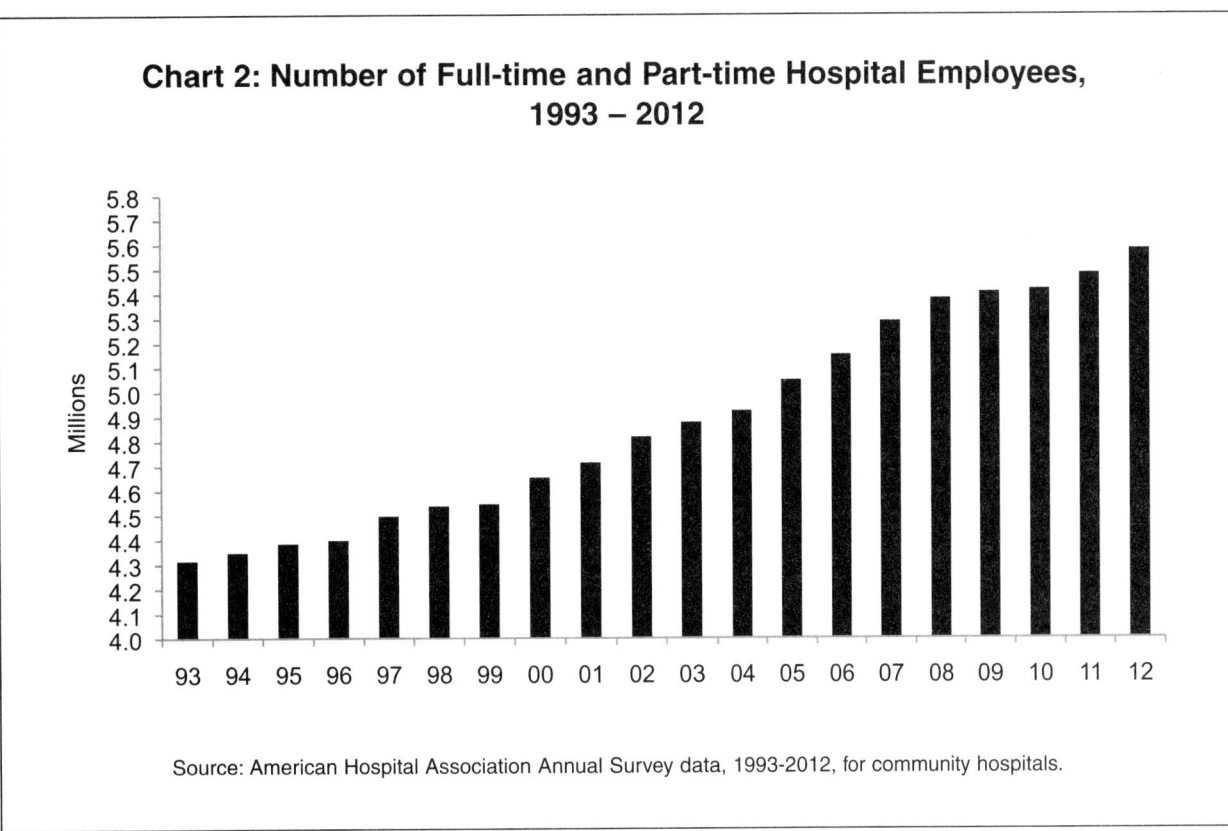

Chart 2: Number of Full-time and Part-time Hospital Employees, 1993 – 2012

Source: American Hospital Association Annual Survey data, 1993-2012, for community hospitals.

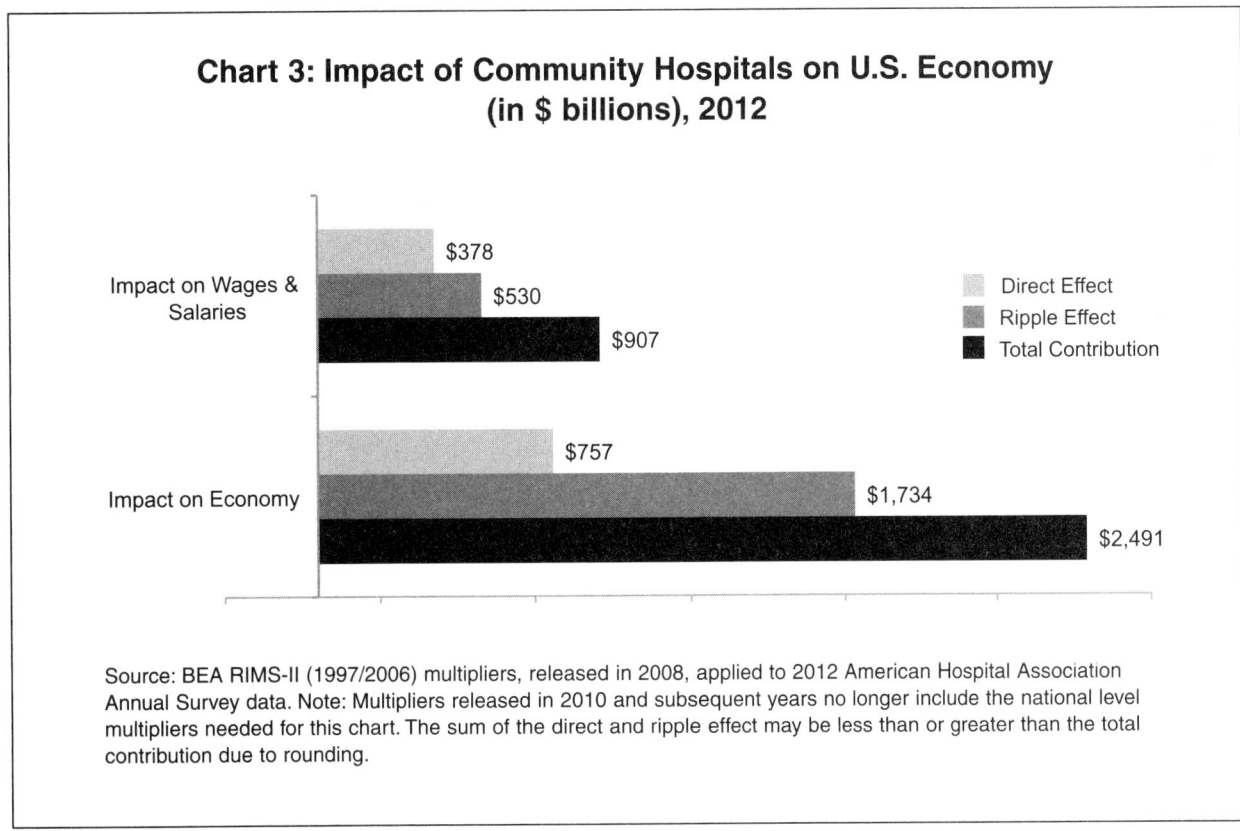

Chart 3: Impact of Community Hospitals on U.S. Economy (in $ billions), 2012

Source: BEA RIMS-II (1997/2006) multipliers, released in 2008, applied to 2012 American Hospital Association Annual Survey data. Note: Multipliers released in 2010 and subsequent years no longer include the national level multipliers needed for this chart. The sum of the direct and ripple effect may be less than or greater than the total contribution due to rounding.

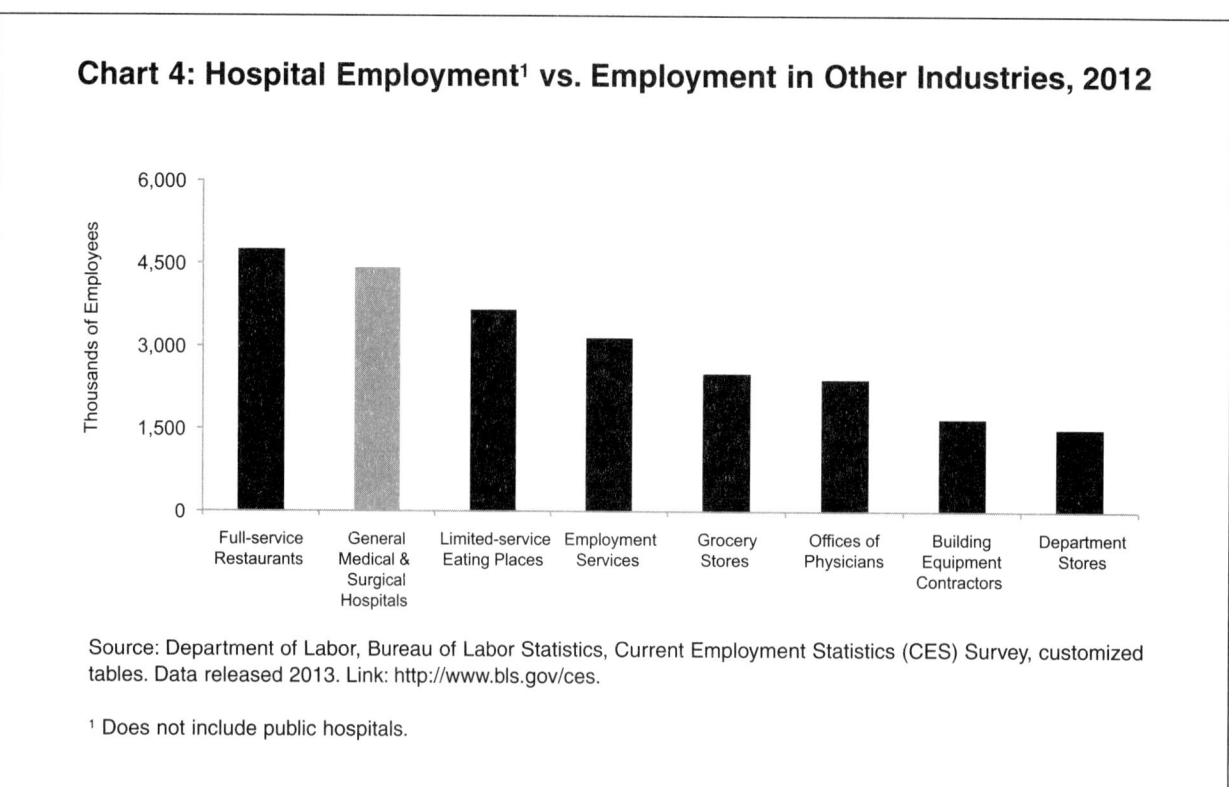

Chart 4: Hospital Employment[1] vs. Employment in Other Industries, 2012

Thousands of Employees

Full-service Restaurants | General Medical & Surgical Hospitals | Limited-service Eating Places | Employment Services | Grocery Stores | Offices of Physicians | Building Equipment Contractors | Department Stores

Source: Department of Labor, Bureau of Labor Statistics, Current Employment Statistics (CES) Survey, customized tables. Data released 2013. Link: http://www.bls.gov/ces.

[1] Does not include public hospitals.

Hospitals Are Among the Largest Employers in Many Communities

More than half of hospital expenses are salaries, wages and benefits. In 2012, U.S. hospitals paid about $378 billion in employee compensation. Hospitals rank second as a source of private sector jobs, behind only full-service restaurants (Chart 4).

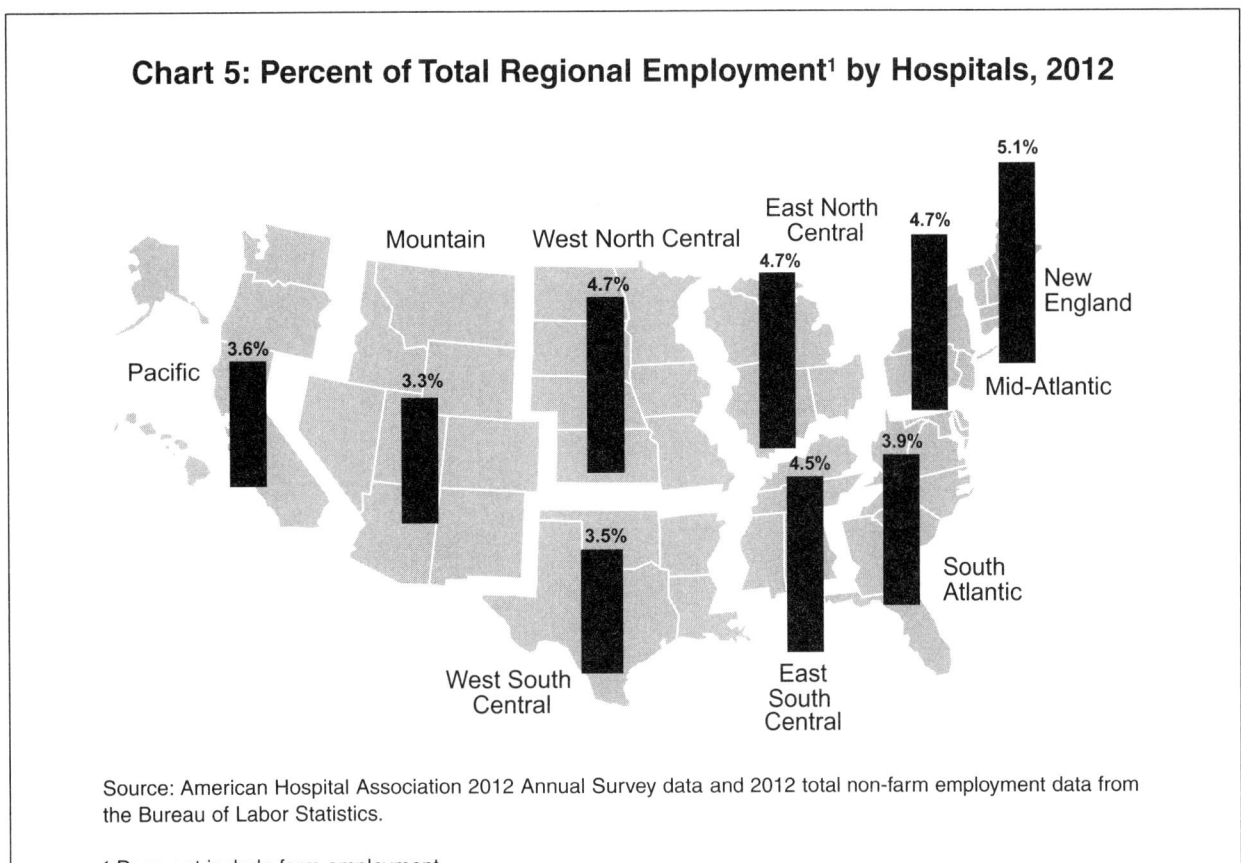

Chart 5: Percent of Total Regional Employment[1] by Hospitals, 2012

Pacific 3.6%

Mountain 3.3%

West North Central 4.7%

East North Central 4.7%

East North Central 4.7%

New England 5.1%

Mid-Atlantic 4.7%

South Atlantic 3.9%

West South Central 3.5%

East South Central 4.5%

Source: American Hospital Association 2012 Annual Survey data and 2012 total non-farm employment data from the Bureau of Labor Statistics.

[1] Does not include farm employment.

Hospitals regularly rank among the top 10 employers in large urban areas, such as Boston, New York and Detroit. The hospitals in the Chicago metropolitan area directly and indirectly support nearly 470,000 jobs.[6] Regionally, hospitals can account for as much as 5 percent of employment (Chart 5).

Hospitals Offer High-quality Jobs and Consistent Job Growth

Hospitals are a large, established source of employment, providing jobs for a wide range of skill levels. Hospitals employ highly-skilled doctors, nurses and therapists, as well as lower-skilled workers in environmental and food services (Chart 6). Earnings of hospital workers, on average, are higher than those of workers in service-producing industries as a whole (Chart 7). Hospitals also furnish benefits, such as health insurance. These benefits are often lacking in other jobs available to lower-skilled workers, such as retail or food service.

Chart 6: Hospital Employment by Occupation Type, 2012[1]

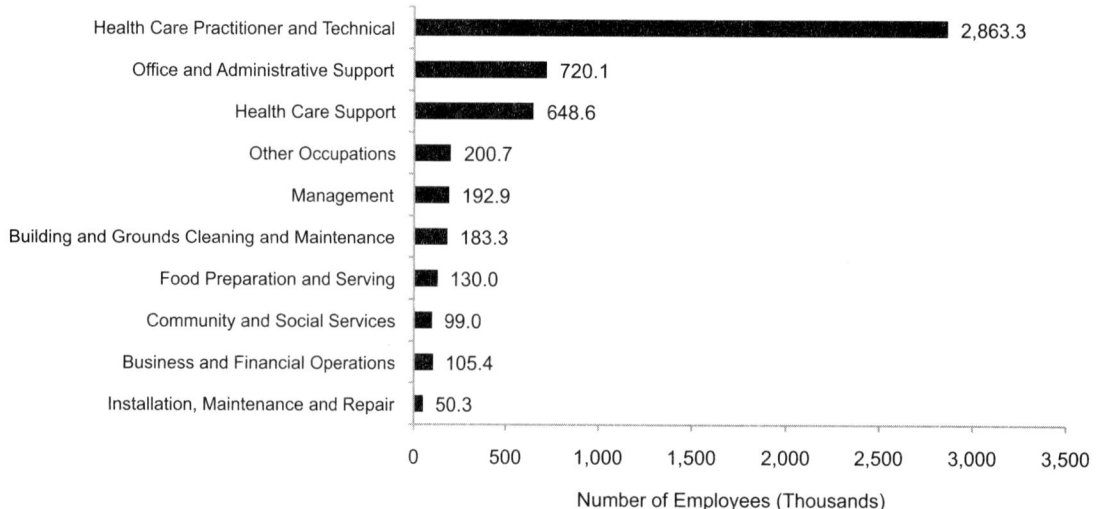

Occupation	Number of Employees (Thousands)
Health Care Practitioner and Technical	2,863.3
Office and Administrative Support	720.1
Health Care Support	648.6
Other Occupations	200.7
Management	192.9
Building and Grounds Cleaning and Maintenance	183.3
Food Preparation and Serving	130.0
Community and Social Services	99.0
Business and Financial Operations	105.4
Installation, Maintenance and Repair	50.3

Source: Department of Labor, Bureau of Labor Statistics, 2012 National Industry-specific Occupational Employment and Wage. Data released March 2013. Link: http://www.bls.gov/oes/current/naics4_622100.htm

[1] Does not include public hospitals.

Chart 7: Average Weekly Earnings of Workers, Hospitals[1,2] vs. All Service-providing Industries, 1992–2012

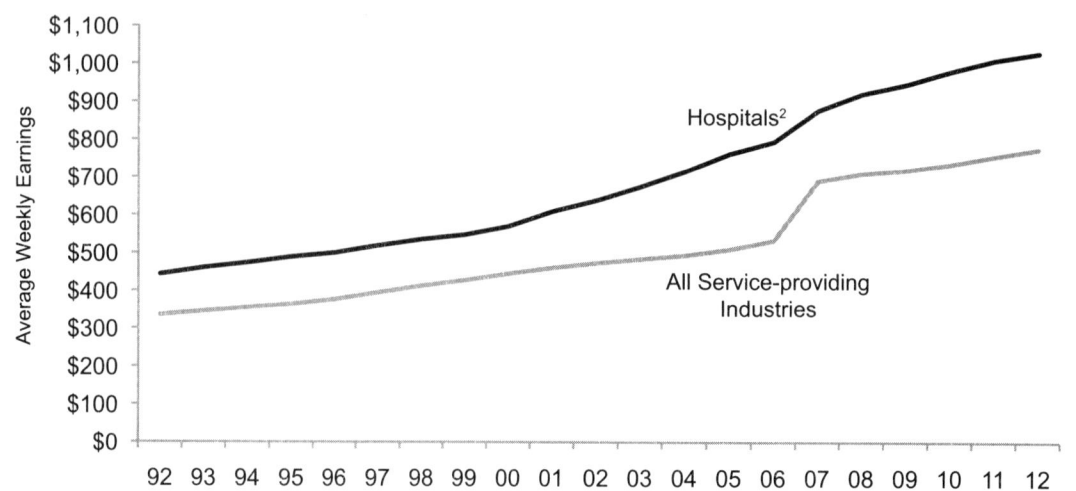

Source: Department of Labor, Bureau of Labor Statistics, Current Employment Statistics (CES) Survey, customized tables. Data released 2013. Link: http://www.bls.gov/ces.

[1] Includes physicians employed by hospitals.
[2] Does not include public hospitals.

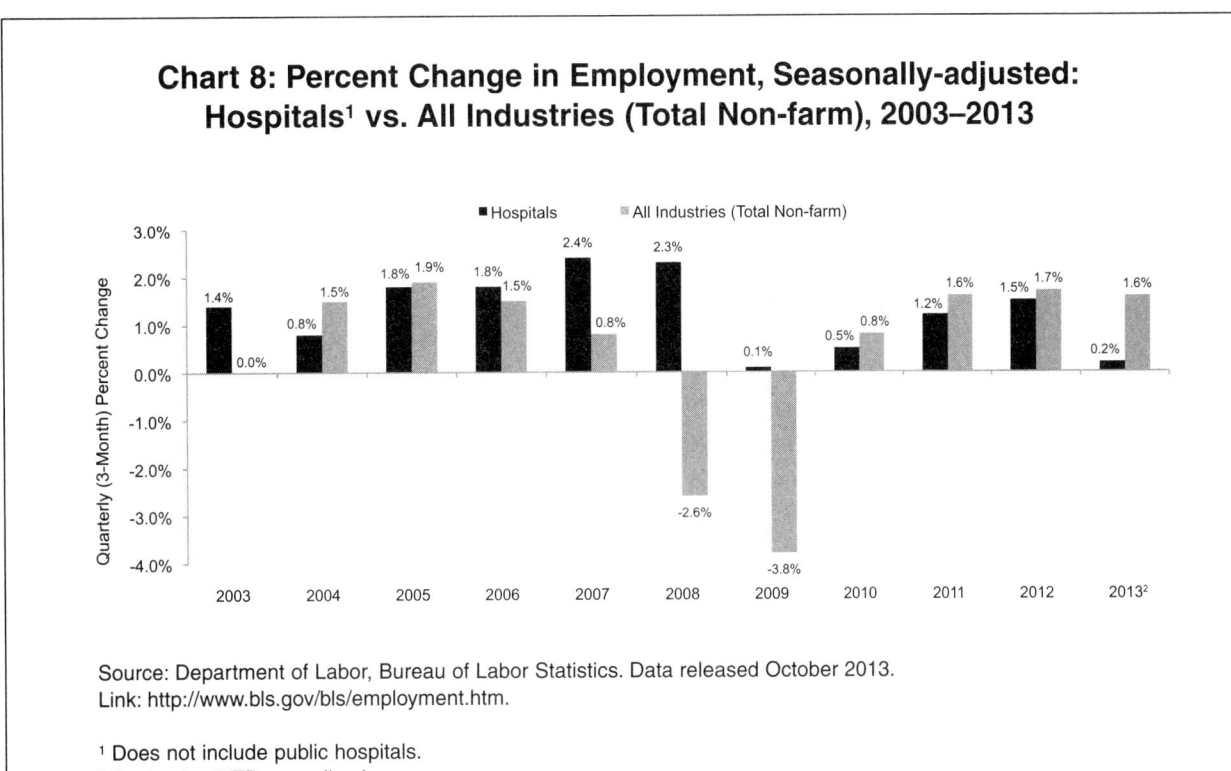

Chart 8: Percent Change in Employment, Seasonally-adjusted: Hospitals[1] vs. All Industries (Total Non-farm), 2003–2013

Source: Department of Labor, Bureau of Labor Statistics. Data released October 2013.
Link: http://www.bls.gov/bls/employment.htm.

[1] Does not include public hospitals.
[2] September YTD annualized.

Hospitals offer a stable source of employment growth, even in times of economic stress. Hospitals had a 2.3 percent increase in employment in 2008, despite the economic downturn, while all non-farm employers experienced a 2.6 percent decline.[7] In 2012, the health care sector overall added more than 320,000 jobs, nearly 15 percent of the job growth in the economy as a whole.[8] However, this stability is at risk with cuts to government health care program payments, such as the sequester, placing increasing stress on hospitals and other providers. In 2013, hospital job growth is down significantly (Chart 8).

Facing a future shortage of skilled workers, hospitals are investing in workforce development and retention activities – another way hospitals contribute to the economic base of communities. Some hospitals offer tuition reimbursement programs, partner with local colleges to provide training programs for employees to update or develop their skills, or implement mentoring programs for less experienced staff.

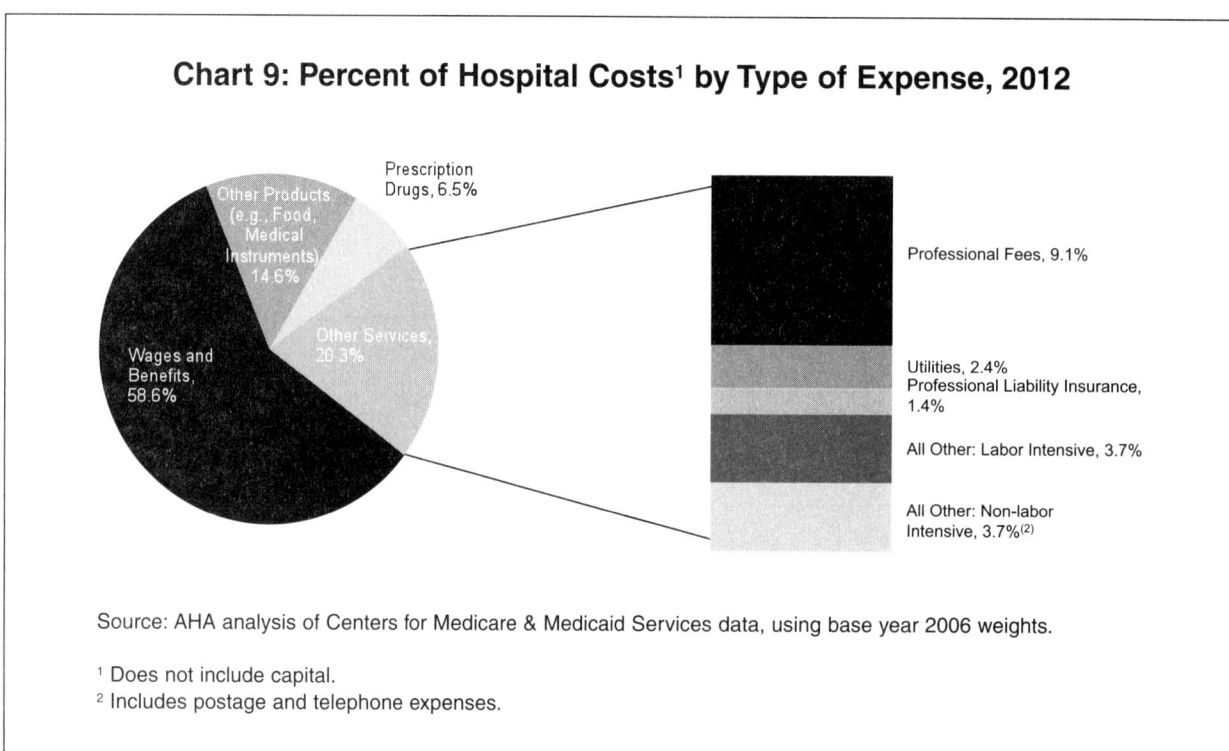

Chart 9: Percent of Hospital Costs[1] by Type of Expense, 2012

Prescription Drugs, 6.5%

Other Products (e.g., Food, Medical Instruments), 14.6%

Wages and Benefits, 58.6%

Other Services, 20.3%

Professional Fees, 9.1%

Utilities, 2.4%
Professional Liability Insurance, 1.4%

All Other: Labor Intensive, 3.7%

All Other: Non-labor Intensive, 3.7%[2]

Source: AHA analysis of Centers for Medicare & Medicaid Services data, using base year 2006 weights.

[1] Does not include capital.
[2] Includes postage and telephone expenses.

Hospital Expenditures Stimulate Economies

The economic contribution of hospitals extends beyond the people they directly employ, the goods and services they purchase and the taxes they pay (Chart 9).

Hospitals also support other businesses through so-called "ripple effects" that are generated in three ways:

- *Hospitals purchase goods and services,* such as drugs, information technology, food, bed linens and "bricks and mortar," from other businesses in their communities. Those purchases create revenue for local businesses and jobs and income for their employees.

- *Hospitals provide income for employees.* Hospital employees spend their paychecks on goods and services, such as cars, household appliances and groceries. These purchases generate income and create jobs for other businesses in the community.

- *Wages and salaries paid by hospitals are subject to federal, state and local taxes (e.g., payroll taxes, sales taxes).*

These ripple effects result in jobs and income for other businesses. In 2012, with ripple effects included, hospitals supported a total of 15.6 million jobs and $2.5 trillion of economic activity (Charts 10, 11 and 12).

Chart 10: Impact of Community Hospitals on U.S. Jobs (in millions), 2012

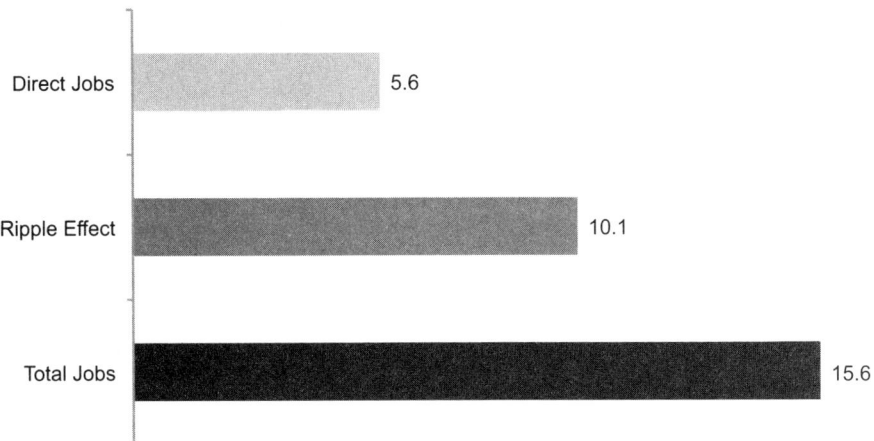

Direct Jobs	5.6
Ripple Effect	10.1
Total Jobs	15.6

Source: BEA RIMS-II (1997/2006) multipliers, released in 2008, applied to 2012 American Hospital Association Annual Survey data. Note: Multipliers released in 2010 and subsequent years no longer include the national level multipliers needed for this chart. The sum of the direct and ripple effect may be less than or greater than the total contribution due to rounding.

Chart 11: Impact of Community Hospitals on U.S. Economy; All States, DC and Total U.S., 2012

State Name	Number of Hospital Jobs (FT and PT)	Multiplier for Employment	Effect of Hospital Jobs on Total Jobs in State Economy	Percent of Total Employment Supported by Hospital Employment	Hospital Payroll and Benefits ($ millions)
Alabama	81,104	2.0293	164,584	8.82%	$4,407
Alaska	11,190	1.8145	20,304	6.18%	$925
Arizona	82,960	2.3261	192,973	8.02%	$5,750
Arkansas	50,683	1.8577	94,154	8.12%	$2,657
California	520,641	2.3233	1,209,605	8.60%	$43,638
Colorado	72,055	2.3607	170,100	7.54%	$5,209
Connecticut	67,078	2.1168	141,991	8.75%	$5,166
Delaware	21,339	2.0789	44,362	10.63%	$1,495
District of Columbia	26,285	1.6374	43,039	5.91%	$2,059
Florida	294,524	2.2413	660,117	9.08%	$19,033
Georgia	138,334	2.3002	318,196	8.20%	$8,646
Hawaii	18,151	2.1635	39,270	6.63%	$1,508
Idaho	28,532	1.886	53,811	8.87%	$1,580
Illinois	241,429	2.2589	545,364	9.63%	$15,533
Indiana	129,882	2.0612	267,713	9.46%	$8,390
Iowa	68,257	1.7103	116,740	7.90%	$3,871
Kansas	54,967	1.7657	97,055	7.27%	$3,347
Kentucky	81,522	2.0314	165,604	9.25%	$4,831
Louisiana	88,300	1.9489	172,088	9.03%	$4,860
Maine	35,789	2.1174	75,780	12.77%	$2,400
Maryland	103,627	2.0626	213,741	8.39%	$6,630
Massachusetts	182,811	2.1805	398,619	12.42%	$11,758
Michigan	210,019	2.2037	462,819	11.76%	$13,312
Minnesota	120,905	2.235	270,223	10.10%	$8,369
Mississippi	58,450	1.8678	109,173	10.02%	$3,511
Missouri	140,819	2.1876	308,056	11.62%	$8,506
Montana	23,463	1.8443	43,273	10.12%	$1,390
Nebraska	42,828	1.7205	73,686	7.81%	$2,394
Nevada	26,196	2.2397	58,671	5.21%	$2,018
New Hampshire	31,965	2.0467	65,423	10.44%	$2,237
New Jersey	143,927	2.2526	324,210	8.41%	$10,390
New Mexico	28,198	2.0145	56,805	7.06%	$1,958
New York	439,222	1.9938	875,721	10.08%	$35,532
North Carolina	175,654	2.2429	393,974	10.04%	$11,044
North Dakota	25,478	1.6142	41,127	10.43%	$1,290
Ohio	282,039	2.2008	620,711	12.21%	$18,228
Oklahoma	60,049	1.9603	117,714	7.59%	$3,393
Oregon	58,244	2.3049	134,247	8.30%	$4,667
Pennsylvania	285,487	2.2071	630,098	11.08%	$17,494
Rhode Island	20,718	2.1003	43,514	9.46%	$1,682
South Carolina	73,990	2.2139	163,806	8.94%	$4,434
South Dakota	23,350	1.5601	36,428	8.97%	$1,395
Tennessee	117,026	2.164	253,244	9.53%	$6,769
Texas	343,203	2.2946	787,514	7.46%	$23,728
Utah	41,007	2.3204	95,153	7.88%	$2,346
Vermont	14,557	1.9799	28,821	9.62%	$1,113
Virginia	113,880	2.0564	234,183	6.36%	$7,756
Washington	113,054	2.2617	255,694	9.07%	$8,590
West Virginia	44,397	1.8046	80,119	10.63%	$2,465
Wisconsin	112,110	2.0695	232,012	8.47%	$7,278
Wyoming	9,712	1.6148	15,683	5.49%	$649
United States*	5,579,407	2.8048	15,649,121	11.70%	$377,633

Source: BEA RIMS-II (2002/2010) multipliers for hospital NAICS Code 622, released 2012, applied to American Hospital Association Annual Survey data for 2012. Hospital jobs are total part-time and full-time jobs. Hospital labor income is defined as payroll plus benefits. The percent of total employment supported by direct and indirect hospital employment is based on 2012 BLS data. Expenditures are defined as total expenditures minus bad debt. In previous years, expenditures were defined as net patient revenue plus other operating revenue.

* Multipliers released in 2010 and subsequent years no longer include the national level multipliers needed for the U.S. summary row. BEA RIMS-II (1997/2006) multipliers released in 2008 and applied to 2012 AHA annual survey data were used instead.

(continued)

State Name	Multiplier for Earnings	Effect of Hospital Payroll and Benefits on Total Labor Income ($ millions)	Hospital Expenditures ($ millions)	Multiplier for Output	Effect of Hospital Expenditures on Total State Economic Output ($ millions)
Alabama	1.6538	$7,288	$9,010	1.9782	$17,823
Alaska	1.4829	$1,372	$1,766	1.7423	$3,076
Arizona	1.7473	$10,047	$12,113	2.0921	$25,341
Arkansas	1.5592	$4,143	$5,759	1.8417	$10,607
California	1.8782	$81,961	$83,357	2.3155	$193,013
Colorado	1.8929	$9,860	$10,942	2.3212	$25,398
Connecticut	1.7191	$8,881	$9,795	2.0802	$20,376
Delaware	1.5948	$2,384	$2,662	1.8967	$5,050
District of Columbia	1.3241	$2,726	$3,938	1.3378	$5,268
Florida	1.7906	$34,081	$40,816	2.1546	$87,943
Georgia	1.8813	$16,265	$17,664	2.3035	$40,689
Hawaii	1.6503	$2,489	$2,856	1.9679	$5,620
Idaho	1.5086	$2,384	$3,128	1.7539	$5,486
Illinois	1.9129	$29,713	$31,915	2.3704	$75,651
Indiana	1.7103	$14,350	$17,927	2.0808	$37,302
Iowa	1.4704	$5,692	$7,710	1.7231	$13,284
Kansas	1.5244	$5,102	$6,514	1.8186	$11,846
Kentucky	1.6948	$8,187	$10,401	2.0341	$21,156
Louisiana	1.6285	$7,915	$10,147	1.8985	$19,264
Maine	1.6767	$4,024	$4,422	1.9987	$8,838
Maryland	1.7266	$11,448	$13,808	2.0773	$28,684
Massachusetts	1.8188	$21,386	$24,081	2.2142	$53,319
Michigan	1.7709	$23,574	$27,293	2.139	$58,380
Minnesota	1.8076	$15,128	$15,069	2.2165	$33,401
Mississippi	1.5474	$5,433	$6,983	1.8228	$12,728
Missouri	1.8001	$15,311	$17,024	2.1788	$37,092
Montana	1.474	$2,049	$2,661	1.7012	$4,527
Nebraska	1.4993	$3,589	$4,972	1.7508	$8,705
Nevada	1.6295	$3,289	$4,200	1.9298	$8,105
New Hampshire	1.7353	$3,882	$4,025	2.007	$8,078
New Jersey	1.8654	$19,382	$19,791	2.3092	$45,701
New Mexico	1.5475	$3,030	$4,003	1.7898	$7,165
New York	1.6732	$59,453	$62,123	2.0617	$128,079
North Carolina	1.8107	$19,998	$22,660	2.212	$50,123
North Dakota	1.4083	$1,816	$2,666	1.6154	$4,307
Ohio	1.8469	$33,665	$35,772	2.2541	$80,634
Oklahoma	1.6445	$5,579	$7,463	1.9496	$14,549
Oregon	1.7395	$8,118	$9,103	2.082	$18,952
Pennsylvania	1.8641	$32,611	$37,279	2.2768	$84,878
Rhode Island	1.7022	$2,863	$3,068	2.0206	$6,199
South Carolina	1.7258	$7,652	$9,730	2.1104	$20,533
South Dakota	1.3914	$1,941	$2,495	1.6058	$4,006
Tennessee	1.8163	$12,295	$14,708	2.2215	$32,674
Texas	1.8783	$44,568	$51,154	2.3343	$119,409
Utah	1.847	$4,332	$5,117	2.2759	$11,647
Vermont	1.551	$1,726	$1,931	1.7831	$3,444
Virginia	1.7199	$13,340	$16,505	2.1081	$34,795
Washington	1.7321	$14,879	$16,740	2.1029	$35,202
West Virginia	1.5245	$3,758	$5,151	1.7444	$8,986
Wisconsin	1.7308	$12,598	$15,602	2.0677	$32,260
Wyoming	1.3738	$891	$1,182	1.5703	$1,856
United States*	**2.4031**	**$907,489**	**$757,200**	**3.2896**	**$2,490,884**

Chart 12: Hospital Impact on Sectors of the U.S. Economy (in $ billions), 2012

Industry	Economic Impact
Health care and social assistance	$876.2
Manufacturing	373.1
Real estate, rental and leasing	235.9
Finance and insurance	159.2
Professional, scientific and technical services	103.5
Retail trade	101.8
Wholesale trade	81.6
Information	81.5
Transportation and warehousing	77.5
Administrative and waste management services	77.2
Accommodation and food services	64.0
Other services	62.4
Management of companies and enterprises	50.1
Utilities	44.3
Agriculture, forestry, fishing and hunting	36.6
Educational services	20.1
Arts, entertainment and recreation	17.8
Mining	15.7
Construction	12.3
Total	**$2,490.7**

Source: BEA RIMS-II (1997/2006) multipliers, released in 2008, applied to 2012 American Hospital Association Annual Survey data. Note: Multipliers released in 2010 and subsequent years no longer include the national level multipliers needed for this chart.

Hospitals Support Their Communities in Many Additional Ways

In addition to providing traditional health care services and supporting their local economies, hospitals offer an array of special programs and activities to help meet communities' broader health and social needs.

Hospitals offer services that aid in disease prevention, promote health awareness, contribute to advances in medicine, and address other societal needs. Examples of community programs that hospitals offer are:

- Health programs such as educational outreach, health screenings and support groups;

- Subsidized health services (e.g., free clinics, vaccinations);

- Programs to address the social needs of communities (e.g., Meals on Wheels and various shelters);

- Health professions training programs for physicians, nurses and technical staff;

- Continuing education for health professionals; and

- Clinical research.

Hospital charity care programs provide care for free or on a sliding scale for patients with limited financial means. Hospitals have specific criteria to identify patients eligible for this care. In 2012, hospitals provided nearly $46 billion in uncompensated care – a mixture of charity care and other care for which payment was expected but not received.

Hospitals also offer services to needy patients through Medicaid, a federal-state program that does not fully reimburse community hospitals for the services provided to these patients. In 2012, Medicaid payments fell short of the actual costs of care by $13.7 billion, a number that includes disproportionate share payments intended to subsidize the costs of caring for other low-income populations.

Summary

Hospitals contribute to the economic viability of local and regional communities by serving as the anchors of local health care networks and stimulating demand for goods and services produced by local businesses. Hospitals continue to provide jobs and job growth during recessions. However, when investors, policymakers and the public think about industries that promote economic stability and growth, most do not think about hospitals. Indeed, increases in expenditures on manufacturing or technology inspire optimism about the nation's fiscal health, while increases in expenditures on health care are typically viewed with concern. But, the fact remains that hospitals are strong contributors to the U.S. economy.

Hospitals create a steady source of employment even in economic downturns. Hospitals offer:

- High pay relative to other service sectors;
- Jobs across a wide spectrum of skill levels; and
- Jobs not easily "outsourced" abroad.

Hospital – and hospital employee – purchases of goods and services support other community businesses. With "ripple effects" included, hospitals:

- Support more than one of 9 jobs in the U.S.; and
- Support nearly $2.5 trillion in economic activity.

Endnotes

[1] Health Forum. (2014). *AHA Hospital Statistics.* Chicago, IL.

[2] Centers for Medicare & Medicaid Services, Office of the Actuary, National Health Statistics Group. Data released January 2013.

[3] *Ibid.*

[4] Department of Labor, Bureau of Labor Statistics, *Current Employment Statistics Survey.* Data released October 2013. Washington, DC.

[5] Avalere Health, using BEA RIMS-II (1997/2006) multipliers applied to 2012 American Hospital Association Annual Survey data.

[6] The Metropolitan Chicago Healthcare Council. (2012). *The Economic Impact of Chicago's Hospitals on the Metropolitan Chicago Area.* Chicago, IL.

[7] Department of Labor, Bureau of Labor Statistics. (2013). *Current Employment Statistics,* Data released October 2013. Washington, DC.

[8] *Ibid.*

How to Use this Book

For more than seven decades, *AHA Hospital Statistics*™ has reported aggregate hospital data derived from the AHA Annual Survey and is the definitive source when doing trend analysis with data by bed size category, U.S. Census Divisions, States, and Metropolitan Statistical Areas (MSAs). As the health care delivery system changes, so have the data tracked by the survey and presented in this report. Recent additions include:

- **Community health indicators** that offer readers a connection to the community for their analysis and planning: the data are broken down into beds, admissions, inpatient days, ER outpatient visits, and other indicators per 1000 population, as well as expense per capita.

- **Utilization, personnel and finance** by all MSAs in the United States.

- **Five-year trend data** on physician models, insurance products, and managed care contracts enable you to identify changes in relationships between hospitals and other health care systems and providers.

- **Tables 3 through 6 have been organized** to show breakdowns between inpatient and outpatient care to better reflect market shifts toward outpatient-centered care. Additional clarity is gained by the breakdown between total facility data (which includes nursing home type units under the control of the hospital) and hospital units (which exclude the nursing home data).

TABLE 6   **Sample State**

U.S. Registered Community Hospitals
(Nonfederal, short-term general and other special hospitals)

Overview 2008-2012

	2012	2011	2010	2009	2008
Physician Models					
Independent Practice Association	14	17	17	17	14
Group Practice without Walls	4	5	5	8	4
Open Physician-Hospital Organization	20	21	24	23	18
Closed Physician-Hospital Organization . . .	21	17	18	17	11
Management Service Organization	14	18	20	14	9
Integrated Salary Model	35	29	30	26	24
Equity Model	4	3	4	6	3
Foundation	9	8	23	21	19
Insurance Products					
Health Maintenance Organization	20	22	23	24	19
Preferred Provider Organization	39	47	52	53	37
Indemnity Fee for Service.	7	12	14	12	6
Managed Care Contracts					
Health Maintenance Organization	64	67	62	49	42
Preferred Provider Organization	97	93	92	87	72

Example of five-year trend data

- **Facilities and Services information** on more than 100 categories of hospital facilities and services in Table 7. At a glance, you can determine the number and percentage of hospitals offering a specific service such as Oncology, Palliative Care Program, Complementary Medicine, Women's Health Services and Tobacco Cessation.

- **Plus, System and Network involvement along with Group Purchasing Organizations** that demonstrate ways in which organizations are linked.

The survey instrument and the glossary

A good place to begin your analysis is the AHA Annual Survey instrument. Found on page 215, it includes the instructions, questions, and terms that were used to gather the data for fiscal year 2012. This can be extremely valuable for a clearer understanding of the data we collect and the tables presented in *AHA Hospital Statistics*.

Please also review the glossary in the back of the book. The glossary contains complete definitions for specific terms used in the tables and text of *AHA Hospital Statistics*. These definitions will clarify how terminology is being used.

As mentioned above, it is important to note that the primary focus of the most detailed data contained in *AHA Hospital Statistics* is community hospitals. As defined, community hospitals are all non-federal, short-term general and special hospitals whose facilities and services are available to the public. If the majority of a hospital's patients are admitted to units where the average length of stay is 30 days or less, a hospital may still be classified as short-term even if it includes a nursing- home-type unit. (For a more complete definition of community hospitals, please see the glossary definition, located on page 201.)

Getting the most out of
AHA Hospital Statistics
This section of the book provides an introduction for getting the most out of your *AHA Hospital Statistics* 2014 edition. Here, you'll find a guide to the book, with insights into each table.

Equity model: An arrangement that allows established practitioners to become shareholders in a professional corporation in exchange for tangible and intangible assets of their existing practices.

Expenses: Includes all expenses for the reporting period including payroll, non-payroll, and all nonoperating expenses. *Payroll expenses* include all salaries and wages. *Non-payroll expenses* are all professional fees and those salary expenditures excluded from payroll. *Labor related expenses* are defined as payroll expenses plus employee benefits. *Non-labor related expenses* are all other non-payroll expenses. *Bad debt* has been reclassified from a "reduction in revenue" to an expense in accordance with the revised AICPA Audit Guide. However, for purposes of historical consistency, the expense total that appears throughout *AHA Hospital Statistics does not include "bad debt" as an expense item.* Note: Financial data may not add due to rounding.

Extracorporeal shock wave lithotripter (ESWL): A medical device used for treating stones in the kidney or urethra. The device disintegrates kidney stones noninvasively through the transmission of acoustic shock waves directed at the stones.

Fitness center: Provides exercise, testing, or evaluation programs and fitness activities to the community and hospital employees.

Example of Glossary definitions.

Table 1 — Historical Trends in Utilization, Personnel and Finances for Selected Years from 1946 through 2012

Table 1	Historical Trends in Utilization, Personnel, and Finances for Selected Years from 1946 through 2012

CLASSIFICATION	YEAR	HOSPITALS	BEDS (in thousands)	ADMISSIONS (in thousands)	AVERAGE DAILY CENSUS (in thousands)	ADJUSTED AVERAGE DAILY CENSUS (in thousands)
Total United States	1946	6,125	1,436	15,675	1,142	—
	1950	6,788	1,456	18,483	1,253	—
	1955	6,956	1,604	21,073	1,363	—
	1960	6,876	1,658	25,027	1,402	—
	1965	7,123	1,704	28,812	1,403	—
	1970	7,123	1,616	31,759	1,298	—
	1971	7,097	1,556	32,664	1,237	—
	1972	7,061	1,550	33,265	1,209	—
	1973	7,123	1,535	34,352	1,189	—
	1974	7,174	1,513	35,506	1,167	—
	1975	7,156	1,466	36,157	1,125	—
	1976	7,082	1,434	36,776	1,090	—
	1977	7,099	1,407	37,060	1,066	—
	1978	7,015	1,381	37,243	1,042	—
	1979	6,988	1,372	37,802	1,043	—
	1980	6,965	1,365	38,892	1,060	—
	1981	6,933	1,362	39,169	1,061	—
	1982	6,915	1,360	39,095	1,053	—
	1983	6,888	1,350	38,887	1,028	—
	1984	6,872	1,339	37,938	970	—
	1985	6,872	1,318	36,304	910	—
	1986	6,841	1,290	35,219	883	—
	1987	6,821	1,267	34,439	873	—
	1988	6,780	1,248	34,107	863	—
	1989	6,720	1,226	33,742	853	—
	1990	6,649	1,213	33,774	844	—
	1991	6,634	1,202	33,567	827	—
	1992	6,539	1,178	33,536	807	—
	1993	6,467	1,163	33,201	783	—
	1994	6,374	1,128	33,125	745	—
	1995	6,291	1,081	33,282	710	—
	1996	6,201	1,062	33,307	685	—
	1997	6,097	1,035	33,624	673	—
	1998	6,021	1,013	33,766	662	—
	1999	5,890	994	34,181	657	—
	2000	5,810	984	34,891	650	—
	2001	5,801	987	35,644	658	—
	2002	5,794	976	36,326	662	—
	2003	5,764	965	36,611	657	—
	2004	5,759	956	36,942	658	—
	2005	5,756	947	37,006	656	—

Example of Table 1

Table 1 at a Glance

This table is used to evaluate historical data and allows you to examine long-term trends in health care with data dating back more than sixty years. Table 1 reports on all AHA registered hospitals in the United States. One important note: To be considered an AHA-registered hospital, a hospital does not need to be an AHA member. Rather, the hospital must meet particular certification or satisfy a number of requirements. These Registration Requirements immediately follow this section and begin on page (xxviii.)

This table segments the data into various organizational structure categories. Here's a brief look at these different classifications:

- Total United States Hospitals
- Total Non-Federal Short-term and other special hospitals
- Community hospitals
- Non-government not-for-profit community hospitals
- Investor-owned (for-profit) community hospitals
- State and local government community hospitals

Table 1 also provides input on nationwide utilization, personnel and finance trends. You'll find answers to questions such as: *Over the past 25 years, what trends do I see comparing the average length of stay at government and non-government not-for-profit community hospitals and investor-owned for-profit community hospitals?* or *What has been the trend in outpatient visits?*

Table 2 — 2012 U.S. Registered Hospitals: Utilization, Personnel and Finances

Table 2 at a Glance

This table takes a closer look at U.S. Registered Hospitals for 2012. It offers a snapshot of utilization, personnel and finance statistics, and breaks down this information for specialty hospitals. In addition, this is the only table that outlines data on federal hospitals. You'll be able to use this table to better understand the number of beds set-up and staffed, how many personnel and trainees are on the payroll, and what the financial implications of these may be.

TABLE 3

TOTAL UNITED STATES

U.S. Registered Community Hospitals
(Nonfederal, short-term general and other special hospitals)

Utilization, Personnel, Revenue and Expenses, Community Health Indicators 2008-2012

	2012	2011	2010	2009	2008
TOTAL FACILITY (Includes Hospital and Nursing Home Units)					
Utilization - Inpatient					
Beds	839,988	853,287	862,352	872,736	902,061
Admissions	31,811,673	31,576,960	31,098,959	30,945,357	30,718,136
Inpatient Days	191,430,450	192,504,015	193,747,004	199,876,367	207,180,278
Average Length of Stay	6.0	6.1	6.2	6.5	6.7
Inpatient Surgeries	9,735,705	9,509,081	9,545,612	9,700,613	9,833,938
Births	3,726,233	3,742,191	3,723,871	3,764,698	3,809,367
HOSPITAL UNIT (Excludes Separate Nursing Home Units)					
Utilization - Inpatient					
Beds	758,186	769,505	782,504	794,502	824,969
Admissions	31,265,867	31,047,930	30,652,820	30,577,564	30,403,766
Inpatient Days	165,644,176	165,605,620	168,189,130	174,898,504	182,702,882
Average Length of Stay	5.3	5.3	5.5	5.7	6.0
Personnel					
Total Full Time	3,235,153	3,183,730	3,154,603	3,166,729	3,147,922
Total Part Time	1,213,426	1,214,232	1,153,790	1,146,082	1,122,957
Revenue and Expenses - Totals					
(Includes Inpatient and Outpatient)					
Total Net Revenue	$333,054,828,642	$322,459,942,930	$310,513,291,998	$298,519,717,355	$285,858,018,951
Total Expenses	314,709,758,455	301,905,101,393	290,128,641,153	282,372,557,487	272,840,121,437

Example of Table 3. Helps contrast acute and long-term care

Table 3 — Total United States

Table 3 at a Glance

This table provides a look at all U .S. Registered Community Hospitals, in terms of general overview with utilization by inpatient and outpatient, personnel, revenue, expenses and community health indicators. It provides a snapshot of the past five years, allowing you to track emerging trends.

This national information can be compared to local or regional trends, for benchmarking:

- Both inpatient and outpatient information is included, for better evaluation of data.

- Reporting by total facility *Includes hospital and Nursing Home Units* and hospital unit only *Excludes Separate Nursing Home Units* helps contrast acute and long-term care.

- Community health indicators can help uncover trends and help determine future facility needs.

TABLE 4   BED SIZE CATEGORY 25-49

	2012	2011	2010	2009	2008
Total U.S. Community Hospitals in Bed Size Category 25-49	900	890	906	922	900

Location
Hospitals Urban
Hospitals Rural

Control
State and Local Gover
Not for Profit
Investor owned

Physician Models
Independent Practice
Group Practice without
Open Physician-Hospi
Closed Physician-Hosp
Management Service
Integrated Salary Mod
Equity Model
Foundation

Insurance Products
Health Maintenance
Preferred Provider Org
Indemnity Fee for Serv

Managed Care Contract
Health Maintenance
Preferred Provider Org

TABLE 4   BED SIZE CATEGORY 100-199

	2012	2011	2010	2009	2008
Total U.S. Community Hospitals in Bed Size Category 100-199	1,304	1,289	1,338	1,324	1,331

TABLE 4   BED SIZE CATEGORY 500 +

	2012	2011	2010	2009	2008
Total U.S. Community Hospitals in Bed Size Category 500 +	254	255	251	264	273
Location					
Hospitals Urban	251	251	247	260	270
Hospitals Rural	3	4	4	4	3
Control					
State and Local Government	42	43	48	53	56
Not for Profit	198	197	186	197	208
Investor owned	14	15	17	14	9
Physician Models					
Independent Practice Association	85	86	93	93	93
Group Practice without Walls	25	28	38	34	35
Open Physician-Hospital Organization	79	87	79	83	82
Closed Physician-Hospital Organization	53	50	61	68	53
Management Service Organization	80	93	108	90	90
Integrated Salary Model	103	97	96	97	94
Equity Model	17	17	18	17	16
Foundation	35	41	52	53	49
Insurance Products					
Health Maintenance Organization	138	130	121	115	116
Preferred Provider Organization	122	127	119	121	122
Indemnity Fee for Service	34	37	35	35	35
Managed Care Contracts					
Health Maintenance Organization	197	206	199	213	217
Preferred Provider Organization	193	202	199	215	211

Example of Table 4. Compares facilities with peers.

Table 4 — Bed Size Categories

Table 4 at a Glance

This table provides a look at all U.S. Registered Community Hospitals, broken down by bed size. The table includes general overview, utilization, personnel, and revenue and expense information. These categories of bed sizes were developed by the AHA, and have become an industry standard. By categorizing each facility into a peer group, this table provides a snapshot of the past five years allowing you to compare facilities with their peers.

TABLE 5 — U.S. CENSUS DIVISION 2: MIDDLE ATLANTIC

U.S. Registered Community Hospitals
(Nonfederal, short-term general and other special hospitals)

Utilization, Personnel, Revenue and Expenses, Community Health Indicators 2008-2012

	2012	2011	2010	2009	2008
COMMUNITY HEALTH INDICATORS PER 1000 POPULATION					
Total Population (in thousands)....	38,292	38,216	38,184	38,147	38,108
Inpatient					
Beds.........................	3.6	3.8	3.9	4.0	4.1
Admissions....................	135.8	136.7	136.2	138.3	137.4
Inpatient Days................	963.5	988.8	1,019.0	1,093.8	1,145.0
Inpatient Surgeries.............	42.2	41.4	41.2	42.7	43.6
Births........................	13.0	13.2	13.6	13.7	14.3
Outpatient					
Emergency Outpatient Visits......	367.7	362.0	363.4	379.5	360.1
Other Outpatient Visits..........	1,970.9	1,802.3	1,767.7	1,680.3	1,573.9
Total Outpatient Visits..........	2,338.6	2,164.3	2,131.1	2,059.8	1,934.0
Outpatient Surgeries............	67.8	62.4	59.9	55.4	53.5
Expense per Capita (per person)....	$1,494.9	$1,462.7	$1,428.6	$1,429.8	$1,369.2

Example of Table 5. Uncovers trends to determine future facility needs.

Table 5 — U.S. Census Divisions

Table 5 at a Glance
This table provides a look at all U.S. Registered Community Hospitals, broken down by Census Division. The table includes general overview, utilization, personnel, and expenses, and community health indicator information. It provides a snapshot of the past five years, allowing you to track trends on a regional level. In addition, this allows you to compare this data to other population based health indicators, offering a more comprehensive look than the survey data alone. Community health indicators can help uncover trends and help determine future facility needs.

Table 6 — States

Table 6 at a Glance
This table provides a look at all U.S. Registered Community Hospitals, broken down by State. The table includes general overview, utilization, personnel, revenue and expenses, and community health indicator information. It provides a snapshot of the past five years, allowing you to track trends on a state level.

Note:
You can use the information in tables 3, 4, 5 and 6 to make accurate comparisons across Total U.S., Bed Size Category, Census Division and State.

Table 7 at a Glance

This table examines facilities and services by both Census Division and State. A comprehensive alphabetical guide helps make each facility or service easy to find. This table will allow you to better understand what service lines are emerging and how many facilities offer a particular service in a discrete state or region.

This collection of facilities and services information data is unique to *AHA Hospital Statistics* and the list is continually growing. Recent additions include:

- Pediatric Emergency Department
- Psychiatric Residential Treatment
- Magneotoencephalography (MEG)

These new categories reflect the trends as hospitals expand their service lines to mirror the needs of their patients. For example, services such as acupuncture or massage therapy are now accounted for in the Complementary Medicine service item.

Example of Table 7.

This table can answer questions such as: *What percentage of hospitals in the United States offer complementary medicine or wound management?* or *How are these new services distributed by state?*

Table 8 at a Glance

This table provides a look at all U.S. Registered Community Hospitals, broken down by Metropolitan Statistical Area (MSA). The table includes general overview, utilization, personnel, and finance information. It provides a snapshot of the past year.

Additional Resources

Again, in the back of the book you will find the comprehensive glossary and the 2011 annual survey questionnaire. The survey itself can be a valuable resource to understanding what was asked in order to gather the data in the book. This survey is also used to produce the *AHA Guide*® and AHA Annual Survey Database™.

AHA-Registered Hospitals

Any institution that can be classified as a hospital according to the requirements may be registered if it so desires. Membership in the American Hospital Association is not a prerequisite.

The American Hospital Association may, at the sole discretion of the Executive Committee of the Board of Trustees, grant, deny, or withdraw the registration of an institution.

An institution may be registered by the American Hospital Association as a hospital if it is accredited as a hospital by The Joint Commission or is certified as a provider of acute services under Title 18 of the Social Security Act and has provided the Association with documents verifying the accreditation or certification.

In lieu of the preceding accreditation or certification, an institution licensed as a hospital by the appropriate state agency may be registered by AHA as a hospital by meeting the following alternative requirements:

Function: The primary function of the institution is to provide patient services, diagnostic and therapeutic, for particular or general medical conditions.

1. The institution shall maintain at least six inpatient beds, which shall be continuously available for the care of patients who are nonrelated and who stay on the average in excess of 24 hours per admission.

2. The institution shall be constructed, equipped, and maintained to ensure the health and safety of patients and to provide uncrowded, sanitary facilities for the treatment of patients.

3. There shall be an identifiable governing authority legally and morally responsible for the conduct of the hospital.

4. There shall be a chief executive to whom the governing authority delegates the continuous responsibility for the operation of the hospital in accordance with established policy.

5. There shall be an organized medical staff of fully licensed physicians* that may include other licensed individuals permitted by law and by the hospital to provide patient care services independently in the hospital. The medical staff shall be accountable to the governing authority for maintaining proper standards of medical care, and it shall be governed by bylaws adopted by said staff and approved by the governing authority.

6. Each patient shall be admitted on the authority of a member of the medical staff who has been granted the privilege to admit patients to inpatient services in accordance with state law and criteria for standards of medical care established by the individual medical staff. Each patient's general medical condition is the responsibility of a qualified physician member of the medical staff. When nonphysician members of the medical staff are granted privileges to admit patients, provision is made for prompt medical evaluation of these patients by a qualified physician. Any graduate of a foreign medical school who is permitted to assume responsibilities for patient care shall possess a valid license to practice medicine, or shall be certified by the Educational Commission for Foreign Medical Graduates, or shall have qualified for and have successfully completed an academic year of supervised clinical training under the direction of a medical school approved by the Liaison Committee on GAT Medical Education.

7. Registered nurse supervision and other nursing services are continuous.

8. A current and complete‡ medical record shall be maintained by the institution for each patient and shall be available for reference.

9. Pharmacy service shall be maintained in the institution and shall be supervised by a registered pharmacist.

10. The institution shall provide patients with food service that meets their nutritional and therapeutic requirements; special diets shall also be available.

Types of Hospitals

In addition to meeting these 10 general registration requirements, hospitals are registered as one of four types of hospitals: general, special, rehabilitation and chronic disease, or psychiatric. The following type of hospital and special requirements for registration are employed:

General

The primary function of the institution is to provide patient services, diagnostic and therapeutic, for a variety of medical conditions. A general hospital also shall provide:

- diagnostic x-ray services with facilities and staff for a variety of procedures
- clinical laboratory service with facilities and staff for a variety of procedures and with anatomical pathology services regularly and conveniently available
- operating room service with facilities and staff.

Special

The primary function of the institution is to provide diagnostic and treatment services for patients who have specified medical conditions, both surgical and nonsurgical. A special hospital also shall provide:

- such diagnostic and treatment services as may be determined by the Executive Committee of the Board of Trustees of the American Hospital Association to be appropriate for the specified medical conditions for which medical services are provided shall be maintained in the institution with suitable facilities and staff. If such conditions do not normally require diagnostic x-ray service, laboratory service, or operating room service, and if any such services are therefore not maintained in the institution, there shall be written arrangements to make them available to patients requiring them.
- clinical laboratory services capable of providing tissue diagnosis when offering pregnancy termination services.

Rehabilitation and Chronic Disease

The primary function of the institution is to provide diagnostic and treatment services to handicapped or disabled individuals requiring restorative and adjustive services. A rehabilitation and chronic disease hospital also shall provide:

- arrangements for diagnostic x-ray services, as required, on a regular and conveniently available basis
- arrangements for clinical laboratory service, as required on a regular and conveniently available basis
- arrangements for operating room service, as required, on a regular and conveniently available basis
- a physical therapy service with suitable facilities and staff in the institution
- an occupational therapy service with suitable facilities and staff in the institution
- arrangements for psychological and social work services on a regular and conveniently available basis

---

* Physician—Term used to describe an individual with an M.D. or D.O. degree who is fully licensed to practice medicine in all its phases.

‡ The completed records in general shall contain at least the following: the patient's identifying data and consent forms, medical history, record of physical examination, physicians' progress notes, operative notes, nurses' notes, routine x-ray and laboratory reports, doctors' orders, and final diagnosis.

- arrangements for educational and vocational services on a regular and conveniently available basis
- written arrangements with a general hospital for the transfer of patients who require medical, obstetrical, or surgical services not available in the institution.

Psychiatric

The primary function of the institution is to provide diagnostic and treatment services for patients who have psychiatric-related illnesses. A psychiatric hospital also shall provide:

- arrangements for clinical laboratory service, as required, on a regular and conveniently available basis
- arrangements for diagnostic x-ray services, as required on a regular and conveniently available basis
- psychiatric, psychological, and social work service with facilities and staff in the institution
- arrangements for electroencephalograph services, as required, on a regular and conveniently available basis.
- written arrangements with a general hospital for the transfer of patients who require medical, obstetrical, or surgical services not available in the institution.

The American Hospital Association may, at the sole discretion of the Executive Committee of the Board of Trustees, grant, deny, or withdraw the registration of an institution.

Data Comparability

The economic climate, demographic characteristics, personnel issues, and health care financing and payment policies differ by region, state, and city across the country. *Differences in these factors must be taken into account when using the data.* In addition, the profiles of hospitals across comparison groups vary. For example, states will differ in terms of the number and percentage of hospitals by size, ownership, services provided, types of patients treated, and so forth. *Differences in these variables also must be taken into consideration when doing a comparative analysis.*

Notes on the Survey

The 2014 edition of *AHA Hospital Statistics*™ draws its data from the 2012 AHA Annual Survey of Hospitals. It is the statistical complement to the 2014 edition of the *AHA Guide*®, which contains selected data about individual hospitals.

The AHA Survey was mailed to all hospitals, both AHA-registered and nonregistered, in the U.S. and its associated areas: American Samoa, Guam, the Marshall Islands, Puerto Rico, and the Virgin Islands. U.S. government hospitals located outside the U.S. were not included. Overall, the average response rate over the past five years has been approximately 83 percent.

Reporting Period

In completing the survey, hospitals were requested to report data for a full year, in accord with their fiscal year, ending in 2012. The statistical table present data reported or estimated for a 12-month period, except for data on personnel, which represent situations as they existed at the end of the reporting period.

Respondents

Data for Tables 1 and 2 include 5,723 AHA-registered hospitals in the U.S. Data on community hospitals (nonfederal, short-term general and other special hospitals) only are presented in Tables 3-6, and Table 8.

It is important to note that the AHA-registered hospitals included in *AHA Hospital Statistics* are not necessarily identical to those included in *AHA Guide*. The institutions listed in the 2014 edition of AHA Guide include all of those institutions CMS certified, Joint Commission accredited, or AHA registered as of September 2011. Tables 1-6 in *AHA Hospital Statistics* present data for AHA-registered hospitals that were in operation during the 12-month reporting period ending 2012.

Estimates

Estimates were made of data for nonreporting hospitals and for reporting hospitals that submitted incomplete AHA Annual Survey questionnaires. Estimates were not made for beds, bassinets and facilities and services. Data for beds and bassinets of nonreporting hospitals were based on the most recent information from those hospitals. (Note that in all statistical tables, whenever bed-size categories are listed, all eight categories appear, whether or not there are hospitals in every category.)

Missing revenue, expenses, admissions, births, inpatient days, surgical operations, outpatient visits, and full-time-equivalent personnel values are estimates from regression models. For all other variables the estimates were based on ratios such as per bed averages derived from data reported by hospitals similar in size, control, major service provided, length of stay, and geographical characteristics to the hospitals that did not report this information.

Tables 1–2

Table

1

Historical Trends in Utilization, Personnel, and Finances for Selected Years from 1946 through 2012

Data are for all AHA-registered hospitals in the United States. Data are estimated for nonreporting hospitals with the exception of newborn and outpatient data before 1972. Personnel data exclude residents, interns, and students from 1952 on; personnel data include full-time personnel and full-time equivalents for part-time personnel from 1954 on. As a result of the AHA Annual Survey validation process, the New York state expense data from 1976 were revised after the 1977 edition was published. The revised figures are included below. In order to provide trend data on a consistent basis, the 1970 and 1971 psychiatric and long-term data have been slightly modified. The 1982 FTE figures have updated to provide the most accurate data possible.

Total United States

YEAR	HOSPITALS	BEDS (in thousands)	ADMISSIONS (in thousands)	AVERAGE DAILY CENSUS (in thousands)	ADJUSTED AVERAGE DAILY CENSUS (in thousands)	AVERAGE STAY (days)	OUTPATIENT VISITS (in thousands)	NEWBORNS Bassinets	NEWBORNS Births	FTE PERSONNEL Number (in thousands)	FTE PERSONNEL Per 100 Adjusted Census	TOTAL EXPENSES Amount (In Millions of dollars)	TOTAL EXPENSES Adjusted per Inpatient Stay (dollars)	TOTAL EXPENSES Adjusted per Inpatient Day (dollars)
1946	6,125	1,436	15,675	1,142	—	—	—	85,585	2,135,327	830	—	$1,963	—	—
1950	6,788	1,456	18,483	1,253	—	—	—	90,101	2,742,780	1,058	—	$3,651	—	—
1955	6,956	1,604	21,073	1,363	—	—	—	98,823	3,476,753	1,301	—	$5,594	—	—
1960	6,876	1,658	25,027	1,402	—	—	—	102,764	3,835,735	1,598	—	$8,421	—	—
1965	7,123	1,704	28,812	1,403	—	—	125,793	101,287	3,565,344	1,952	—	$12,948	—	—
1970	7,123	1,616	31,759	1,298	—	—	181,370	97,128	3,537,000	2,537	—	$25,556	—	—
1971	7,097	1,556	32,664	1,237	—	—	199,725	94,344	3,464,513	2,589	—	$28,812	—	—
1972	7,061	1,550	33,265	1,209	—	—	219,182	92,960	3,231,875	2,671	—	$32,667	—	—
1973	7,123	1,535	34,352	1,189	—	—	233,555	90,071	3,087,210	2,769	—	$36,290	—	—
1974	7,174	1,513	35,506	1,167	—	—	250,481	88,269	3,043,386	2,919	—	$41,406	—	—
1975	7,156	1,466	36,157	1,125	—	—	254,844	86,875	3,091,629	3,023	—	$48,706	—	—
1976	7,082	1,434	36,776	1,090	—	—	270,951	85,284	3,067,063	3,108	—	$56,005	—	—
1977	7,099	1,407	37,060	1,066	—	—	263,775	83,193	3,223,699	3,213	—	$63,630	—	—
1978	7,015	1,381	37,243	1,042	—	—	263,606	80,650	3,250,373	3,280	—	$70,927	—	—
1979	6,988	1,372	37,802	1,043	—	—	262,009	79,720	3,376,467	3,382	—	$79,796	—	—
1980	6,965	1,365	38,892	1,060	—	—	262,951	79,842	3,500,043	3,492	—	$91,886	—	—
1981	6,933	1,362	39,169	1,061	—	—	265,332	78,823	3,558,274	3,661	—	$107,146	—	—
1982	6,915	1,360	39,095	1,053	—	—	313,667	77,998	3,615,751	3,746	—	$123,219	—	—
1983	6,888	1,350	38,887	1,028	—	—	273,168	77,837	3,596,146	3,707	—	$136,315	—	—
1984	6,872	1,339	37,938	970	—	—	276,566	77,845	3,563,106	3,630	—	$144,114	—	—
1985	6,872	1,318	36,304	910	—	—	282,140	77,202	3,630,961	3,625	—	$153,327	—	—
1986	6,841	1,290	35,219	883	—	—	294,634	76,002	3,680,178	3,647	—	$165,194	—	—
1987	6,821	1,267	34,439	873	—	—	310,707	74,770	3,698,294	3,742	—	$178,662	—	—
1988	6,780	1,248	34,107	863	—	—	336,208	72,568	3,794,369	3,839	—	$196,704	—	—
1989	6,720	1,226	33,742	853	—	—	352,248	71,491	3,920,384	3,937	—	$214,886	—	—
1990	6,649	1,213	33,774	844	—	—	368,184	70,539	4,046,704	4,063	—	$234,870	—	—
1991	6,634	1,202	33,567	827	—	—	387,675	69,464	4,047,504	4,165	—	$258,508	—	—
1992	6,539	1,178	33,536	807	—	—	417,874	69,052	4,007,179	4,236	—	$282,531	—	—
1993	6,467	1,163	33,201	783	—	—	435,619	67,911	3,949,788	4,289	—	$301,538	—	—
1994	6,374	1,128	33,125	745	—	—	453,584	67,311	3,886,667	4,270	—	$310,834	—	—
1995	6,291	1,081	33,282	710	—	—	483,195	66,256	3,833,132	4,273	—	$320,252	—	—
1996	6,201	1,062	33,307	685	—	—	505,455	65,138	3,790,678	4,276	—	$330,531	—	—
1997	6,097	1,035	33,624	673	—	—	520,600	64,649	3,811,522	4,333	—	$342,334	—	—
1998	6,021	1,013	33,766	662	—	—	545,481	63,485	3,795,212	4,407	—	$355,450	—	—
1999	5,890	994	34,181	657	—	—	573,461	62,714	3,829,881	4,369	—	$372,933	—	—
2000	5,810	984	34,891	650	—	—	592,673	61,915	3,940,017	4,454	—	$395,391	—	—
2001	5,801	987	35,644	658	—	—	612,276	61,527	3,929,733	4,535	—	$426,849	—	—
2002	5,794	976	36,326	662	—	—	640,515	62,151	3,934,421	4,610	—	$462,222	—	—
2003	5,764	965	36,611	657	—	—	648,560	60,699	3,976,886	4,651	—	$498,104	—	—
2004	5,759	956	36,942	658	—	—	662,131	59,660	3,965,906	4,696	—	$533,853	—	—
2005	5,756	947	37,006	656	—	—	673,689	59,073	4,048,442	4,791	—	$570,534	—	—
2006	5,747	947	37,189	653	—	—	690,425	58,670	4,126,598	4,907	—	$607,355	—	—
2007	5,708	945	37,120	645	—	—	693,510	58,429	4,128,796	5,024	—	$641,124	—	—
2008	5,815	951	37,529	649	—	—	709,960	58,133	4,109,081	5,116	—	$690,074	—	—
2009	5,795	944	37,480	641	—	—	741,551	58,078	4,001,748	5,178	—	$726,671	—	—
2010	5,754	942	36,915	627	—	—	750,408	57,396	3,871,751	5,184	—	$750,602	—	—
2011	5,724	924	36,565	615	—	—	754,454	57,022	3,767,697	5,196	—	$773,547	—	—
2012	5,723	921	36,156	600	—	—	777,961	56,693	3,754,085	5,258	—	$829,665	—	—

Table 1 (Continued)

CLASSIFICATION: Total nonfederal short-term general and other special

YEAR	HOSPITALS	BEDS (in thousands)	ADMISSIONS (in thousands)	AVERAGE DAILY CENSUS (in thousands)	ADJUSTED AVERAGE DAILY CENSUS (in thousands)	AVERAGE STAY (days)	OUTPATIENT VISITS (in thousands)	NEWBORNS		FTE PERSONNEL		TOTAL EXPENSES		
								Bassinets	Births	Number (in thousands)	Per 100 Adjusted Census	Amount (In Millions of dollars)	Adjusted per Inpatient Stay (dollars)	Adjusted per Inpatient Day (dollars)
1946	4,444	473	13,655	341	—	9.1	—	80,987	2,087,503	505	—	$1,169	—	—
1950	5,031	505	16,663	372	—	8.1	—	86,019	2,660,982	662	—	$2,120	—	—
1955	5,237	568	19,100	407	—	7.8	—	93,868	3,304,451	826	—	$3,434	—	—
1960	5,407	639	22,970	477	—	7.6	—	98,127	3,678,051	1,080	—	$5,617	—	—
1965	5,736	741	26,463	563	620	7.8	92,631	96,782	3,413,370	1,386	224	$9,147	$316.37	$40.56
1970	5,859	848	29,252	662	727	8.2	133,545	93,079	3,403,064	1,929	265	$19,560	$604.59	$73.73
1971	5,865	867	30,142	665	736	8.0	148,423	90,444	3,337,605	1,999	272	$22,400	$667.44	$83.43
1972	5,843	884	30,777	664	739	7.9	166,983	89,315	3,119,446	2,056	278	$25,549	$747.42	$94.61
1973	5,891	903	31,761	681	768	7.8	178,939	86,851	2,987,089	2,149	280	$28,496	$793.88	$101.78
1974	5,977	931	32,943	701	793	7.8	194,838	85,208	2,947,342	2,289	289	$32,751	$883.04	$113.21
1975	5,979	947	33,519	708	806	7.7	196,311	83,834	2,998,590	2,399	298	$39,110	$1,024.72	$133.08
1976	5,956	961	34,068	715	816	7.7	207,725	82,307	2,962,305	2,483	304	$45,402	$1,172.25	$152.24
1977	5,973	974	34,353	717	820	7.6	204,238	80,228	3,117,756	2,581	315	$51,832	$1,316.70	$173.25
1978	5,935	980	34,575	720	841	7.6	204,461	78,090	3,156,570	2,662	323	$58,348	$1,470.13	$193.81
1979	5,923	988	35,160	729	841	7.6	203,873	77,277	3,287,157	2,762	328	$66,184	$1,631.16	$215.75
1980	5,904	992	36,198	748	861	7.6	206,752	77,539	3,408,699	2,879	334	$76,970	$1,844.19	$244.44
1981	5,879	1,007	36,494	764	876	7.6	206,729	76,567	3,465,683	3,039	347	$90,739	$2,167.70	$283.94
1982	5,863	1,015	36,429	763	882	7.6	250,888	75,739	3,514,761	3,110	353	$105,094	$2,493.09	$326.68
1983	5,843	1,021	36,201	750	869	7.6	213,995	75,471	3,490,629	3,102	357	$116,632	$2,775.55	$368.01
1984	5,814	1,020	35,202	703	824	7.3	216,474	75,587	3,456,467	3,023	367	$123,550	$2,984.00	$409.85
1985	5,784	1,003	33,501	650	780	7.1	222,773	74,899	3,521,296	3,003	385	$130,700	$3,238.94	$459.57
1986	5,728	982	32,410	631	774	7.1	234,270	73,688	3,584,530	3,032	392	$140,907	$3,529.60	$499.19
1987	5,659	961	31,633	624	780	7.2	247,704	72,516	3,602,416	3,120	400	$152,909	$3,848.79	$536.96
1988	5,579	949	31,480	622	795	7.2	271,436	70,361	3,706,748	3,209	404	$168,941	$4,194.39	$581.08
1989	5,497	936	31,141	619	805	7.3	287,909	69,436	3,831,051	3,307	411	$185,204	$4,572.23	$630.59
1990	5,420	929	31,203	620	820	7.3	302,691	68,443	3,958,646	3,423	417	$203,927	$4,929.93	$681.52
1991	5,370	926	31,084	612	828	7.2	323,202	67,440	3,965,489	3,539	427	$225,230	$5,345.63	$745.37
1992	5,321	923	31,053	606	832	7.1	349,397	67,095	3,925,024	3,624	436	$248,318	$5,788.52	$815.99
1993	5,289	921	30,770	593	834	7.0	368,358	66,060	3,870,392	3,681	441	$266,382	$6,120.94	$874.98
1994	5,256	904	30,739	569	814	6.8	384,880	65,728	3,809,367	3,697	454	$276,148	$6,230.33	$929.65
1995	5,220	874	30,966	549	811	6.5	415,710	64,742	3,764,756	3,718	458	$286,073	$6,220.54	$966.79
1996	5,160	864	31,116	531	800	6.2	440,845	63,646	3,723,907	3,728	466	$293,920	$6,225.95	$1,005.45
1997	5,082	855	31,595	529	813	6.1	450,907	63,247	3,742,240	3,794	467	$306,088	$6,266.24	$1,031.68
1998	5,039	842	31,830	527	821	6.0	474,366	62,162	3,726,234	3,835	467	$319,035	$6,387.53	$1,064.93
1999	4,977	831	32,377	527	835	5.9	495,850	61,534	3,760,295	3,840	460	$335,405	$6,512.44	$1,101.47
2000	4,934	825	33,102	527	850	5.8	522,970	60,845	3,880,166	3,916	461	$356,757	$6,650.68	$1,147.99
2001	4,927	828	33,834	534	866	5.8	539,316	60,454	3,873,395	3,990	461	$383,911	$6,979.29	$1,216.04
2002	4,949	823	34,501	541	887	5.7	557,336	59,974	3,870,191	4,072	459	$416,791	$7,353.17	$1,288.63
2003	4,918	815	34,800	540	895	5.7	563,804	59,662	3,915,842	4,112	459	$450,403	$7,798.19	$1,378.78
2004	4,942	810	35,098	542	910	5.6	573,126	58,710	3,931,508	4,151	456	$481,517	$8,168.06	$1,449.90
2005	4,956	804	35,265	542	930	5.6	587,296	58,195	3,987,766	4,260	458	$516,172	$8,538.30	$1,521.58
2006	4,947	805	35,403	540	940	5.6	599,597	57,832	4,075,193	4,347	462	$552,276	$8,972.85	$1,610.76
2007	4,915	803	35,370	535	944	5.5	603,411	57,546	4,077,962	4,468	473	$583,550	$9,377.82	$1,694.38
2008	5,026	810	35,776	538	963	5.5	624,185	57,301	4,073,724	4,552	473	$626,823	$9,789.69	$1,780.45
2009	5,023	807	35,603	529	973	5.4	643,420	57,302	3,960,432	4,594	472	$657,242	$10,042.56	$1,851.44
2010	4,995	806	35,160	520	974	5.4	651,617	56,610	3,818,399	4,603	473	$678,254	$10,316.07	$1,908.59
2011	4,983	799	34,852	514	983	5.4	657,071	56,290	3,730,342	4,654	473	$702,822	$10,542.09	$1,959.69
2012	5,010	802	34,438	508	992	5.4	675,223	55,987	3,715,479	4,732	477	$757,213	$11,222.23	$2,089.07

Table 1 (Continued)

CLASSIFICATION: Total community hospitals

YEAR	HOSPITALS	BEDS (in thousands)	ADMISSIONS (in thousands)	AVERAGE DAILY CENSUS (in thousands)	ADJUSTED AVERAGE DAILY CENSUS (in thousands)	AVERAGE LENGTH OF STAY (days)	OUTPATIENT VISITS (in thousands)	NEWBORNS		FTE PERSONNEL		EXPENSES		
								Bassinets	Births	Number (in thousands)	Per 100 Adjusted Census	Amount (In Millions of dollars)	Adjusted per Inpatient Stay (dollars)	Adjusted per Inpatient Day (dollars)
1975	5,875	942	33,435	706	798	7.7	190,672	83,829	2,998,552	2,392	300	$38,962	$1,030.34	$133.81
1976	5,857	956	33,979	713	810	7.7	201,247	82,296	2,962,216	2,475	306	$45,240	$1,176.25	$152.76
1979	5,842	984	35,099	727	833	7.6	198,778	77,266	3,287,012	2,756	331	$66,004	$1,641.67	$217.34
1980	5,830	988	36,143	747	857	7.6	202,310	77,522	3,408,482	2,873	335	$76,851	$1,851.04	$245.12
1981	5,813	1,003	36,438	763	873	7.6	202,768	76,561	3,465,401	3,033	347	$90,572	$2,171.20	$284.33
1982	5,801	1,012	36,379	762	878	7.6	248,124	75,733	3,514,457	3,103	353	$104,876	$2,500.52	$327.37
1983	5,783	1,018	36,152	749	864	7.6	210,044	75,465	3,490,254	3,096	358	$116,438	$2,789.18	$369.49
1984	5,759	1,017	35,155	702	820	7.3	211,961	75,581	3,456,308	3,017	368	$123,336	$2,995.38	$411.10
1985	5,732	1,001	33,449	649	777	7.1	218,716	74,893	3,521,135	2,997	386	$130,499	$3,244.74	$460.19
1986	5,678	978	32,379	629	770	7.1	231,912	73,682	3,584,408	3,025	393	$140,654	$3,532.51	$500.81
1987	5,611	958	31,601	622	776	7.2	245,524	72,510	3,602,296	3,114	401	$152,585	$3,850.16	$538.96
1988	5,533	947	31,453	620	787	7.2	269,129	70,325	3,706,402	3,205	407	$168,722	$4,206.73	$586.33
1989	5,455	933	31,116	618	796	7.2	285,712	69,405	3,830,615	3,303	415	$184,898	$4,587.87	$636.96
1990	5,384	927	31,181	619	813	7.2	301,329	68,412	3,958,263	3,420	421	$203,693	$4,946.68	$686.83
1991	5,342	924	31,064	611	820	7.2	322,048	67,434	3,965,396	3,535	431	$225,023	$5,359.56	$752.10
1992	5,292	921	31,034	604	827	7.1	348,522	67,089	3,924,944	3,620	437	$248,095	$5,794.43	$819.83
1993	5,261	919	30,748	592	828	7.0	366,885	66,054	3,870,376	3,677	444	$266,089	$6,132.06	$880.52
1994	5,229	902	30,718	568	812	6.7	382,924	65,722	3,809,367	3,692	455	$275,779	$6,229.83	$930.71
1995	5,194	873	30,945	548	809	6.5	414,345	64,736	3,764,698	3,714	459	$285,588	$6,215.51	$967.69
1996	5,134	862	31,099	531	799	6.2	439,863	63,640	3,723,871	3,725	466	$293,755	$6,224.94	$1,006.14
1997	5,057	853	31,577	528	811	6.1	450,140	63,241	3,742,191	3,790	467	$305,763	$6,261.93	$1,032.70
1998	5,015	840	31,812	525	819	6.0	474,193	62,156	3,726,233	3,831	468	$318,834	$6,385.99	$1,066.96
1999	4,956	830	32,359	526	833	5.9	495,346	61,528	3,760,295	3,838	461	$335,246	$6,511.72	$1,102.61
2000	4,915	824	33,089	526	849	5.8	521,404	60,839	3,880,166	3,911	461	$356,564	$6,648.82	$1,149.40
2001	4,908	826	33,814	533	865	5.7	538,480	60,448	3,873,395	3,987	461	$383,735	$6,979.53	$1,217.27
2002	4,927	821	34,478	540	886	5.7	556,404	59,974	3,870,191	4,069	459	$416,591	$7,354.60	$1,289.87
2003	4,895	813	34,783	539	894	5.7	563,186	59,662	3,915,842	4,109	460	$450,124	$7,796.41	$1,379.48
2004	4,919	808	35,086	541	909	5.6	571,569	58,710	3,931,508	4,148	456	$481,247	$8,165.55	$1,450.35
2005	4,936	802	35,239	540	929	5.6	584,429	58,195	3,987,766	4,257	458	$515,740	$8,534.90	$1,522.42
2006	4,927	803	35,378	538	939	5.6	599,553	57,832	4,075,193	4,343	463	$551,835	$8,970.31	$1,612.23
2007	4,897	801	35,346	533	943	5.5	603,300	57,546	4,077,962	4,465	474	$583,252	$9,377.17	$1,696.10
2008	5,010	808	35,761	536	962	5.5	624,098	57,301	4,073,724	4,550	473	$626,577	$9,788.25	$1,782.28
2009	5,008	806	35,527	528	970	5.4	641,953	57,282	3,959,605	4,585	472	$656,156	$10,045.15	$1,852.59
2010	4,985	805	35,149	520	973	5.4	651,424	56,610	3,818,399	4,600	473	$677,968	$10,313.44	$1,909.64
2011	4,973	797	34,843	513	982	5.4	656,079	56,290	3,730,342	4,650	473	$702,091	$10,532.52	$1,959.58
2012	4,999	801	34,422	507	991	5.4	674,971	55,987	3,715,479	4,731	477	$756,917	$11,220.70	$2,090.01

Table 1 (Continued)

CLASSIFICATION: Nongovernment not-for-profit community hospitals

YEAR	HOSPITALS	BEDS (in thousands)	ADMISSIONS (in thousands)	AVERAGE DAILY CENSUS (in thousands)	ADJUSTED AVERAGE DAILY CENSUS (in thousands)	AVERAGE LENGTH OF STAY (days)	OUTPATIENT VISITS (in thousands)	NEWBORNS Bassinets	NEWBORNS Births	FTE PERSONNEL Number (in thousands)	FTE PERSONNEL Per 100 Adjusted Census	EXPENSES Amount (In Millions of dollars)	EXPENSES Adjusted per Inpatient Stay (dollars)	EXPENSES Adjusted per Inpatient Day (dollars)
1975	3,339	658	23,722	510	574	7.8	131,435	57,496	2,131,057	1,712	298	$27,938	$1,040.21	$133.36
1976	3,345	670	24,082	517	586	7.9	140,914	56,442	2,100,917	1,791	306	$32,764	$1,208.23	$152.94
1979	3,330	690	24,874	528	603	7.7	139,565	52,859	2,308,548	1,999	332	$47,937	$1,684.40	$218.06
1980	3,322	692	25,566	542	621	7.7	142,156	52,659	2,389,478	2,086	336	$55,780	$1,901.64	$245.74
1981	3,340	706	25,945	555	636	7.8	143,380	52,302	2,455,033	2,213	399	$66,267	$2,225.17	$285.64
1982	3,338	712	25,898	553	637	7.8	176,245	51,566	2,483,345	2,265	355	$76,806	$2,572.93	$330.41
1983	3,347	718	25,827	544	629	7.7	150,839	51,649	2,465,604	2,270	362	$85,637	$2,868.80	$373.78
1984	3,351	716	25,236	512	598	7.4	153,281	51,491	2,446,540	2,222	372	$90,814	$3,072.51	$415.04
1985	3,349	707	24,179	476	569	7.2	158,953	51,424	2,507,288	2,216	389	$96,150	$3,307.41	$462.69
1986	3,323	689	23,483	460	563	7.2	167,633	50,885	2,547,170	2,241	398	$103,524	$3,589.64	$503.64
1987	3,274	673	22,937	455	566	7.2	177,413	50,133	2,557,294	2,298	406	$112,325	$3,914.23	$543.67
1988	3,242	668	22,939	456	577	7.3	195,363	48,828	2,653,794	2,373	412	$124,703	$4,272.95	$591.13
1989	3,220	661	22,792	455	584	7.3	209,191	48,305	2,751,426	2,454	420	$136,889	$4,649.22	$642.45
1990	3,191	657	22,878	455	596	7.3	221,073	47,441	2,833,204	2,533	424	$150,673	$5,001.24	$692.36
1991	3,175	656	22,964	451	603	7.2	238,204	47,229	2,845,995	2,624	435	$166,806	$5,393.30	$758.21
1992	3,173	656	23,056	445	606	7.1	257,887	47,185	2,846,386	2,692	443	$183,793	$5,808.80	$828.44
1993	3,154	651	22,749	432	602	6.9	270,138	46,214	2,802,164	2,711	451	$197,187	$6,177.69	$897.70
1994	3,139	637	22,704	413	589	6.6	282,653	46,381	2,792,116	2,719	462	$204,219	$6,256.72	$950.31
1995	3,092	610	22,557	393	578	6.4	303,851	45,198	2,725,641	2,702	468	$209,614	$6,279.17	$994.39
1996	3,045	598	22,542	379	567	6.1	320,746	44,650	2,683,750	2,711	478	$215,950	$6,344.05	$1,042.04
1997	3,000	591	22,905	376	575	6.0	330,215	44,484	2,698,086	2,765	481	$225,287	$6,392.74	$1,074.26
1998	3,026	588	23,282	377	587	5.9	352,114	44,087	2,715,958	2,834	483	$237,978	$6,525.68	$1,110.50
1999	3,012	587	23,871	381	605	5.8	370,784	44,172	2,746,453	2,862	473	$251,534	$6,607.51	$1,139.89
2000	3,003	583	24,452	382	618	5.7	393,168	43,655	2,833,615	2,919	472	$267,051	$6,717.48	$1,182.32
2001	2,998	585	24,983	385	628	5.6	404,901	43,640	2,829,691	2,971	473	$287,250	$7,051.76	$1,255.25
2002	3,025	582	25,425	391	646	5.6	416,910	43,241	2,820,159	3,039	471	$312,726	$7,457.84	$1,328.81
2003	2,984	575	25,668	389	647	5.5	424,215	42,965	2,854,764	3,059	473	$337,696	$7,904.93	$1,429.62
2004	2,967	568	25,757	388	655	5.5	430,262	41,968	2,844,617	3,077	470	$359,414	$8,266.64	$1,501.09
2005	2,958	561	25,881	388	667	5.5	441,653	41,585	2,876,677	3,155	473	$385,993	$8,670.83	$1,585.34
2006	2,919	559	25,798	385	671	5.4	453,501	40,888	2,905,275	3,207	478	$412,868	$9,189.58	$1,685.62
2007	2,913	554	25,752	380	673	5.4	455,825	40,681	2,907,002	3,286	488	$436,319	$9,592.93	$1,776.06
2008	2,923	557	25,899	380	683	5.4	469,804	40,567	2,901,854	3,340	489	$468,080	$10,080.50	$1,875.78
2009	2,918	556	25,783	375	690	5.3	485,935	40,467	2,822,527	3,369	488	$492,853	$10,379.09	$1,956.71
2010	2,904	556	25,532	368	691	5.3	494,178	39,946	2,750,163	3,388	490	$510,744	$10,651.81	$2,025.05
2011	2,903	548	25,185	362	694	5.2	496,643	39,651	2,692,577	3,427	494	$528,303	$10,932.55	$2,088.05
2012	2,894	545	24,751	354	697	5.2	512,237	39,778	2,684,600	3,477	499	$563,960	$11,563.17	$2,214.26

Table 1 (Continued)

Investor-owned (for-profit) community hospitals

CLASSIFICATION YEAR	HOSPITALS	BEDS (in thousands)	ADMISSIONS (in thousands)	AVERAGE DAILY CENSUS (in thousands)	ADJUSTED AVERAGE DAILY CENSUS (in thousands)	AVERAGE LENGTH OF STAY (days)	OUTPATIENT VISITS (in thousands)	NEWBORNS Bassinets	NEWBORNS Births	FTE PERSONNEL Number (in thousands)	FTE PERSONNEL Per 100 Adjusted Census	EXPENSES Amount (in Millions of dollars)	EXPENSES Adjusted per Inpatient Stay (dollars)	EXPENSES Adjusted per Inpatient Day (dollars)
1975	775	73	2,646	48	53	6.6	7,713	4,062	141,392	139	263	$2,561	$876.48	$132.80
1976	752	76	2,734	50	54	6.6	8,048	4,044	144,751	147	272	$3,085	$1,031.91	$156.35
1979	727	83	2,963	53	59	6.6	9,289	4,110	174,843	174	300	$4,820	$1,476.42	$225.87
1980	730	87	3,165	57	62	6.5	9,696	4,439	199,722	189	304	$5,847	$1,675.85	$257.12
1981	729	88	3,239	58	63	6.5	9,961	4,523	207,405	203	322	$6,856	$1,952.56	$299.02
1982	748	91	3,316	60	66	6.6	13,193	4,736	219,675	212	320	$8,177	$2,224.75	$340.03
1983	757	94	3,299	59	66	6.5	10,389	5,039	228,883	213	323	$9,208	$2,517.53	$385.42
1984	786	100	3,314	57	64	6.3	11,090	5,807	242,088	214	335	$10,251	$2,748.51	$438.30
1985	805	104	3,242	54	63	6.1	12,378	6,117	266,839	221	350	$11,486	$3,033.06	$500.48
1986	834	107	3,231	54	65	6.1	14,896	6,305	291,112	229	354	$12,987	$3,341.79	$552.40
1987	828	106	3,157	54	66	6.2	16,566	6,391	306,492	242	367	$14,067	$3,617.19	$585.01
1988	790	104	3,090	53	66	6.2	17,926	6,254	308,828	249	379	$15,545	$4,022.77	$649.33
1989	769	102	3,071	53	67	6.3	19,341	6,354	325,711	261	390	$17,240	$4,406.20	$707.90
1990	749	101	3,066	54	69	6.4	20,110	6,261	340,555	273	396	$18,822	$4,727.27	$751.55
1991	738	100	3,016	52	69	6.3	21,174	6,358	359,115	281	409	$20,516	$5,133.53	$820.19
1992	723	99	2,969	51	69	6.3	22,900	6,519	357,776	285	412	$22,496	$5,548.24	$888.73
1993	717	99	2,946	51	69	6.2	24,936	6,395	363,358	289	417	$23,077	$5,643.21	$914.39
1994	719	101	3,035	50	70	6.1	26,443	6,329	354,477	302	434	$23,445	$5,528.91	$923.90
1995	752	106	3,428	55	77	5.8	31,940	7,164	408,339	343	443	$26,653	$5,425.20	$946.99
1996	759	109	3,684	56	82	5.6	37,347	7,441	444,697	359	437	$28,385	$5,207.44	$945.49
1997	797	115	3,953	60	89	5.5	40,919	8,026	465,919	385	433	$31,179	$5,218.69	$961.96
1998	771	113	3,971	60	90	5.5	42,072	7,895	466,025	383	425	$31,732	$5,262.44	$968.00
1999	747	107	3,905	58	86	5.5	39,896	7,486	467,585	362	422	$31,179	$5,350.07	$999.03
2000	749	110	4,141	61	90	5.4	43,378	7,792	503,497	378	418	$34,969	$5,642.18	$1,057.32
2001	754	109	4,197	63	92	5.4	44,706	7,413	494,669	379	413	$37,348	$5,971.81	$1,121.31
2002	766	108	4,365	64	93	5.3	45,215	7,467	496,988	380	407	$40,082	$6,161.44	$1,180.83
2003	790	110	4,481	65	95	5.3	44,246	7,491	515,693	391	411	$43,953	$6,589.91	$1,264.50
2004	835	113	4,599	68	100	5.4	44,962	7,763	534,503	406	406	$48,971	$7,139.13	$1,362.42
2005	868	114	4,618	68	101	5.3	46,016	7,714	546,307	421	418	$51,833	$7,351.96	$1,412.74
2006	890	115	4,735	68	103	5.2	44,237	8,012	574,113	423	413	$55,030	$7,422.08	$1,471.53
2007	873	116	4,626	66	101	5.2	43,943	7,760	555,670	432	429	$56,405	$7,823.44	$1,535.98
2008	982	121	4,839	70	109	5.3	44,897	7,791	562,711	450	414	$61,762	$7,984.62	$1,555.55
2009	998	122	4,887	70	112	5.3	47,281	7,965	553,233	464	414	$64,367	$8,037.18	$1,573.64
2010	1,013	125	4,925	71	113	5.3	48,201	7,965	525,427	474	420	$67,168	$8,336.16	$1,628.90
2011	1,025	128	5,060	73	119	5.3	50,013	8,137	508,330	485	409	$70,340	$8,262.74	$1,627.65
2012	1,068	135	5,224	77	124	5.3	53,854	8,192	530,941	515	414	$79,114	$8,860.94	$1,746.85

Table 1 (Continued)

CLASSIFICATION

State and local government community hospitals

YEAR	HOSPITALS	BEDS (in thousands)	ADMISSIONS (in thousands)	AVERAGE DAILY CENSUS (in thousands)	ADJUSTED AVERAGE DAILY CENSUS (in thousands)	AVERAGE LENGTH OF STAY (days)	OUTPATIENT VISITS (in thousands)	NEWBORNS Bassinets	NEWBORNS Births	FTE PERSONNEL Number (in thousands)	FTE PERSONNEL Per 100 Adjusted Census	EXPENSES Amount (In Millions of dollars)	EXPENSES Adjusted per Inpatient Stay (dollars)	EXPENSES Adjusted per Inpatient Day (dollars)
1975	1,761	210	7,067	148	171	7.6	51,525	22,271	726,103	540	316	$8,463	$1,030.86	$135.64
1976	1,760	210	7,163	146	170	7.5	52,286	21,810	716,548	537	315	$9,391	$1,132.50	$151.00
1979	1,785	211	7,262	146	171	7.4	49,924	20,297	803,621	583	341	$13,247	$1,561.04	$211.89
1980	1,778	209	7,413	149	174	7.3	50,459	20,424	819,282	598	343	$15,204	$1,750.13	$238.63
1981	1,744	210	7,255	150	174	7.6	49,427	19,736	802,963	618	354	$17,449	$2,071.57	$274.25
1982	1,715	210	7,165	149	175	7.6	58,685	19,431	811,437	627	320	$19,893	$2,364.09	$311.56
1983	1,679	207	7,025	145	170	7.6	48,816	18,777	795,767	613	360	$21,593	$2,621.28	$347.56
1984	1,622	201	6,606	133	158	7.3	47,590	18,283	767,680	581	368	$22,271	$2,823.13	$385.17
1985	1,578	189	6,028	119	145	7.2	47,386	17,352	747,008	561	387	$22,863	$3,106.14	$432.84
1986	1,521	182	5,665	114	142	7.4	49,383	16,492	746,126	555	391	$24,143	$3,404.69	$466.17
1987	1,509	180	5,507	113	144	7.5	51,544	15,986	738,510	573	399	$26,192	$3,717.77	$499.33
1988	1,501	175	5,424	112	145	7.6	55,840	15,243	743,780	583	403	$28,474	$4,033.67	$538.63
1989	1,466	170	5,253	110	145	7.7	57,179	14,746	753,478	589	406	$30,769	$4,430.12	$582.15
1990	1,444	169	5,236	111	148	7.7	60,146	14,710	784,504	614	415	$34,198	$4,837.76	$634.45
1991	1,429	168	5,084	108	148	7.8	62,670	13,847	760,286	630	424	$37,701	$5,339.75	$695.89
1992	1,396	166	5,008	108	152	7.9	67,734	13,385	720,782	643	424	$41,806	$5,870.76	$753.92
1993	1,390	169	5,054	109	157	7.8	71,811	13,445	704,854	676	430	$45,825	$6,205.52	$799.73
1994	1,371	164	4,979	104	154	7.6	73,828	13,012	662,774	672	438	$48,115	$6,513.39	$858.62
1995	1,350	157	4,961	100	154	7.4	78,554	12,374	630,718	670	435	$49,322	$6,445.18	$877.85
1996	1,330	155	4,873	96	150	7.2	81,770	11,549	595,424	654	437	$49,420	$6,418.65	$903.41
1997	1,260	148	4,720	92	148	7.1	79,007	10,731	578,186	640	433	$49,298	$6,475.07	$913.62
1998	1,218	139	4,559	87	142	7.0	80,008	10,174	544,250	614	433	$49,123	$6,612.23	$949.36
1999	1,197	136	4,583	86	143	6.9	84,667	9,870	546,257	614	430	$52,534	$6,923.35	$1,006.91
2000	1,163	131	4,496	83	140	6.7	84,858	9,392	543,054	614	438	$54,544	$7,106.05	$1,063.75
2001	1,156	132	4,634	85	145	6.7	88,873	9,395	549,035	637	438	$59,137	$7,400.01	$1,113.79
2002	1,136	130	4,688	84	147	6.6	94,280	9,266	553,044	651	442	$63,783	$7,772.93	$1,188.12
2003	1,121	129	4,634	84	152	6.6	94,725	9,206	545,385	658	434	$68,475	$8,205.10	$1,237.64
2004	1,117	128	4,730	85	154	6.5	96,345	8,979	552,388	666	431	$72,861	$8,473.18	$1,291.06
2005	1,110	128	4,740	85	161	6.5	96,760	8,896	564,782	681	424	$77,914	$8,793.26	$1,329.64
2006	1,119	128	4,848	86	165	6.5	101,845	8,932	595,805	713	433	$83,974	$9,147.40	$1,400.09
2007	1,111	131	4,967	87	169	6.4	103,532	9,105	615,290	747	443	$90,528	$9,523.22	$1,472.26
2008	1,105	131	5,023	86	170	6.3	109,398	8,943	609,159	760	446	$96,735	$9,826.94	$1,552.32
2009	1,092	127	4,857	83	168	6.2	108,738	8,850	583,845	751	447	$98,937	$10,067.96	$1,611.31
2010	1,068	125	4,693	80	169	6.2	109,045	8,699	542,809	738	437	$100,056	$10,283.35	$1,624.93
2011	1,045	121	4,598	78	170	6.2	109,423	8,502	529,435	738	434	$103,448	$10,531.65	$1,666.96
2012	1,037	120	4,447	77	170	6.3	108,880	8,017	499,938	739	435	$113,843	$11,668.15	$1,831.00

Table 2

2012 U.S. Registered Hospitals: Utilization, Personnel, and Finances

Excludes U.S.-Associated Areas, Puerto Rico, and nonregistered hospitals.

CLASSIFICATION	HOSPITALS	BEDS	ADMISSIONS	INPATIENT DAYS	ADJUSTED INPATIENT DAYS	AVERAGE DAILY CENSUS	ADJUSTED AVERAGE DAILY CENSUS	AVERAGE STAY (days)	SURGICAL OPERATIONS	OUTPATIENT VISITS Emergency	OUTPATIENT VISITS Total	NEWBORNS Bassinets	NEWBORNS Births
UNITED STATES	5,723	920,829	36,156,245	219,355,794	—	600,217	—	—	27,476,567	137,281,696	777,960,574	56,693	3,754,085
6-24 Beds	508	8,557	227,801	1,048,536	—	2,858	—	—	352,885	2,323,009	16,606,241	529	23,313
25-49	1,298	42,216	1,214,299	6,942,713	—	19,015	—	—	1,447,155	9,047,343	55,311,025	3,100	124,153
50-99	1,145	81,901	2,367,929	17,419,562	—	47,666	—	—	2,163,896	12,274,557	73,476,044	5,179	232,030
100-199	1,205	172,535	6,446,743	38,572,100	—	105,625	—	—	5,081,648	28,200,488	144,774,491	11,622	658,802
200-299	661	161,353	6,647,600	38,303,465	—	104,895	—	—	4,829,114	25,222,343	133,394,955	10,438	676,325
300-399	390	135,310	5,803,338	32,881,377	—	90,070	—	—	3,982,219	19,755,426	103,796,418	8,851	635,069
400-499	204	90,763	4,030,805	22,624,831	—	61,834	—	—	2,828,028	13,127,334	75,860,830	5,690	427,993
500 or more	312	228,194	9,417,730	61,563,210	—	168,254	—	—	6,791,622	27,331,196	174,740,570	11,284	976,400
Psychiatric	422	72,062	798,083	22,390,025	—	61,355	—	—	13,200	142,414	11,017,439	0	0
Hospitals	416	69,677	797,991	21,527,744	—	58,994	—	—	13,200	142,414	11,017,439	0	0
Institutions for mentally retarded	6	2,385	92	862,281	—	2,361	—	—	0	0	0	0	0
General	4,673	797,473	34,528,856	184,377,894	—	504,416	—	—	26,997,896	136,739,333	750,984,962	55,936	3,701,139
Hospitals	4,659	795,769	34,510,907	183,898,892	—	503,104	—	—	26,995,508	136,691,945	750,176,350	55,936	3,701,139
Hospital units of institutions	14	1,704	17,949	479,002	—	1,312	—	—	2,388	47,388	808,612	0	0
TB and other respiratory diseases	1	42	81	15,172	—	41	—	—	0	0	0	0	0
Obstetrics and gynecology	8	1,497	73,814	327,748	—	895	—	—	55,824	58,456	804,611	584	48,733
Eye, ear, nose and throat	4	139	2,427	7,465	—	20	—	—	73,509	35,774	785,635	0	0
Rehabilitation	202	15,540	275,896	3,944,350	—	10,811	—	—	7,745	16,867	5,932,658	16	0
Orthopedic	26	1,210	53,200	190,008	—	520	—	—	115,009	5,301	1,064,200	0	0
Chronic Disease	5	403	1,391	99,267	—	273	—	—	191	40,897	96,978	0	0
Surgical	8	259	6,037	40,259	—	109	—	—	16,860	24,766	168,143	0	0
Cancer	9	1,976	87,747	602,635	—	1,647	—	—	76,663	12,408	3,968,411	0	0
Heart	7	521	26,392	95,185	—	261	—	—	12,484		102,053	0	830
Acute long-term care hospital	319	24,410	231,922	5,986,851	—	16,370	—	—	57,261	69,637	1,428,574	25	3,383
All other	39	5,297	70,399	1,278,935	—	3,499	—	—	49,925	135,843	1,606,268	132	0
Federal	211	38,557	900,550	8,957,994	—	24,502	—	—	645,422	3,868,438	92,890,602	702	38,605
Psychiatric	9	2,215	15,941	631,699	—	1,728	—	—	1,447	882	2,070,361	0	0
General and other special	202	36,342	884,609	8,326,295	—	22,774	—	—	643,975	3,867,556	90,820,241	702	38,605
Nonfederal	5,512	882,272	35,255,695	210,397,800	—	575,715	—	—	26,831,145	133,413,258	685,069,972	55,991	3,715,480
Psychiatric	413	69,847	782,142	21,758,326	—	59,627	—	—	11,753	141,532	8,947,078	0	0
Hospitals	407	67,462	782,050	20,896,045	—	57,266	—	—	11,753	141,532	8,947,078	0	0
Institutions for mentally retarded	6	2,385	92	862,281	—	2,361	—	—	0	0	0	0	0
TB and other respiratory diseases	1	42	81	15,172	15,172	41	41	187.0	0	0	642	0	0
Long-term general and other special	88	10,633	35,602	2,901,462	3,131,157	7,933	8,557	82.0	8,157	44,460	899,667	4	1
Short-term general and other special	5,010	801,750	34,437,870	185,722,840	362,464,557	508,114	991,836	5.4	26,811,235	133,227,266	675,222,585	55,987	3,715,479
Hospital units of institutions	11	1,184	15,799	299,805	305,291	822	837	19.0	4	6,236	251,254	0	0
Community Hospitals	4,999	800,566	34,422,071	185,423,035	362,159,266	507,292	990,999	5.4	26,811,231	133,221,030	674,971,331	55,987	3,715,479
6-24 Beds	462	7,791	197,448	879,985	3,887,733	2,399	10,630	4.5	327,243	1,929,787	10,627,772	463	18,058
25-49	1,192	38,338	1,128,446	6,029,293	19,208,354	16,514	52,613	5.3	1,383,696	8,566,426	46,693,058	2,948	115,996
50-99	954	67,879	2,017,239	13,678,515	34,519,349	37,443	94,458	6.8	1,985,306	11,275,005	56,799,952	4,930	222,207
100-199	1,012	145,556	5,920,309	30,892,477	66,965,400	84,609	183,463	5.2	4,968,051	27,668,989	123,765,040	11,530	658,328
200-299	570	139,212	6,297,821	32,150,843	60,988,277	87,964	166,920	5.1	4,692,499	24,468,359	111,663,614	10,291	661,428
300-399	348	120,554	5,659,683	28,628,393	51,194,765	78,436	140,258	5.1	3,924,988	19,494,322	93,787,068	8,851	635,069
400-499	189	84,007	3,966,019	20,755,259	36,921,362	56,721	100,900	5.2	2,806,876	12,993,712	72,412,649	5,690	427,993
500 or more	272	197,229	9,235,106	52,408,270	88,474,206	143,206	241,757	5.7	6,722,572	26,824,430	159,222,178	11,284	976,400
Nongovernment not-for-profit	2,894	545,287	24,751,485	129,413,780	254,694,610	353,953	696,730	5.2	19,598,704	94,302,219	512,237,001	39,778	2,684,600
Investor-owned (for profit)	1,068	135,008	5,223,992	27,944,662	45,289,380	76,626	124,324	5.3	3,831,208	19,261,151	53,854,465	8,192	530,941
State and Local Government	1,037	120,271	4,446,594	28,064,593	62,175,276	76,713	169,945	6.3	3,381,319	19,657,660	108,879,865	8,017	499,938

Table 2 (Continued)

CLASSIFICATION	FULL-TIME EQUIVALENT PERSONNEL					FULL-TIME EQUIVALENT TRAINEES			EXPENSES — LABOR			EXPENSES		TOTAL	
	Physicians and Dentists	Registered Nurses	Licensed Practical Nurses	Other Salaried Personnel	Total Personnel	Medical and Dental Residents	Other Trainees	Total Trainees	Payroll (in thousands)	Employee Benefits (in thousands)	Total (in thousands)	Percent of Total	Amount (in thousands)	Adjusted per Admission	Adjusted per Inpatient Day
UNITED STATES	143,642	1,448,676	112,430	3,552,801	5,257,549	109,860	12,001	121,862	$331,565,933	$91,193,301	$422,759,234	51.0	$829,665,386	—	—
6-24 Beds	1,651	13,581	3,386	47,529	66,147	23	35	58	$3,444,564	$896,584	$4,341,148	50.8	$8,541,649	—	—
25-49	7,359	60,020	10,825	199,060	277,264	505	760	1,265	$14,614,577	$3,823,719	$18,438,296	53.3	$34,614,101	—	—
50-99	9,073	95,244	14,761	275,647	394,725	1,077	539	1,616	$22,657,347	$6,024,055	$28,681,402	52.4	$54,689,347	—	—
100-199	19,794	232,737	21,186	590,967	864,684	6,616	1,800	8,416	$52,816,952	$14,436,777	$67,253,729	52.0	$129,338,200	—	—
200-299	23,722	244,450	23,731	594,728	886,631	11,589	1,950	13,539	$56,456,224	$15,207,610	$71,663,834	50.7	$141,325,939	—	—
300-399	17,134	214,002	12,213	499,753	743,102	11,573	1,040	12,613	$47,307,341	$13,438,319	$60,745,659	50.5	$120,361,847	—	—
400-499	14,577	163,968	7,892	362,326	548,763	15,691	974	16,666	$36,404,360	$9,922,592	$46,326,952	50.9	$91,067,612	—	—
500 or more	50,332	424,674	18,436	982,791	1,476,233	62,786	4,903	67,689	$97,864,569	$27,443,645	$125,308,214	50.2	$249,726,691	—	—
Psychiatric	4,258	27,332	6,316	140,480	178,386	385	624	1,009	$8,932,622	$3,005,148	$11,937,769	71.0	$16,813,109	—	—
Hospitals	4,233	27,143	6,002	134,966	172,344	385	498	883	$8,669,398	$2,873,652	$11,543,050	70.6	$16,347,312	—	—
Institutions for mentally retarded	25	189	314	5,514	6,042	0	126	126	$263,224	$131,496	$394,720	84.7	$465,797	—	—
General	133,992	1,372,032	98,635	3,257,220	4,861,879	108,217	10,222	118,439	$309,441,660	$84,700,009	$394,141,669	50.4	$781,640,838	—	—
Hospitals	133,802	1,371,720	98,347	3,254,447	4,858,316	108,217	10,190	118,407	$309,222,898	$84,632,119	$393,855,017	50.4	$781,118,781	—	—
Hospital units of institutions	190	312	288	2,773	3,563	0	32	32	$218,763	$67,890	$286,653	54.9	$522,057	—	—
TB and other respiratory diseases	0	26	19	125	170	0	0	0	$5,975	$1,930	$7,905	60.8	$13,009	—	—
Obstetrics and gynecology	169	3,130	44	4,830	8,173	60	4	64	$564,038	$146,420	$710,458	50.5	$1,407,991	—	—
Eye, ear, nose and throat	191	388	18	2,822	3,419	84	43	127	$163,168	$50,368	$213,537	45.6	$468,455	—	—
Rehabilitation	587	11,575	2,055	43,972	58,189	166	37	203	$2,975,567	$699,307	$3,674,874	58.3	$6,304,512	—	—
Orthopedic	488	2,293	101	7,290	10,172	60	8	68	$804,931	$238,855	$1,043,786	50.3	$2,074,255	—	—
Chronic Disease	13	228	35	1,197	1,473	0	13	13	$75,207	$21,394	$96,600	59.8	$161,443	—	—
Surgical	6	419	24	907	1,356	0	13	13	$75,196	$17,417	$92,613	39.6	$233,757	—	—
Cancer	2,819	8,777	173	33,315	45,084	720	949	1,669	$3,425,365	$995,413	$4,420,778	50.5	$8,745,971	—	—
Heart	17	889	23	1,290	2,219	5	0	5	$151,038	$35,986	$187,024	41.9	$446,070	—	—
Acute long-term care hospital	256	16,749	4,354	44,784	66,143	38	1	40	$3,541,724	$861,927	$4,403,651	53.0	$8,307,640	—	—
All other	846	4,838	633	14,569	20,886	125	100	225	$1,409,442	$419,128	$1,828,570	60.0	$3,048,338	—	—
Federal	24,973	66,952	22,939	216,062	330,926	6,521	4,153	10,674	$25,545,598	$6,800,964	$32,346,562	59.6	$54,261,745	—	—
Psychiatric	483	1,724	397	7,115	9,719	10	60	70	$722,024	$209,942	$931,965	64.3	$1,448,612	—	—
General and other special	24,490	65,228	22,542	208,947	321,207	6,511	4,093	10,604	$24,823,574	$6,591,022	$31,414,596	59.5	$52,813,133	—	—
Nonfederal	118,669	1,381,724	89,491	3,336,739	4,926,623	103,339	7,848	111,188	$306,020,335	$84,392,337	$390,412,673	50.3	$775,403,641	—	—
Psychiatric	3,775	25,608	5,919	133,365	168,667	375	564	939	$8,210,598	$2,795,206	$11,005,804	71.6	$15,364,497	—	—
Hospitals	3,750	25,419	5,605	127,851	162,625	375	438	813	$7,947,374	$2,663,711	$10,611,085	71.2	$14,898,700	—	—
Institutions for mentally retarded	25	189	314	5,514	6,042	0	126	126	$263,224	$131,496	$394,720	84.7	$465,797	—	—
TB and other respiratory diseases	0	26	19	125	170	0	0	0	$5,975	$1,930	$7,905	60.8	$13,009	$160,606.31	$857.44
Long-term general and other special	300	4,790	1,147	19,338	25,575	60	47	108	$1,362,231	$416,153	$1,778,384	63.2	$2,813,176	$70,354.03	$898.45
Short-term general and other special	114,594	1,351,300	82,406	3,183,911	4,732,211	102,904	7,237	110,141	$296,441,531	$81,179,049	$377,620,580	49.9	$757,212,959	$11,222.23	$2,089.07
Hospital units of institutions	115	136	138	874	1,263	0	7	7	$105,600	$25,252	$130,852	44.2	$296,203	$17,194.10	$970.23
Community Hospitals	114,479	1,351,164	82,268	3,183,037	4,730,948	102,904	7,230	110,134	$296,335,931	$81,153,797	$377,489,728	49.1	$756,916,757	$11,220.70	$2,090.01
6-24 Beds	920	11,822	2,504	37,938	53,184	4	21	25	$2,732,368	$704,902	$3,437,270	49.2	$6,984,977	$7,626.39	$1,796.67
25-49	5,709	55,302	10,085	173,401	244,497	260	729	989	$13,103,619	$3,430,762	$16,534,381	51.5	$32,080,809	$7,922.10	$1,670.15
50-99	5,732	80,412	10,359	225,881	322,384	400	35	435	$17,713,227	$4,615,427	$22,328,654	51.3	$43,488,786	$8,253.60	$1,259.84
100-199	13,530	210,290	16,477	509,472	749,769	5,066	436	5,502	$45,032,578	$12,238,745	$57,271,323	50.8	$112,758,082	$8,968.22	$1,683.83
200-299	16,702	223,610	12,700	520,301	773,313	8,984	508	9,492	$48,541,128	$13,228,858	$61,769,985	49.5	$124,808,644	$10,523.92	$2,046.44
300-399	14,174	204,577	9,410	457,816	685,977	11,364	789	12,153	$44,008,096	$12,370,558	$56,378,654	49.4	$114,103,096	$11,276.85	$2,228.80
400-499	12,878	159,340	6,707	347,525	526,450	14,844	859	15,703	$34,899,168	$9,439,136	$44,338,304	50.5	$87,804,965	$12,453.84	$2,378.16
500 or more	44,834	405,811	14,026	910,703	1,375,374	61,982	3,853	65,835	$90,305,747	$25,125,409	$115,431,156	49.1	$234,887,398	$15,036.35	$2,654.87
Nongovernment not-for-profit	94,285	983,833	49,285	2,349,913	3,477,316	72,804	5,333	78,137	$220,301,581	$60,278,203	$280,579,784	49.8	$563,960,296	$11,563.17	$2,214.26
Investor-owned (for profit)	3,980	171,419	14,755	324,820	514,974	4,741	131	4,872	$30,034,044	$6,771,137	$36,805,181	46.5	$79,113,760	$8,860.94	$1,746.85
State and Local Government	16,214	195,912	18,228	508,304	738,658	25,359	1,766	27,125	$46,000,306	$14,104,456	$60,104,762	52.8	$113,842,700	$11,668.15	$1,831.00

U.S. Registered Hospitals

Tables 3–6

Total U.S.

TABLE **3**

TOTAL UNITED STATES

U.S. Registered Community Hospitals
(Nonfederal, short-term general and other special hospitals)

Overview 2008–2012

	2012	2011	2010	2009	2008
TOTAL U.S. Community Hospitals	**4,999**	**4,973**	**4,985**	**5,008**	**5,010**
Bed Size Category					
6-24	462	445	424	402	389
25-49	1,192	1,177	1,167	1,164	1,151
50-99	954	955	970	991	995
100-199	1,012	1,005	1,029	1,063	1,070
200-299	570	582	585	582	596
300-399	348	353	352	348	355
400-499	189	184	185	192	184
500 + ...	272	272	273	266	270
Location					
Hospitals Urban.	3,019	2,989	2,998	3,011	2,838
Hospitals Rural	1,980	1,984	1,987	1,997	2,172
Control					
State and Local Government.	1,037	1,045	1,068	1,092	1,105
Not for Profit	2,894	2,903	2,904	2,918	2,923
Investor owned	1,068	1,025	1,013	998	982
Physician Models					
Independent Practice Association	496	514	563	579	597
Group Practice without Walls.	165	161	159	175	160
Open Physician-Hospital Organization	620	622	630	649	672
Closed Physician-Hospital Organization	219	210	203	207	213
Management Service Organization	441	446	454	449	436
Integrated Salary Model	1,844	1,795	1,728	1,664	1,583
Equity Model	84	76	80	92	97
Foundation.	269	263	261	237	248
Insurance Products					
Health Maintenance Organization	627	640	614	587	597
Preferred Provider Organization.	576	744	740	693	685
Indemnity Fee for Service	210	253	260	235	250
Managed Care Contracts					
Health Maintenance Organization	2,697	2,665	2,677	2,702	2,670
Preferred Provider Organization.	3,030	3,045	3,074	3,137	3,125
Affiliations					
Hospitals in a System.	3,100	3,007	2,941	2,921	2,868
Hospitals in a Network	1,508	1,535	1,508	1,485	1,490
Hospitals in a Group Purchasing Organization. .	3,519	3,562	3,595	3,674	3,677

TABLE 3

TOTAL UNITED STATES

U.S. Registered Community Hospitals
(Nonfederal, short-term general and other special hospitals)

Utilization, Personnel, Revenue and Expenses, Community Health Indicators 2008–2012

	2012	2011	2010	2009	2008
TOTAL FACILITY (Includes Hospital and Nursing Home Units)					
Utilization - Inpatient					
Beds	800,566	797,403	804,943	805,593	808,069
Admissions	34,422,071	34,843,085	35,149,427	35,527,377	35,760,750
Inpatient Days	185,423,035	187,072,013	189,593,349	192,656,804	196,078,468
Average Length of Stay	5.4	5.4	5.4	5.4	5.5
Inpatient Surgeries	9,513,598	9,638,467	9,954,821	10,100,980	10,105,156
Births	3,715,479	3,730,342	3,818,399	3,959,605	4,073,724
Utilization - Outpatient					
Emergency Outpatient Visits	133,221,030	129,461,658	127,249,317	127,298,193	123,024,024
Other Outpatient Visits	541,750,301	526,617,284	524,174,400	514,655,249	501,074,272
Total Outpatient Visits	674,971,331	656,078,942	651,423,717	641,953,442	624,098,296
Outpatient Surgeries	17,297,633	17,269,245	17,357,177	17,357,534	17,354,282
Personnel					
Full Time RNs	1,103,906	1,071,952	1,055,118	1,029,828	984,649
Full Time LPNs	69,318	72,641	76,503	82,159	86,750
Part Time RNs	494,530	483,351	477,739	477,699	487,480
Part Time LPNs	25,892	26,448	29,164	31,647	35,602
Total Full Time	4,105,295	4,034,205	3,989,587	3,971,118	3,919,415
Total Part Time	1,471,619	1,446,076	1,427,136	1,434,492	1,460,487
Revenue - Inpatient					
Gross Inpatient Revenue	$1,355,940,534,641	$1,275,806,742,970	$1,224,790,498,627	$1,154,085,466,645	$1,090,598,012,951
Revenue - Outpatient					
Gross Outpatient Revenue	$1,075,704,443,658	$968,928,635,990	$887,419,059,972	$802,893,402,009	$711,918,761,681
Revenue and Expenses - Totals					
(Includes Inpatient and Outpatient)					
Total Gross Revenue	$2,431,644,978,299	$2,244,735,378,960	$2,112,209,558,599	$1,956,978,868,654	$1,802,516,774,632
Deductions from Revenue	1,669,437,831,803	1,545,016,281,249	1,435,826,277,742	1,309,916,141,834	1,191,615,889,365
Net Patient Revenue	762,207,146,496	699,719,097,711	676,383,280,857	647,062,726,820	610,900,885,267
Other Operating Revenue	47,528,382,573	43,297,884,991	41,269,017,419	38,997,453,520	37,136,577,114
Other Nonoperating Revenue	11,599,107,141	12,267,965,061	13,251,393,842	4,467,480,534	-4,453,107,631
Total Net Revenue	821,334,636,210	755,284,947,763	730,903,692,118	690,527,660,874	643,584,354,750
Total Expenses	756,916,756,696	702,091,033,815	677,968,038,012	656,156,258,314	626,576,957,912
HOSPITAL UNIT (Excludes Separate Nursing Home Units)					
Utilization - Inpatient					
Beds	751,490	749,181	755,091	755,286	753,905
Admissions	34,217,866	34,636,454	34,935,503	35,304,455	35,522,351
Inpatient Days	169,860,722	171,803,076	173,686,925	176,511,062	179,043,949
Average Length of Stay	5.0	5.0	5.0	5.0	5.0
Personnel					
Total Full Time	4,068,209	4,002,112	3,955,083	3,930,304	3,875,073
Total Part Time	1,452,480	1,428,754	1,407,838	1,413,237	1,436,850
Revenue and Expenses - Totals					
(Includes Inpatient and Outpatient)					
Total Net Revenue	$817,155,645,229	$751,284,115,404	$726,685,542,179	$686,454,003,753	$639,389,781,304
Total Expenses	753,064,177,148	698,572,269,130	674,188,184,839	652,470,080,058	622,828,801,705
COMMUNITY HEALTH INDICATORS PER 1000 POPULATION					
Total Population (in thousands)	313,914	311,592	309,051	307,007	304,375
Inpatient					
Beds	2.6	2.6	2.6	2.6	2.7
Admissions	109.7	111.8	113.7	115.7	117.5
Inpatient Days	590.7	600.4	613.5	627.5	644.2
Inpatient Surgeries	30.3	30.9	32.2	32.9	33.2
Births	11.8	12.0	12.4	12.9	13.4
Outpatient					
Emergency Outpatient Visits	424.4	415.5	411.7	414.6	404.2
Other Outpatient Visits	1,725.8	1,690.1	1,696.1	1,676.4	1,646.2
Total Outpatient Visits	2,150.2	2,105.6	2,107.8	2,091.0	2,050.4
Outpatient Surgeries	55.1	55.4	56.2	56.5	57.0
Expense per Capita (per person)	$2,411.2	$2,253.2	$2,193.7	$2,137.3	$2,058.6

Total U.S.

TABLE 4

BED SIZE CATEGORY 6-24

U.S. Registered Community Hospitals
(Nonfederal, short-term general and other special hospitals)

Overview 2008–2012

	2012	2011	2010	2009	2008
Total Community Hospitals in					
Bed Size Category 6-24	**462**	**445**	**424**	**402**	**389**
Location					
Hospitals Urban.	120	114	113	111	86
Hospitals Rural	342	331	311	291	303
Control					
State and Local Government.	176	178	165	154	148
Not for Profit	235	216	207	194	186
Investor owned	51	51	52	54	55
Physician Models					
Independent Practice Association	46	46	51	57	49
Group Practice without Walls.	12	12	10	13	11
Open Physician-Hospital Organization	31	32	29	31	34
Closed Physician-Hospital Organization	8	8	5	6	9
Management Service Organization	18	16	17	20	18
Integrated Salary Model	163	149	120	116	110
Equity Model	9	5	3	2	6
Foundation.	16	14	10	11	7
Insurance Products					
Health Maintenance Organization	42	37	40	36	34
Preferred Provider Organization.	39	44	44	38	39
Indemnity Fee for Service	13	13	13	11	15
Managed Care Contracts					
Health Maintenance Organization	181	163	156	151	137
Preferred Provider Organization.	244	231	218	210	203
Affiliations					
Hospitals in a System.	207	185	172	166	158
Hospitals in a Network	133	138	129	122	116
Hospitals in a Group Purchasing Organization. .	317	306	291	286	263

TABLE **4**

BED SIZE CATEGORY 6-24

U.S. Registered Community Hospitals
(Nonfederal, short-term general and other special hospitals)

Utilization, Personnel, Revenue and Expenses, Community Health Indicators 2008–2012

	2012	2011	2010	2009	2008
TOTAL FACILITY (Includes Hospital and Nursing Home Units)					
Utilization - Inpatient					
Beds	7,791	7,616	7,261	6,894	6,726
Admissions	197,448	197,272	198,692	196,599	204,522
Inpatient Days	879,985	888,064	854,226	846,228	835,702
Average Length of Stay	4.5	4.5	4.3	4.3	4.1
Inpatient Surgeries	41,274	35,479	36,003	33,615	36,519
Births	18,058	14,880	13,839	14,161	13,938
Utilization - Outpatient					
Emergency Outpatient Visits	1,929,787	1,702,152	1,658,487	1,558,802	1,505,235
Other Outpatient Visits	8,697,985	8,828,732	8,275,935	7,553,921	6,877,919
Total Outpatient Visits	10,627,772	10,530,884	9,934,422	9,112,723	8,383,154
Outpatient Surgeries	285,969	271,645	271,260	250,113	249,528
Personnel					
Full Time RNs	9,066	8,052	7,587	6,790	6,382
Full Time LPNs	2,044	2,104	2,113	1,992	1,996
Part Time RNs	5,508	4,752	4,701	4,212	3,931
Part Time LPNs	903	1,012	886	918	859
Total Full Time	42,797	40,408	38,328	34,290	32,101
Total Part Time	20,824	19,087	17,746	16,301	14,933
Revenue - Inpatient					
Gross Inpatient Revenue	$3,344,514,225	$2,808,082,491	$2,786,370,995	$2,627,018,044	$2,459,057,974
Revenue - Outpatient					
Gross Outpatient Revenue	$10,460,225,077	$8,967,777,277	$8,039,286,106	$7,310,737,048	$6,343,851,906
Revenue and Expenses - Totals					
(Includes Inpatient and Outpatient)					
Total Gross Revenue	$13,804,739,302	$11,775,859,768	$10,825,657,101	$9,937,755,092	$8,802,909,880
Deductions from Revenue	6,997,808,590	6,019,723,826	5,474,162,402	5,035,910,207	4,391,015,802
Net Patient Revenue	6,806,930,712	5,756,135,942	5,351,494,699	4,901,844,885	4,411,894,078
Other Operating Revenue	611,148,966	620,276,695	540,121,094	436,638,024	343,522,682
Other Nonoperating Revenue	154,545,670	107,732,522	103,852,868	70,082,709	69,707,381
Total Net Revenue	7,572,625,348	6,484,145,159	5,995,468,661	5,408,565,618	4,825,124,141
Total Expenses	6,984,976,928	6,128,099,984	5,644,509,939	5,099,918,468	4,510,451,244
HOSPITAL UNIT (Excludes Separate Nursing Home Units)					
Utilization - Inpatient					
Beds	7,738	7,610	7,225	6,852	6,693
Admissions	197,163	197,272	198,651	196,571	204,445
Inpatient Days	854,715	885,028	841,349	829,135	823,878
Average Length of Stay	4.3	4.5	4.2	4.2	4.0
Personnel					
Total Full Time	42,674	40,404	38,313	34,160	31,993
Total Part Time	20,730	19,087	17,743	16,225	14,902
Revenue and Expenses - Totals					
(Includes Inpatient and Outpatient)					
Total Net Revenue	$7,561,431,638	$6,483,007,236	$5,990,190,925	$5,395,279,787	$4,821,483,710
Total Expenses	6,979,227,864	6,127,873,361	5,642,553,901	5,092,088,584	4,508,680,031

TABLE **4**

BED SIZE CATEGORY 25-49

U.S. Registered Community Hospitals
(Nonfederal, short-term general and other special hospitals)

Overview 2008–2012

	2012	2011	2010	2009	2008
Total Community Hospitals in Bed Size Category 25-49	**1,192**	**1,177**	**1,167**	**1,164**	**1,151**
Location					
Hospitals Urban..........................	420	403	408	411	348
Hospitals Rural	772	774	759	753	803
Control					
State and Local Government...............	367	366	381	391	397
Not for Profit	574	570	547	536	527
Investor owned	251	241	239	237	227
Physician Models					
Independent Practice Association	97	96	102	108	104
Group Practice without Walls...............	25	30	32	32	27
Open Physician-Hospital Organization	79	80	82	94	92
Closed Physician-Hospital Organization	23	25	23	23	24
Management Service Organization	55	56	54	56	54
Integrated Salary Model...................	358	353	344	350	309
Equity Model...........................	9	13	17	15	14
Foundation.............................	44	41	39	40	42
Insurance Products					
Health Maintenance Organization	90	93	86	90	83
Preferred Provider Organization.............	94	142	134	123	112
Indemnity Fee for Service	31	47	44	41	39
Managed Care Contracts					
Health Maintenance Organization	502	477	471	488	474
Preferred Provider Organization.............	636	631	636	658	649
Affiliations					
Hospitals in a System.....................	639	620	598	593	580
Hospitals in a Network....................	309	305	302	296	296
Hospitals in a Group Purchasing Organization..	780	781	791	805	795

TABLE 4

BED SIZE CATEGORY 25-49

U.S. Registered Community Hospitals
(Nonfederal, short-term general and other special hospitals)

Utilization, Personnel, Revenue and Expenses, Community Health Indicators 2008–2012

	2012	2011	2010	2009	2008
TOTAL FACILITY (Includes Hospital and Nursing Home Units)					
Utilization - Inpatient					
Beds	38,338	37,680	37,446	37,338	37,142
Admissions	1,128,446	1,173,246	1,168,665	1,217,233	1,218,123
Inpatient Days	6,029,293	6,091,172	6,116,350	6,265,180	6,342,577
Average Length of Stay	5.3	5.2	5.2	5.1	5.2
Inpatient Surgeries	235,988	241,364	256,940	266,047	242,142
Births	115,996	112,584	107,380	113,460	106,334
Utilization - Outpatient					
Emergency Outpatient Visits	8,566,426	8,170,484	7,923,353	8,004,368	7,781,578
Other Outpatient Visits	38,126,632	36,927,369	35,175,869	34,456,501	32,947,438
Total Outpatient Visits	46,693,058	45,097,853	43,099,222	42,460,869	40,729,016
Outpatient Surgeries	1,147,708	1,084,955	1,092,740	1,067,767	1,022,034
Personnel					
Full Time RNs	42,864	39,915	37,943	37,289	34,935
Full Time LPNs	8,417	8,460	8,776	8,901	9,165
Part Time RNs	24,910	23,665	22,187	21,865	20,005
Part Time LPNs	3,356	3,365	3,605	3,815	3,809
Total Full Time	201,196	194,434	187,568	184,562	178,257
Total Part Time	88,578	86,421	81,895	80,350	76,222
Revenue - Inpatient					
Gross Inpatient Revenue	$26,339,586,346	$23,060,034,924	$21,382,867,485	$20,489,409,044	$18,764,220,947
Revenue - Outpatient					
Gross Outpatient Revenue	$47,719,363,855	$43,836,287,394	$39,164,706,833	$36,064,974,499	$31,292,050,672
Revenue and Expenses - Totals					
(Includes Inpatient and Outpatient)					
Total Gross Revenue	$74,058,950,201	$66,896,322,318	$60,547,574,318	$56,554,383,543	$50,056,271,619
Deductions from Revenue	42,336,288,207	38,545,311,880	34,313,307,874	31,432,916,209	26,923,199,398
Net Patient Revenue	31,722,661,994	28,351,010,438	26,234,266,444	25,121,467,334	23,133,072,221
Other Operating Revenue	2,679,807,646	2,558,100,321	2,209,537,503	2,229,830,552	1,982,012,610
Other Nonoperating Revenue	466,597,263	465,541,424	523,520,663	299,120,900	142,977,449
Total Net Revenue	34,869,066,903	31,374,652,183	28,967,324,610	27,650,418,786	25,258,062,280
Total Expenses	32,080,809,215	29,219,811,844	27,075,731,145	26,281,664,624	24,074,708,651
HOSPITAL UNIT (Excludes Separate Nursing Home Units)					
Utilization - Inpatient					
Beds	36,965	36,335	35,924	35,726	35,230
Admissions	1,126,060	1,171,231	1,166,430	1,213,515	1,215,522
Inpatient Days	5,586,318	5,661,438	5,638,505	5,745,424	5,747,460
Average Length of Stay	5.0	4.8	4.8	4.7	4.7
Personnel					
Total Full Time	200,121	193,678	186,670	182,894	176,408
Total Part Time	87,785	85,897	81,286	79,370	75,100
Revenue and Expenses - Totals					
(Includes Inpatient and Outpatient)					
Total Net Revenue	$34,771,427,302	$31,292,864,199	$28,881,412,934	$27,550,727,504	$25,153,457,365
Total Expenses	31,999,027,638	29,151,001,828	27,009,348,946	26,216,346,135	23,996,899,302

Bed Size Categories

TABLE 4

BED SIZE CATEGORY 50-99

U.S. Registered Community Hospitals
(Nonfederal, short-term general and other special hospitals)

Overview 2008–2012

	2012	2011	2010	2009	2008
Total Community Hospitals in Bed Size Category 50-99	**954**	**955**	**970**	**991**	**995**
Location					
Hospitals Urban.	489	484	483	483	440
Hospitals Rural	465	471	487	508	555
Control					
State and Local Government	185	190	194	210	215
Not for Profit	470	478	485	501	508
Investor owned	299	287	291	280	272
Physician Models					
Independent Practice Association	61	66	84	86	97
Group Practice without Walls.	21	21	21	20	25
Open Physician-Hospital Organization	98	89	93	94	112
Closed Physician-Hospital Organization	29	32	33	29	34
Management Service Organization	49	48	54	54	61
Integrated Salary Model	296	292	288	280	277
Equity Model	9	10	12	13	14
Foundation.	34	35	40	35	45
Insurance Products					
Health Maintenance Organization	94	98	89	80	94
Preferred Provider Organization.	98	129	128	124	135
Indemnity Fee for Service	37	40	49	44	56
Managed Care Contracts					
Health Maintenance Organization	434	426	444	435	456
Preferred Provider Organization.	512	508	533	548	564
Affiliations					
Hospitals in a System.	604	588	584	576	559
Hospitals in a Network	254	256	260	257	271
Hospitals in a Group Purchasing Organization. .	628	635	649	672	682

Bed Size Categories

TABLE 4

BED SIZE CATEGORY 50-99

U.S. Registered Community Hospitals
(Nonfederal, short-term general and other special hospitals)

Utilization, Personnel, Revenue and Expenses, Community Health Indicators 2008–2012

	2012	2011	2010	2009	2008
TOTAL FACILITY (Includes Hospital and Nursing Home Units)					
Utilization - Inpatient					
Beds	67,879	67,844	69,470	71,012	71,477
Admissions	2,017,239	2,104,041	2,173,195	2,255,591	2,318,730
Inpatient Days	13,678,515	13,720,587	13,960,874	14,494,367	14,775,775
Average Length of Stay	6.8	6.5	6.4	6.4	6.4
Inpatient Surgeries	477,962	498,804	543,313	557,900	573,876
Births	222,207	223,326	228,035	245,282	252,752
Utilization - Outpatient					
Emergency Outpatient Visits	11,275,005	11,503,565	11,667,902	11,702,839	11,523,593
Other Outpatient Visits	45,524,947	44,622,553	46,033,464	45,633,323	45,219,692
Total Outpatient Visits	56,799,952	56,126,118	57,701,366	57,336,162	56,743,285
Outpatient Surgeries	1,507,344	1,542,936	1,592,532	1,625,749	1,608,622
Personnel					
Full Time RNs	63,278	61,781	60,774	59,702	58,276
Full Time LPNs	8,560	8,721	9,718	10,384	10,739
Part Time RNs	34,249	33,998	33,585	33,613	33,996
Part Time LPNs	3,584	3,685	4,125	4,537	4,911
Total Full Time	261,529	260,825	260,463	263,865	264,056
Total Part Time	122,577	120,605	118,372	119,501	121,026
Revenue - Inpatient					
Gross Inpatient Revenue	$55,035,035,760	$53,109,381,343	$52,180,741,692	$48,434,688,539	$46,010,068,854
Revenue - Outpatient					
Gross Outpatient Revenue	$69,635,311,624	$66,009,645,599	$60,748,431,980	$57,539,780,471	$51,849,631,924
Revenue and Expenses - Totals					
(Includes Inpatient and Outpatient)					
Total Gross Revenue	$124,670,347,384	$119,119,026,942	$112,929,173,672	$105,974,469,010	$97,859,700,778
Deductions from Revenue	79,025,510,314	76,709,358,028	71,250,437,701	65,093,252,794	59,144,961,432
Net Patient Revenue	45,644,837,070	42,409,668,914	41,678,735,971	40,881,216,216	38,714,739,346
Other Operating Revenue	1,974,942,100	1,689,476,095	1,566,850,196	1,628,159,436	1,598,169,545
Other Nonoperating Revenue	927,504,094	625,595,709	677,949,955	358,788,581	248,970,994
Total Net Revenue	48,547,283,264	44,724,740,718	43,923,536,122	42,868,164,233	40,561,879,885
Total Expenses	43,488,785,543	41,141,854,495	40,509,092,623	39,918,181,789	38,332,175,201
HOSPITAL UNIT (Excludes Separate Nursing Home Units)					
Utilization - Inpatient					
Beds	59,055	58,517	60,417	60,783	60,983
Admissions	1,999,782	2,086,226	2,152,715	2,233,384	2,293,835
Inpatient Days	10,929,906	10,790,706	11,108,738	11,303,044	11,528,634
Average Length of Stay	5.5	5.2	5.2	5.1	5.0
Personnel					
Total Full Time	256,240	255,669	255,262	257,466	257,784
Total Part Time	118,696	116,620	114,674	115,249	116,770
Revenue and Expenses - Totals					
(Includes Inpatient and Outpatient)					
Total Net Revenue	$47,999,122,812	$44,157,904,896	$43,379,453,757	$42,231,656,619	$39,967,178,977
Total Expenses	43,042,562,713	40,660,522,689	40,049,446,577	39,405,302,301	37,833,276,129

TABLE **4**

BED SIZE CATEGORY 100-199

U.S. Registered Community Hospitals
(Nonfederal, short-term general and other special hospitals)

Overview 2008–2012

	2012	2011	2010	2009	2008
Total Community Hospitals in					
Bed Size Category 100-199	**1,012**	**1,005**	**1,029**	**1,063**	**1,070**
Location					
Hospitals Urban	717	707	707	726	699
Hospitals Rural	295	298	322	337	371
Control					
State and Local Government	135	135	149	159	162
Not for Profit	617	623	633	656	660
Investor owned	260	247	247	248	248
Physician Models					
Independent Practice Association	97	107	120	122	124
Group Practice without Walls	36	35	36	44	33
Open Physician-Hospital Organization	142	144	152	166	167
Closed Physician-Hospital Organization	48	51	47	53	53
Management Service Organization	106	102	103	102	91
Integrated Salary Model	345	343	332	317	308
Equity Model	21	20	17	25	26
Foundation	62	59	56	49	43
Insurance Products					
Health Maintenance Organization	125	132	124	116	108
Preferred Provider Organization	122	142	136	134	122
Indemnity Fee for Service	52	58	52	46	44
Managed Care Contracts					
Health Maintenance Organization	566	578	587	621	591
Preferred Provider Organization	606	624	641	675	668
Affiliations					
Hospitals in a System	686	667	655	665	661
Hospitals in a Network	281	280	278	298	296
Hospitals in a Group Purchasing Organization . .	688	705	724	779	792

TABLE **4**

BED SIZE CATEGORY 100-199

U.S. Registered Community Hospitals
(Nonfederal, short-term general and other special hospitals)

Utilization, Personnel, Revenue and Expenses, Community Health Indicators 2008–2012

	2012	2011	2010	2009	2008
TOTAL FACILITY (Includes Hospital and Nursing Home Units)					
Utilization - Inpatient					
Beds	145,556	143,843	148,090	152,655	153,488
Admissions	5,920,309	6,022,274	6,124,987	6,337,184	6,304,036
Inpatient Days	30,892,477	31,348,118	32,616,034	34,162,392	34,742,992
Average Length of Stay	5.2	5.2	5.3	5.4	5.5
Inpatient Surgeries	1,546,794	1,520,872	1,602,340	1,687,965	1,670,856
Births	658,328	677,253	706,284	747,784	765,495
Utilization - Outpatient					
Emergency Outpatient Visits	27,668,989	26,551,709	26,433,098	27,527,025	26,601,799
Other Outpatient Visits	96,096,051	94,003,431	94,469,225	99,739,947	93,178,685
Total Outpatient Visits	123,765,040	120,555,140	120,902,323	127,266,972	119,780,484
Outpatient Surgeries	3,421,257	3,466,539	3,551,479	3,694,985	3,653,497
Personnel					
Full Time RNs	167,593	162,016	163,437	161,715	154,376
Full Time LPNs	13,807	14,534	15,414	16,777	17,825
Part Time RNs	85,380	84,492	87,526	90,352	89,500
Part Time LPNs	5,356	5,653	6,135	6,982	7,788
Total Full Time	622,757	612,257	624,072	634,361	623,645
Total Part Time	265,049	265,264	270,145	275,686	274,371
Revenue - Inpatient					
Gross Inpatient Revenue	$196,130,283,474	$181,129,764,497	$177,873,737,781	$172,022,467,282	$161,279,571,502
Revenue - Outpatient					
Gross Outpatient Revenue	$190,830,856,203	$172,268,570,520	$160,748,748,573	$148,908,204,845	$131,980,398,456
Revenue and Expenses - Totals **(Includes Inpatient and Outpatient)**					
Total Gross Revenue	$386,961,139,677	$353,398,335,017	$338,622,486,354	$320,930,672,127	$293,259,969,958
Deductions from Revenue	269,772,483,763	245,217,347,870	231,276,346,434	216,014,370,801	195,921,601,786
Net Patient Revenue	117,188,655,914	108,180,987,147	107,346,139,920	104,916,301,326	97,338,368,172
Other Operating Revenue	5,062,039,669	4,265,506,812	4,194,548,704	3,845,471,488	3,635,678,864
Other Nonoperating Revenue	1,638,797,895	1,324,614,718	1,589,574,499	773,148,510	-86,795,995
Total Net Revenue	123,889,493,478	113,771,108,677	113,130,263,123	109,534,921,324	100,887,251,041
Total Expenses	112,758,082,370	105,195,692,008	104,618,604,747	103,165,948,166	96,955,948,353
HOSPITAL UNIT (Excludes Separate Nursing Home Units)					
Utilization - Inpatient					
Beds	132,541	131,102	134,182	138,351	137,233
Admissions	5,876,426	5,976,691	6,074,709	6,284,177	6,247,190
Inpatient Days	26,855,548	27,367,543	28,160,867	29,540,921	29,546,134
Average Length of Stay	4.6	4.6	4.6	4.7	4.7
Personnel					
Total Full Time	613,726	604,314	614,788	624,258	612,571
Total Part Time	259,764	260,194	264,091	269,719	267,530
Revenue and Expenses - Totals **(Includes Inpatient and Outpatient)**					
Total Net Revenue	$122,970,772,210	$112,746,343,253	$112,109,514,588	$108,564,165,998	$99,832,442,896
Total Expenses	111,908,745,686	104,375,763,548	103,732,105,185	102,320,666,510	95,982,012,829

Bed Size Categories

TABLE 4

BED SIZE CATEGORY 200-299

U.S. Registered Community Hospitals
(Nonfederal, short-term general and other special hospitals)

Overview 2008–2012

	2012	2011	2010	2009	2008
Total Community Hospitals in Bed Size Category 200-299...............	570	582	585	582	596
Location					
Hospitals Urban..........................	487	498	505	503	496
Hospitals Rural	83	84	80	79	100
Control					
State and Local Government...............	62	58	63	58	62
Not for Profit	393	410	422	427	435
Investor owned	115	114	100	97	99
Physician Models					
Independent Practice Association	56	60	67	68	72
Group Practice without Walls...............	22	23	18	23	26
Open Physician-Hospital Organization	98	108	111	104	110
Closed Physician-Hospital Organization	30	26	28	26	27
Management Service Organization	69	81	76	74	84
Integrated Salary Model....................	238	225	223	211	206
Equity Model	15	13	17	17	14
Foundation...............................	34	38	40	35	35
Insurance Products					
Health Maintenance Organization	90	95	93	89	93
Preferred Provider Organization..............	77	105	105	88	95
Indemnity Fee for Service	32	37	35	36	33
Managed Care Contracts					
Health Maintenance Organization	373	379	380	382	400
Preferred Provider Organization..............	383	399	402	406	421
Affiliations					
Hospitals in a System......................	390	392	386	381	377
Hospitals in a Network.....................	185	194	192	185	195
Hospitals in a Group Purchasing Organization..	424	443	448	452	475

TABLE **4**

BED SIZE CATEGORY 200-299

U.S. Registered Community Hospitals
(Nonfederal, short-term general and other special hospitals)

Utilization, Personnel, Revenue and Expenses, Community Health Indicators 2008–2012

	2012	2011	2010	2009	2008
TOTAL FACILITY (Includes Hospital and Nursing Home Units)					
Utilization - Inpatient					
Beds	139,212	141,308	142,616	141,920	144,895
Admissions	6,297,821	6,463,753	6,569,492	6,684,169	6,866,533
Inpatient Days	32,150,843	32,799,097	33,301,779	33,902,236	35,165,769
Average Length of Stay	5.1	5.1	5.1	5.1	5.1
Inpatient Surgeries	1,728,626	1,749,337	1,896,663	1,871,675	1,945,775
Births	661,428	660,610	681,848	739,459	794,470
Utilization - Outpatient					
Emergency Outpatient Visits	24,468,359	24,513,239	24,171,792	24,181,322	24,185,692
Other Outpatient Visits	87,195,255	85,387,424	86,489,482	83,087,309	83,791,081
Total Outpatient Visits	111,663,614	109,900,663	110,661,274	107,268,631	107,976,773
Outpatient Surgeries	2,963,873	3,017,123	3,001,309	3,015,075	3,224,033
Personnel					
Full Time RNs	178,938	179,617	178,567	172,868	171,515
Full Time LPNs	10,635	11,593	12,698	13,435	14,215
Part Time RNs	89,327	86,739	84,923	85,762	88,610
Part Time LPNs	4,108	4,315	5,133	5,396	6,221
Total Full Time	654,260	655,559	657,452	650,138	651,645
Total Part Time	257,126	255,998	252,299	256,501	265,981
Revenue - Inpatient					
Gross Inpatient Revenue	$240,835,907,576	$222,460,322,498	$216,302,711,528	$203,207,782,786	$197,533,594,288
Revenue - Outpatient					
Gross Outpatient Revenue	$185,911,616,840	$167,530,250,112	$152,845,016,955	$136,999,646,724	$124,669,613,502
Revenue and Expenses - Totals (Includes Inpatient and Outpatient)					
Total Gross Revenue	$426,747,524,416	$389,990,572,610	$369,147,728,483	$340,207,429,510	$322,203,207,790
Deductions from Revenue	300,061,387,153	272,710,512,076	254,962,232,713	230,420,211,811	215,803,795,922
Net Patient Revenue	126,686,137,263	117,280,060,534	114,185,495,770	109,787,217,699	106,399,411,868
Other Operating Revenue	5,987,888,496	5,683,916,062	5,345,831,411	4,960,901,489	5,082,400,440
Other Nonoperating Revenue	1,814,706,798	2,168,529,841	2,413,672,808	869,665,589	-782,268,587
Total Net Revenue	134,488,732,557	125,132,506,437	121,944,999,989	115,617,784,777	110,699,543,721
Total Expenses	124,808,644,131	116,575,732,582	113,049,739,427	109,876,595,200	108,021,530,166
HOSPITAL UNIT (Excludes Separate Nursing Home Units)					
Utilization - Inpatient					
Beds	130,652	133,352	133,765	133,463	136,050
Admissions	6,248,381	6,414,383	6,516,545	6,624,904	6,806,537
Inpatient Days	29,421,703	30,290,801	30,497,421	31,155,392	32,384,629
Average Length of Stay	4.7	4.7	4.7	4.7	4.8
Personnel					
Total Full Time	647,761	649,600	650,650	642,802	642,916
Total Part Time	254,363	253,312	248,794	252,441	261,723
Revenue and Expenses - Totals (Includes Inpatient and Outpatient)					
Total Net Revenue	$133,703,328,242	$124,426,000,759	$121,195,426,366	$114,847,552,059	$109,893,167,266
Total Expenses	124,088,653,959	115,962,048,197	112,407,841,598	109,171,734,399	107,333,326,624

TABLE **4**

BED SIZE CATEGORY 300-399

U.S. Registered Community Hospitals
(Nonfederal, short-term general and other special hospitals)

Overview 2008–2012

	2012	2011	2010	2009	2008
Total Community Hospitals in					
Bed Size Category 300-399................	**348**	**353**	**352**	**348**	**355**
Location					
Hospitals Urban...........................	331	332	329	327	325
Hospitals Rural	17	21	23	21	30
Control					
State and Local Government...............	37	44	41	49	47
Not for Profit............................	255	258	261	252	259
Investor owned	56	51	50	47	49
Physician Models					
Independent Practice Association	47	49	52	55	65
Group Practice without Walls...............	21	15	15	11	11
Open Physician-Hospital Organization	67	71	66	60	61
Closed Physician-Hospital Organization	30	28	28	29	29
Management Service Organization	49	49	57	54	50
Integrated Salary Model...................	168	165	161	143	140
Equity Model............................	6	4	5	5	8
Foundation..............................	30	27	27	20	25
Insurance Products					
Health Maintenance Organization	60	63	61	62	69
Preferred Provider Organization.............	47	65	66	65	67
Indemnity Fee for Service	14	19	18	19	22
Managed Care Contracts					
Health Maintenance Organization	254	264	263	251	250
Preferred Provider Organization.............	260	273	269	266	260
Affiliations					
Hospitals in a System.....................	241	237	234	228	227
Hospitals in a Network....................	128	146	147	139	141
Hospitals in a Group Purchasing Organization..	278	291	296	287	287

TABLE 4

BED SIZE CATEGORY 300-399

U.S. Registered Community Hospitals
(Nonfederal, short-term general and other special hospitals)

Utilization, Personnel, Revenue and Expenses, Community Health Indicators 2008–2012

	2012	2011	2010	2009	2008
TOTAL FACILITY (Includes Hospital and Nursing Home Units)					
Utilization - Inpatient					
Beds	120,554	122,269	121,749	120,201	122,363
Admissions	5,659,683	5,850,631	5,835,325	5,761,848	5,894,366
Inpatient Days	28,628,393	29,754,662	29,931,672	29,771,668	31,089,796
Average Length of Stay.	5.1	5.1	5.1	5.2	5.3
Inpatient Surgeries.	1,505,394	1,577,523	1,594,088	1,638,540	1,679,276
Births.	635,069	661,840	669,356	669,093	678,865
Utilization - Outpatient					
Emergency Outpatient Visits	19,494,322	19,606,197	18,788,786	18,319,154	17,724,755
Other Outpatient Visits.	74,292,746	75,676,049	71,726,267	68,364,695	72,894,987
Total Outpatient Visits	93,787,068	95,282,246	90,515,053	86,683,849	90,619,742
Outpatient Surgeries	2,419,594	2,450,334	2,401,308	2,371,683	2,340,405
Personnel					
Full Time RNs	167,220	166,975	159,878	157,652	151,208
Full Time LPNs	8,157	8,862	8,875	10,238	10,864
Part Time RNs	74,735	75,111	73,727	71,718	75,014
Part Time LPNs	2,519	2,778	3,090	3,461	4,125
Total Full Time	592,655	589,570	572,775	571,380	575,521
Total Part Time	210,937	212,248	211,094	206,711	215,729
Revenue - Inpatient					
Gross Inpatient Revenue	$230,446,967,570	$216,619,573,502	$209,508,102,124	$192,767,208,267	$188,790,420,618
Revenue - Outpatient					
Gross Outpatient Revenue	$164,159,129,172	$149,199,860,634	$133,493,602,189	$118,085,940,332	$107,500,249,231
Revenue and Expenses - Totals					
(Includes Inpatient and Outpatient)					
Total Gross Revenue.	$394,606,096,742	$365,819,434,136	$343,001,704,313	$310,853,148,599	$296,290,669,849
Deductions from Revenue	277,863,090,524	256,798,261,828	239,740,752,936	213,449,294,445	201,399,629,121
Net Patient Revenue	116,743,006,218	109,021,172,308	103,260,951,377	97,403,854,154	94,891,040,728
Other Operating Revenue	6,414,161,778	6,181,177,363	5,624,897,632	5,833,232,696	5,496,095,330
Other Nonoperating Revenue	1,472,292,314	1,684,050,046	2,187,362,723	421,501,249	-735,779,905
Total Net Revenue.	124,629,460,310	116,886,399,717	111,073,211,732	103,658,588,099	99,651,356,153
Total Expenses.	114,103,095,511	107,750,738,297	102,319,306,727	97,985,067,095	96,680,861,169
HOSPITAL UNIT (Excludes Separate Nursing Home Units)					
Utilization - Inpatient					
Beds	115,302	116,402	115,138	114,177	115,956
Admissions	5,626,701	5,812,423	5,794,184	5,722,480	5,852,894
Inpatient Days	27,018,257	27,951,385	27,890,368	27,966,432	29,131,108
Average Length of Stay.	4.8	4.8	4.8	4.9	5.0
Personnel					
Total Full Time	588,298	585,534	567,683	565,928	570,294
Total Part Time	209,136	210,406	208,623	204,570	212,975
Revenue and Expenses - Totals					
(Includes Inpatient and Outpatient)					
Total Net Revenue.	$124,094,300,216	$116,327,869,334	$110,402,770,436	$102,987,034,415	$98,992,882,329
Total Expenses.	113,626,750,271	107,307,019,085	101,715,147,145	97,429,327,288	96,149,983,308

TABLE **4**

BED SIZE CATEGORY 400-499

U.S. Registered Community Hospitals
(Nonfederal, short-term general and other special hospitals)

Overview 2008–2012

	2012	2011	2010	2009	2008
Total Community Hospitals in					
Bed Size Category 400-499	**189**	**184**	**185**	**192**	**184**
Location					
Hospitals Urban.	186	181	182	187	178
Hospitals Rural	3	3	3	5	6
Control					
State and Local Government	29	26	28	23	24
Not for Profit	142	141	139	148	142
Investor owned	18	17	18	21	18
Physician Models					
Independent Practice Association	32	31	27	28	34
Group Practice without Walls.	14	14	13	16	15
Open Physician-Hospital Organization	44	40	35	41	39
Closed Physician-Hospital Organization	16	12	13	15	15
Management Service Organization	33	35	30	30	29
Integrated Salary Model	96	90	94	86	79
Equity Model	6	4	4	4	4
Foundation.	24	24	24	22	23
Insurance Products					
Health Maintenance Organization	38	37	38	33	36
Preferred Provider Organization.	37	40	41	37	40
Indemnity Fee for Service	8	13	15	9	12
Managed Care Contracts					
Health Maintenance Organization	151	148	149	147	134
Preferred Provider Organization.	152	150	147	149	135
Affiliations					
Hospitals in a System.	137	127	128	128	122
Hospitals in a Network	88	86	78	70	65
Hospitals in a Group Purchasing Organization. .	159	160	158	159	154

TABLE **4**

BED SIZE CATEGORY 400-499

U.S. Registered Community Hospitals
(Nonfederal, short-term general and other special hospitals)

Utilization, Personnel, Revenue and Expenses, Community Health Indicators 2008–2012

	2012	2011	2010	2009	2008
TOTAL FACILITY (Includes Hospital and Nursing Home Units)					
Utilization - Inpatient					
Beds	84,007	81,699	82,071	84,783	80,815
Admissions	3,966,019	3,862,877	3,869,124	4,049,002	3,895,152
Inpatient Days	20,755,259	20,364,896	20,521,474	21,675,972	20,830,426
Average Length of Stay	5.2	5.3	5.3	5.4	5.3
Inpatient Surgeries	1,137,327	1,150,202	1,178,350	1,220,457	1,133,598
Births	427,993	410,117	408,256	431,706	435,954
Utilization - Outpatient					
Emergency Outpatient Visits	12,993,712	11,929,789	11,546,221	12,078,252	10,828,538
Other Outpatient Visits	59,418,937	54,498,516	53,996,342	51,649,202	46,814,290
Total Outpatient Visits	72,412,649	66,428,305	65,542,563	63,727,454	57,642,828
Outpatient Surgeries	1,669,549	1,623,929	1,665,216	1,804,693	1,739,961
Personnel					
Full Time RNs	131,578	123,351	121,762	123,770	113,628
Full Time LPNs	5,571	5,525	6,176	6,578	7,035
Part Time RNs	55,526	53,067	53,293	55,922	52,946
Part Time LPNs	2,269	1,972	2,317	2,330	2,903
Total Full Time	462,528	439,370	441,431	458,527	435,911
Total Part Time	159,252	149,644	146,459	155,793	152,140
Revenue - Inpatient					
Gross Inpatient Revenue	$165,404,143,916	$158,709,548,655	$150,837,747,313	$154,483,680,751	$134,562,622,630
Revenue - Outpatient					
Gross Outpatient Revenue	$119,532,259,113	$105,408,223,039	$98,160,076,960	$94,037,031,898	$77,496,854,013
Revenue and Expenses - Totals					
(Includes Inpatient and Outpatient)					
Total Gross Revenue	$284,936,403,029	$264,117,771,694	$248,997,824,273	$248,520,712,649	$212,059,476,643
Deductions from Revenue	197,528,264,702	184,087,484,155	172,382,284,117	170,485,791,464	144,218,038,992
Net Patient Revenue	87,408,138,327	80,030,287,539	76,615,540,156	78,034,921,185	67,841,437,651
Other Operating Revenue	5,272,639,678	4,601,079,434	4,922,929,664	4,809,356,943	4,570,160,760
Other Nonoperating Revenue	1,325,875,743	1,374,562,424	1,471,629,299	576,751,753	-823,396,082
Total Net Revenue	94,006,653,748	86,005,929,397	83,010,099,119	83,421,029,881	71,588,202,329
Total Expenses	87,804,964,580	80,196,968,394	77,854,509,046	79,447,824,942	70,515,262,080
HOSPITAL UNIT (Excludes Separate Nursing Home Units)					
Utilization - Inpatient					
Beds	80,458	78,997	79,722	82,330	77,661
Admissions	3,947,024	3,848,071	3,854,485	4,034,937	3,878,278
Inpatient Days	19,600,701	19,494,041	19,770,661	20,873,864	19,817,710
Average Length of Stay	5.0	5.1	5.1	5.2	5.1
Personnel					
Total Full Time	459,192	437,087	439,282	455,941	431,434
Total Part Time	157,372	148,452	145,585	154,827	150,412
Revenue and Expenses - Totals					
(Includes Inpatient and Outpatient)					
Total Net Revenue	$93,581,430,291	$85,724,707,161	$82,724,653,206	$83,143,956,566	$71,316,876,706
Total Expenses	87,395,944,309	79,940,658,386	77,613,265,522	79,186,633,408	70,261,647,760

Bed Size Categories

TABLE 4

BED SIZE CATEGORY 500 +

U.S. Registered Community Hospitals
(Nonfederal, short-term general and other special hospitals)

Overview 2008–2012

	2012	2011	2010	2009	2008
Total Community Hospitals in Bed Size Category 500 +..................	**272**	**272**	**273**	**266**	**270**
Location					
Hospitals Urban............................	269	270	271	263	266
Hospitals Rural	3	2	2	3	4
Control					
State and Local Government................	46	48	47	48	50
Not for Profit	208	207	210	204	206
Investor owned	18	17	16	14	14
Physician Models					
Independent Practice Association	60	59	60	55	52
Group Practice without Walls................	14	11	14	16	12
Open Physician-Hospital Organization	61	58	62	59	57
Closed Physician-Hospital Organization	35	28	26	26	22
Management Service Organization	62	59	63	59	49
Integrated Salary Model....................	180	178	166	161	154
Equity Model	9	7	5	11	11
Foundation................................	25	25	25	25	28
Insurance Products					
Health Maintenance Organization	88	85	83	81	80
Preferred Provider Organization..............	62	77	86	84	75
Indemnity Fee for Service	23	26	34	29	29
Managed Care Contracts					
Health Maintenance Organization	236	230	227	227	228
Preferred Provider Organization..............	237	229	228	225	225
Affiliations					
Hospitals in a System......................	196	191	184	184	184
Hospitals in a Network	130	130	122	118	110
Hospitals in a Group Purchasing Organization..	245	241	238	234	229

TABLE 4

BED SIZE CATEGORY 500 +

U.S. Registered Community Hospitals
(Nonfederal, short-term general and other special hospitals)

Utilization, Personnel, Revenue and Expenses, Community Health Indicators 2008–2012

	2012	2011	2010	2009	2008
TOTAL FACILITY (Includes Hospital and Nursing Home Units)					
Utilization - Inpatient					
Beds	197,229	195,144	196,240	190,790	191,163
Admissions	9,235,106	9,168,991	9,209,947	9,025,751	9,059,288
Inpatient Days	52,408,270	52,105,417	52,290,940	51,538,761	52,295,431
Average Length of Stay	5.7	5.7	5.7	5.7	5.8
Inpatient Surgeries	2,840,233	2,864,886	2,847,124	2,824,781	2,823,114
Births	976,400	969,732	1,003,401	998,660	1,025,916
Utilization - Outpatient					
Emergency Outpatient Visits	26,824,430	25,484,523	25,059,678	23,926,431	22,872,834
Other Outpatient Visits	132,397,748	126,673,210	128,007,816	124,170,351	119,350,180
Total Outpatient Visits	159,222,178	152,157,733	153,067,494	148,096,782	142,223,014
Outpatient Surgeries	3,882,339	3,811,784	3,781,333	3,527,469	3,516,202
Personnel					
Full Time RNs	343,369	330,245	325,170	310,042	294,329
Full Time LPNs	12,127	12,842	12,733	13,854	14,911
Part Time RNs	124,895	121,527	117,797	114,255	123,478
Part Time LPNs	3,797	3,668	3,873	4,208	4,986
Total Full Time	1,267,573	1,241,782	1,207,498	1,173,995	1,158,279
Total Part Time	347,276	336,809	329,126	323,649	340,085
Revenue - Inpatient					
Gross Inpatient Revenue	$438,404,095,774	$417,910,035,060	$393,918,219,709	$360,053,211,932	$341,198,456,138
Revenue - Outpatient					
Gross Outpatient Revenue	$287,455,681,774	$255,708,021,415	$234,219,190,376	$203,947,086,192	$180,786,111,977
Revenue and Expenses - Totals					
(Includes Inpatient and Outpatient)					
Total Gross Revenue	$725,859,777,548	$673,618,056,475	$628,137,410,085	$564,000,298,124	$521,984,568,115
Deductions from Revenue	495,852,998,550	464,928,281,586	426,426,753,565	377,984,394,103	343,813,646,912
Net Patient Revenue	230,006,778,998	208,689,774,889	201,710,656,520	186,015,904,021	178,170,921,203
Other Operating Revenue	19,525,754,240	17,698,352,209	16,864,301,215	15,253,862,892	14,428,536,883
Other Nonoperating Revenue	3,798,787,364	4,517,338,377	4,283,831,027	1,098,421,243	-2,486,522,886
Total Net Revenue	253,331,320,602	230,905,465,475	222,858,788,762	202,368,188,156	190,112,935,200
Total Expenses	234,887,398,418	215,882,136,211	206,896,544,358	194,381,058,030	187,486,021,048
HOSPITAL UNIT (Excludes Separate Nursing Home Units)					
Utilization - Inpatient					
Beds	188,779	186,866	188,718	183,604	184,099
Admissions	9,196,329	9,130,157	9,177,784	8,994,487	9,023,650
Inpatient Days	49,593,574	49,362,134	49,779,016	49,096,850	50,064,396
Average Length of Stay	5.4	5.4	5.4	5.5	5.5
Personnel					
Total Full Time	1,260,197	1,235,826	1,202,435	1,166,855	1,151,673
Total Part Time	344,634	334,786	327,042	320,836	337,438
Revenue and Expenses - Totals					
(Includes Inpatient and Outpatient)					
Total Net Revenue	$252,473,832,518	$230,125,418,566	$222,002,119,967	$201,733,630,805	$189,412,292,055
Total Expenses	234,023,264,708	215,047,382,036	206,018,475,965	193,647,981,433	186,762,975,722

Census Divisions

Census Division 1

New England
Connecticut, Maine, Massachusetts, New Hampshire, Rhode Island, Vermont

Census Division 2

Middle Atlantic
New Jersey, New York, Pennsylvania

Census Division 3

South Atlantic
Delaware, District of Columbia, Florida, Georgia, Maryland, North Carolina, South Carolina, Virginia, West Virginia

Census Division 4

East North Central
Illinois, Indiana, Michigan, Ohio, Wisconsin

Census Division 5

East South Central
Alabama, Kentucky, Mississippi, Tennessee

Census Division 6

West North Central
Iowa, Kansas, Minnesota, Missouri, Nebraska, North Dakota, South Dakota

Census Division 7

West South Central
Arkansas, Louisiana, Oklahoma, Texas

Census Division 8

Mountain
Arizona, Colorado, Idaho, Montana, Nevada, New Mexico, Utah, Wyoming

Census Division 9

Pacific
Alaska, California, Hawaii, Oregon, Washington

U.S. Census Divisions

TABLE **5**

U.S. CENSUS DIVISION 1: NEW ENGLAND

U.S. Registered Community Hospitals
(Nonfederal, short-term general and other special hospitals)

Overview 2008–2012

	2012	2011	2010	2009	2008
Total Community Hospitals					
in Census Division 1, New England	207	204	203	203	200
Bed Size Category					
6-24	10	10	10	10	10
25-49	43	42	39	40	38
50-99	47	40	40	41	42
100-199	51	56	59	57	54
200-299	26	27	25	22	22
300-399	15	15	14	17	17
400-499	4	3	4	4	5
500 + ...	11	11	12	12	12
Location					
Hospitals Urban.	149	146	145	145	122
Hospitals Rural	58	58	58	58	78
Control					
State and Local Government.	6	4	4	5	5
Not for Profit	176	181	182	184	180
Investor owned	25	19	17	14	15
Physician Models					
Independent Practice Association	32	36	44	40	40
Group Practice without Walls.	7	9	11	8	7
Open Physician-Hospital Organization	43	47	52	51	50
Closed Physician-Hospital Organization	12	12	14	12	11
Management Service Organization	20	21	24	21	20
Integrated Salary Model	101	105	107	98	98
Equity Model	6	4	4	6	6
Foundation.	14	16	13	10	8
Insurance Products					
Health Maintenance Organization	15	18	19	17	19
Preferred Provider Organization.	9	14	9	8	9
Indemnity Fee for Service	4	8	6	4	4
Managed Care Contracts					
Health Maintenance Organization	119	137	141	133	132
Preferred Provider Organization.	119	133	136	132	127
Affiliations					
Hospitals in a System.	102	93	89	77	74
Hospitals in a Network	75	80	75	69	69
Hospitals in a Group Purchasing Organization. .	148	157	166	159	164

TABLE 5

U.S. CENSUS DIVISION 1: NEW ENGLAND

U.S. Registered Community Hospitals
(Nonfederal, short-term general and other special hospitals)

Utilization, Personnel, Revenue and Expenses, Community Health Indicators 2008–2012

	2012	2011	2010	2009	2008
TOTAL FACILITY (Includes Hospital and Nursing Home Units)					
Utilization - Inpatient					
Beds	34,399	33,693	33,974	33,672	33,743
Admissions	1,608,353	1,677,325	1,668,378	1,678,176	1,660,654
Inpatient Days	8,482,806	8,650,119	8,813,799	8,987,254	8,992,337
Average Length of Stay.	5.3	5.2	5.3	5.4	5.4
Inpatient Surgeries.	418,336	429,342	439,721	454,138	457,144
Births.	146,147	159,359	152,389	156,346	163,857
Utilization - Outpatient					
Emergency Outpatient Visits	7,131,256	7,018,233	7,120,183	7,004,583	6,848,347
Other Outpatient Visits.	40,756,179	40,285,469	39,615,363	38,999,668	37,188,267
Total Outpatient Visits	47,887,435	47,303,702	46,735,546	46,004,251	44,036,614
Outpatient Surgeries	960,370	954,123	1,018,591	980,423	996,495
Personnel					
Full Time RNs	46,323	46,138	44,258	44,777	43,571
Full Time LPNs	1,816	1,794	1,811	1,898	1,972
Part Time RNs	41,454	41,003	39,689	38,236	39,421
Part Time LPNs	1,370	1,361	1,359	1,508	1,768
Total Full Time.	226,202	227,567	223,298	223,553	217,995
Total Part Time	126,716	128,182	123,799	118,235	121,345
Revenue - Inpatient					
Gross Inpatient Revenue.	$52,549,975,311	$49,993,866,945	$47,986,647,777	$46,367,979,779	$44,041,639,373
Revenue - Outpatient					
Gross Outpatient Revenue	$60,296,411,970	$55,511,810,142	$52,517,753,883	$49,137,348,602	$43,645,548,924
Revenue and Expenses - Totals					
(Includes Inpatient and Outpatient)					
Total Gross Revenue.	$112,846,387,281	$105,505,677,087	$100,504,401,660	$95,505,328,381	$87,687,188,297
Deductions from Revenue	68,108,106,958	62,731,335,770	59,098,902,583	55,719,745,134	50,488,459,964
Net Patient Revenue	44,738,280,323	42,774,341,317	41,405,499,077	39,785,583,247	37,198,728,333
Other Operating Revenue	4,894,336,432	4,641,150,617	4,151,761,895	3,962,230,864	3,637,620,235
Other Nonoperating Revenue	464,999,614	187,237,842	426,472,039	-167,328,782	-272,745,680
Total Net Revenue.	50,097,616,369	47,602,729,776	45,983,733,011	43,580,485,329	40,563,602,888
Total Expenses.	47,321,636,263	45,537,927,696	44,366,268,718	42,351,771,503	39,734,569,287
HOSPITAL UNIT (Excludes Separate Nursing Home Units)					
Utilization - Inpatient					
Beds	33,332	32,627	32,710	32,524	32,109
Admissions	1,605,312	1,674,145	1,662,431	1,673,090	1,654,586
Inpatient Days	8,161,998	8,384,172	8,377,660	8,601,239	8,442,410
Average Length of Stay.	5.1	5.0	5.0	5.1	5.1
Personnel					
Total Full Time.	224,884	226,972	222,354	222,494	215,906
Total Part Time	125,777	127,672	123,029	117,563	119,472
Revenue and Expenses - Totals					
(Includes Inpatient and Outpatient)					
Total Net Revenue.	$49,974,043,473	$47,525,027,006	$45,855,486,664	$43,455,515,086	$40,395,735,597
Total Expenses.	47,206,585,210	45,467,953,143	44,254,639,824	42,232,006,786	39,589,865,862
COMMUNITY HEALTH INDICATORS PER 1000 POPULATION					
Total Population (in thousands)	14,563	14,492	14,474	14,430	14,363
Inpatient					
Beds	2.4	2.3	2.3	2.3	2.3
Admissions	110.4	115.7	115.3	116.3	115.6
Inpatient Days	582.5	596.9	608.9	622.8	626.1
Inpatient Surgeries.	28.7	29.6	30.4	31.5	31.8
Births.	10.0	11.0	10.5	10.8	11.4
Outpatient					
Emergency Outpatient Visits	489.7	484.3	491.9	485.4	476.8
Other Outpatient Visits.	2,798.7	2,779.8	2,737.0	2,702.7	2,589.2
Total Outpatient Visits	3,288.4	3,264.0	3,228.9	3,188.2	3,066.1
Outpatient Surgeries	65.9	65.8	70.4	67.9	69.4
Expense per Capita (per person).	$3,249.5	$3,142.2	$3,065.2	$2,935.0	$2,766.5

TABLE 5

U.S. CENSUS DIVISION 2: MIDDLE ATLANTIC

U.S. Registered Community Hospitals
(Nonfederal, short-term general and other special hospitals)

Overview 2008–2012

	2012	2011	2010	2009	2008
Total Community Hospitals					
in Census Division 2, Middle Atlantic.......	447	449	454	457	468
Bed Size Category					
6-24.....................................	11	9	8	7	7
25-49....................................	36	36	38	39	41
50-99....................................	63	66	66	64	65
100-199..................................	107	106	102	111	115
200-299..................................	91	91	98	93	95
300-399..................................	52	54	53	53	56
400-499..................................	30	33	33	36	34
500 +....................................	57	54	56	54	55
Location					
Hospitals Urban..........................	362	364	367	369	387
Hospitals Rural	85	85	87	88	81
Control					
State and Local Government................	31	30	30	30	33
Not for Profit............................	354	362	373	381	388
Investor owned	62	57	51	46	47
Physician Models					
Independent Practice Association	61	53	54	54	63
Group Practice without Walls...............	17	12	17	20	20
Open Physician-Hospital Organization	42	39	40	41	55
Closed Physician-Hospital Organization	19	15	15	18	15
Management Service Organization	52	47	51	54	52
Integrated Salary Model...................	182	175	172	158	142
Equity Model............................	7	3	2	5	6
Foundation..............................	15	18	14	12	11
Insurance Products					
Health Maintenance Organization	91	90	80	66	83
Preferred Provider Organization.............	65	69	79	66	80
Indemnity Fee for Service	37	31	42	28	33
Managed Care Contracts					
Health Maintenance Organization	295	284	286	279	283
Preferred Provider Organization.............	285	274	277	264	270
Affiliations					
Hospitals in a System.....................	261	254	242	235	231
Hospitals in a Network	157	163	157	151	154
Hospitals in a Group Purchasing Organization..	323	321	321	305	308

TABLE 5

U.S. CENSUS DIVISION 2: MIDDLE ATLANTIC

U.S. Registered Community Hospitals
(Nonfederal, short-term general and other special hospitals)

Utilization, Personnel, Revenue and Expenses, Community Health Indicators 2008–2012

	2012	2011	2010	2009	2008
TOTAL FACILITY (Includes Hospital and Nursing Home Units)					
Utilization - Inpatient					
Beds	117,624	118,152	120,495	120,666	122,511
Admissions	5,183,982	5,308,422	5,387,182	5,469,937	5,516,053
Inpatient Days	31,440,731	31,927,960	32,429,928	32,905,796	33,922,806
Average Length of Stay	6.1	6.0	6.0	6.0	6.1
Inpatient Surgeries	1,404,460	1,385,212	1,472,258	1,444,280	1,475,219
Births	468,787	473,951	473,143	481,966	493,580
Utilization - Outpatient					
Emergency Outpatient Visits	18,321,971	18,128,050	17,544,922	18,036,427	17,471,705
Other Outpatient Visits	92,940,002	89,610,828	90,638,433	92,532,690	91,694,245
Total Outpatient Visits	111,261,973	107,738,878	108,183,355	110,569,117	109,165,950
Outpatient Surgeries	2,604,246	2,612,230	2,662,613	2,672,246	2,667,312
Personnel					
Full Time RNs	164,025	163,685	159,336	157,599	154,609
Full Time LPNs	8,908	9,399	9,477	10,498	11,135
Part Time RNs	61,911	62,925	61,970	58,758	59,586
Part Time LPNs	2,910	3,059	3,392	3,492	3,915
Total Full Time	667,785	663,442	641,848	649,700	652,192
Total Part Time	200,851	201,876	193,048	188,250	187,630
Revenue - Inpatient					
Gross Inpatient Revenue	$232,928,664,012	$224,663,669,372	$214,875,701,636	$207,428,274,807	$204,106,922,337
Revenue - Outpatient					
Gross Outpatient Revenue	$159,129,515,739	$142,077,957,104	$131,067,665,392	$119,608,818,446	$108,338,945,283
Revenue and Expenses - Totals					
(Includes Inpatient and Outpatient)					
Total Gross Revenue	$392,058,179,751	$366,741,626,476	$345,943,367,028	$327,037,093,253	$312,445,867,620
Deductions from Revenue	276,630,776,133	258,245,571,725	241,791,805,319	226,954,454,439	217,335,551,911
Net Patient Revenue	115,427,403,618	108,496,054,751	104,151,561,709	100,082,638,814	95,110,315,709
Other Operating Revenue	7,842,143,044	7,014,856,042	6,773,917,247	6,240,458,318	5,905,669,784
Other Nonoperating Revenue	1,401,364,085	1,370,628,711	1,636,895,627	1,079,935,145	-522,530,088
Total Net Revenue	124,670,910,747	116,881,539,504	112,562,374,583	107,403,032,277	100,493,455,405
Total Expenses	119,193,201,375	112,027,433,487	107,964,477,816	104,601,314,499	101,341,325,573
HOSPITAL UNIT (Excludes Separate Nursing Home Units)					
Utilization - Inpatient					
Beds	108,572	108,920	112,240	112,737	114,721
Admissions	5,143,373	5,266,742	5,349,564	5,432,647	5,477,486
Inpatient Days	28,351,497	28,745,893	29,691,180	30,267,570	31,398,678
Average Length of Stay	5.5	5.5	5.6	5.6	5.7
Personnel					
Total Full Time	660,600	657,123	636,513	642,529	644,394
Total Part Time	197,298	198,919	189,998	184,726	184,048
Revenue and Expenses - Totals					
(Includes Inpatient and Outpatient)					
Total Net Revenue	$123,724,968,154	$116,030,325,922	$111,642,685,649	$106,605,542,714	$99,744,284,282
Total Expenses	118,279,090,752	111,216,627,510	107,117,179,018	103,815,232,446	100,633,830,609
COMMUNITY HEALTH INDICATORS PER 1000 POPULATION					
Total Population (in thousands)	41,198	41,029	40,943	40,854	40,698
Inpatient					
Beds	2.9	2.9	2.9	3.0	3.0
Admissions	125.8	129.4	131.6	133.9	135.5
Inpatient Days	763.2	778.2	792.1	805.4	833.5
Inpatient Surgeries	34.1	33.8	36.0	35.4	36.2
Births	11.4	11.6	11.6	11.8	12.1
Outpatient					
Emergency Outpatient Visits	444.7	441.8	428.5	441.5	429.3
Other Outpatient Visits	2,255.9	2,184.1	2,213.8	2,265.0	2,253.1
Total Outpatient Visits	2,700.6	2,625.9	2,642.3	2,706.4	2,682.4
Outpatient Surgeries	63.2	63.7	65.0	65.4	65.5
Expense per Capita (per person)	$2,893.2	$2,730.4	$2,636.9	$2,560.4	$2,490.1

U.S. Census Divisions

TABLE **5**

U.S. CENSUS DIVISION 3: SOUTH ATLANTIC

U.S. Registered Community Hospitals
(Nonfederal, short-term general and other special hospitals)

Overview 2008–2012

	2012	2011	2010	2009	2008
Total Community Hospitals					
in Census Division 3, South Atlantic	766	759	758	759	762
Bed Size Category					
6-24	22	22	21	20	18
25-49	139	130	129	127	129
50-99	138	138	133	133	128
100-199	192	193	196	202	209
200-299	109	110	115	115	116
300-399	66	66	65	62	67
400-499	37	33	34	37	30
500 + ...	63	67	65	63	65
Location					
Hospitals Urban..........................	526	515	514	516	473
Hospitals Rural	240	244	244	243	289
Control					
State and Local Government................	135	137	141	144	147
Not for Profit	403	404	398	402	406
Investor owned	228	218	219	213	209
Physician Models					
Independent Practice Association	52	49	52	51	52
Group Practice without Walls...............	30	23	23	26	24
Open Physician-Hospital Organization	77	78	79	77	80
Closed Physician-Hospital Organization	42	37	38	36	39
Management Service Organization	72	66	67	56	51
Integrated Salary Model....................	291	287	287	256	255
Equity Model	19	20	21	20	20
Foundation...............................	17	19	20	16	21
Insurance Products					
Health Maintenance Organization	70	78	74	72	62
Preferred Provider Organization..............	73	95	94	85	75
Indemnity Fee for Service	26	32	29	27	24
Managed Care Contracts					
Health Maintenance Organization	410	428	417	412	402
Preferred Provider Organization..............	432	455	448	452	435
Affiliations					
Hospitals in a System......................	554	527	504	493	479
Hospitals in a Network	220	218	215	205	211
Hospitals in a Group Purchasing Organization..	516	522	538	535	542

TABLE 5

U.S. CENSUS DIVISION 3: SOUTH ATLANTIC

U.S. Registered Community Hospitals
(Nonfederal, short-term general and other special hospitals)

Utilization, Personnel, Revenue and Expenses, Community Health Indicators 2008–2012

	2012	2011	2010	2009	2008
TOTAL FACILITY (Includes Hospital and Nursing Home Units)					
Utilization - Inpatient					
Beds	156,937	156,421	156,678	156,435	156,622
Admissions	6,928,298	6,995,044	6,970,769	7,001,234	6,958,360
Inpatient Days	37,724,388	37,874,666	37,775,346	37,871,460	38,331,279
Average Length of Stay	5.4	5.4	5.4	5.4	5.5
Inpatient Surgeries	1,904,557	1,922,638	1,978,051	2,014,276	2,003,768
Births	690,305	691,803	718,161	736,030	764,298
Utilization - Outpatient					
Emergency Outpatient Visits	26,665,515	25,719,396	25,132,194	25,680,948	24,482,937
Other Outpatient Visits	74,855,137	72,465,338	70,980,844	71,516,908	69,838,160
Total Outpatient Visits	101,520,652	98,184,734	96,113,038	97,197,856	94,321,097
Outpatient Surgeries	3,293,896	3,285,368	3,275,089	3,347,083	3,346,983
Personnel					
Full Time RNs	226,678	218,388	214,222	209,172	195,655
Full Time LPNs	12,717	13,119	14,299	15,153	16,133
Part Time RNs	72,103	71,740	73,321	75,692	79,445
Part Time LPNs	3,438	3,608	4,092	4,515	5,177
Total Full Time	782,368	764,221	753,621	746,119	731,835
Total Part Time	209,662	206,195	204,742	211,449	219,295
Revenue - Inpatient					
Gross Inpatient Revenue	$247,143,243,581	$230,857,582,404	$221,881,724,341	$206,158,157,529	$190,255,383,250
Revenue - Outpatient					
Gross Outpatient Revenue	$191,354,643,518	$171,171,466,560	$156,997,699,889	$141,704,232,345	$123,592,865,886
Revenue and Expenses - Totals **(Includes Inpatient and Outpatient)**					
Total Gross Revenue	$438,497,887,099	$402,029,048,964	$378,879,424,230	$347,862,389,874	$313,848,249,136
Deductions from Revenue	301,779,297,485	278,266,927,544	257,534,395,622	231,360,708,001	204,204,305,242
Net Patient Revenue	136,718,589,614	123,762,121,420	121,345,028,608	116,501,681,873	109,643,943,894
Other Operating Revenue	6,785,768,283	6,233,574,974	5,739,614,294	5,340,444,911	5,395,566,187
Other Nonoperating Revenue	2,215,518,159	1,983,730,368	2,153,138,363	702,305,382	-1,072,116,225
Total Net Revenue	145,719,876,056	131,979,426,762	129,237,781,265	122,544,432,166	113,967,393,856
Total Expenses	132,934,775,278	122,100,282,752	118,053,521,062	115,183,239,713	109,762,268,873
HOSPITAL UNIT (Excludes Separate Nursing Home Units)					
Utilization - Inpatient					
Beds	146,488	145,614	145,304	146,162	145,784
Admissions	6,885,814	6,952,755	6,925,183	6,957,697	6,913,674
Inpatient Days	34,334,087	34,472,561	34,041,050	34,447,166	34,834,753
Average Length of Stay	5.0	5.0	4.9	5.0	5.0
Personnel					
Total Full Time	774,599	756,853	745,348	737,233	723,355
Total Part Time	207,045	203,449	201,603	208,120	216,083
Revenue and Expenses - Totals **(Includes Inpatient and Outpatient)**					
Total Net Revenue	$144,879,731,362	$131,160,884,248	$128,322,166,959	$121,761,391,092	$113,171,813,994
Total Expenses	132,134,543,784	121,286,710,334	117,214,899,415	114,453,158,594	109,002,752,761
COMMUNITY HEALTH INDICATORS PER 1000 POPULATION					
Total Population (in thousands)	61,189	60,514	59,659	59,196	58,607
Inpatient					
Beds	2.6	2.6	2.6	2.6	2.7
Admissions	113.2	115.6	116.8	118.3	118.7
Inpatient Days	616.5	625.9	633.2	639.8	654.0
Inpatient Surgeries	31.1	31.8	33.2	34.0	34.2
Births	11.3	11.4	12.0	12.4	13.0
Outpatient					
Emergency Outpatient Visits	435.8	425.0	421.3	433.8	417.7
Other Outpatient Visits	1,223.4	1,197.5	1,189.8	1,208.1	1,191.6
Total Outpatient Visits	1,659.1	1,622.5	1,611.0	1,642.0	1,609.4
Outpatient Surgeries	53.8	54.3	54.9	56.5	57.1
Expense per Capita (per person)	$2,172.5	$2,017.7	$1,978.8	$1,945.8	$1,872.8

U.S. Census Divisions

TABLE 5

U.S. CENSUS DIVISION 4: EAST NORTH CENTRAL

U.S. Registered Community Hospitals
(Nonfederal, short-term general and other special hospitals)

Overview 2008–2012

	2012	2011	2010	2009	2008
Total Community Hospitals					
in Census Division 4, East North Central....	776	774	777	779	774
Bed Size Category					
6-24	57	45	43	40	37
25-49	204	204	198	196	193
50-99	146	155	163	166	162
100-199	161	155	151	161	159
200-299	84	93	100	96	99
300-399	55	56	56	52	56
400-499	29	27	26	29	29
500 + ...	40	39	40	39	39
Location					
Hospitals Urban..........................	503	501	503	504	486
Hospitals Rural	273	273	274	275	288
Control					
State and Local Government................	90	89	96	99	103
Not for Profit	588	592	590	593	589
Investor owned	98	93	91	87	82
Physician Models					
Independent Practice Association	71	69	73	86	88
Group Practice without Walls................	27	30	25	23	28
Open Physician-Hospital Organization	162	163	164	163	151
Closed Physician-Hospital Organization	46	52	51	45	47
Management Service Organization	65	82	87	93	96
Integrated Salary Model....................	346	321	312	303	295
Equity Model.............................	22	21	22	26	30
Foundation...............................	40	49	59	52	49
Insurance Products					
Health Maintenance Organization	152	151	145	143	140
Preferred Provider Organization..............	141	161	165	167	155
Indemnity Fee for Service	52	54	57	59	57
Managed Care Contracts					
Health Maintenance Organization	527	514	531	552	529
Preferred Provider Organization..............	555	547	568	597	576
Affiliations					
Hospitals in a System......................	492	486	475	467	452
Hospitals in a Network	277	272	277	276	271
Hospitals in a Group Purchasing Organization..	618	608	632	645	643

TABLE 5

U.S. CENSUS DIVISION 4: EAST NORTH CENTRAL

U.S. Registered Community Hospitals
(Nonfederal, short-term general and other special hospitals)

Utilization, Personnel, Revenue and Expenses, Community Health Indicators 2008–2012

	2012	2011	2010	2009	2008
TOTAL FACILITY (Includes Hospital and Nursing Home Units)					
Utilization - Inpatient					
Beds	121,997	122,555	124,528	124,648	124,957
Admissions	5,477,164	5,518,124	5,573,945	5,631,570	5,730,456
Inpatient Days	27,190,027	27,603,703	28,088,741	28,659,008	29,237,134
Average Length of Stay	5.0	5.0	5.0	5.1	5.1
Inpatient Surgeries	1,499,944	1,537,005	1,598,684	1,629,031	1,641,475
Births	524,244	531,487	549,668	569,683	590,869
Utilization - Outpatient					
Emergency Outpatient Visits	22,161,580	21,873,056	21,645,563	21,143,963	20,682,680
Other Outpatient Visits	114,778,170	110,723,087	110,255,848	106,866,440	102,419,976
Total Outpatient Visits	136,939,750	132,596,143	131,901,411	128,010,403	123,102,656
Outpatient Surgeries	3,185,907	3,152,571	3,207,896	3,184,812	3,147,665
Personnel					
Full Time RNs	176,706	171,026	166,190	159,198	154,002
Full Time LPNs	7,987	9,094	8,792	9,506	10,480
Part Time RNs	99,210	97,012	97,309	97,165	96,817
Part Time LPNs	4,590	4,841	5,200	5,538	6,489
Total Full Time	672,905	661,130	656,411	652,503	647,246
Total Part Time	302,574	301,819	305,777	309,198	306,273
Revenue - Inpatient					
Gross Inpatient Revenue	$187,228,187,292	$176,586,489,578	$169,254,285,621	$159,626,875,101	$149,698,495,809
Revenue - Outpatient					
Gross Outpatient Revenue	$185,825,760,037	$167,198,588,978	$153,605,458,204	$139,937,321,698	$125,559,569,848
Revenue and Expenses - Totals (Includes Inpatient and Outpatient)					
Total Gross Revenue	$373,053,947,329	$343,785,078,556	$322,859,743,825	$299,564,196,799	$275,258,065,657
Deductions from Revenue	243,148,787,597	224,785,581,163	206,741,773,300	188,295,725,972	169,876,753,425
Net Patient Revenue	129,905,159,732	118,999,497,393	116,117,970,525	111,268,470,827	105,381,312,232
Other Operating Revenue	7,734,468,170	7,235,875,567	6,838,675,527	6,706,843,261	6,300,528,903
Other Nonoperating Revenue	2,372,671,286	2,481,023,683	2,812,190,226	360,822,911	-2,457,450,887
Total Net Revenue	140,012,299,188	128,716,396,643	125,768,836,278	118,336,136,999	109,224,390,248
Total Expenses	128,508,223,081	118,844,737,908	116,021,099,796	112,388,231,445	108,029,056,637
HOSPITAL UNIT (Excludes Separate Nursing Home Units)					
Utilization - Inpatient					
Beds	116,777	117,051	118,315	118,136	118,085
Admissions	5,443,973	5,480,695	5,532,131	5,587,798	5,687,064
Inpatient Days	25,617,733	25,917,067	26,193,965	26,630,592	27,072,122
Average Length of Stay	4.7	4.7	4.7	4.8	4.8
Personnel					
Total Full Time	669,734	657,862	652,317	647,481	642,131
Total Part Time	299,781	298,789	302,371	305,428	302,441
Revenue and Expenses - Totals (Includes Inpatient and Outpatient)					
Total Net Revenue	$139,565,247,628	$128,223,217,900	$125,272,982,180	$117,798,388,335	$108,726,765,462
Total Expenses	128,116,255,360	118,428,199,417	115,557,672,594	111,947,643,021	107,600,938,852
COMMUNITY HEALTH INDICATORS PER 1000 POPULATION					
Total Population (in thousands)	46,567	46,519	46,522	46,501	46,389
Inpatient					
Beds	2.6	2.6	2.7	2.7	2.7
Admissions	117.6	118.6	119.8	121.1	123.5
Inpatient Days	583.9	593.4	603.8	616.3	630.3
Inpatient Surgeries	32.2	33.0	34.4	35.0	35.4
Births	11.3	11.4	11.8	12.3	12.7
Outpatient					
Emergency Outpatient Visits	475.9	470.2	465.3	454.7	445.8
Other Outpatient Visits	2,464.8	2,380.2	2,370.0	2,298.2	2,207.8
Total Outpatient Visits	2,940.7	2,850.4	2,835.3	2,752.9	2,653.7
Outpatient Surgeries	68.4	67.8	69.0	68.5	67.9
Expense per Capita (per person)	$2,759.7	$2,554.8	$2,493.9	$2,416.9	$2,328.7

U.S. Census Divisions

TABLE 5

U.S. CENSUS DIVISION 5: EAST SOUTH CENTRAL

U.S. Registered Community Hospitals
(Nonfederal, short-term general and other special hospitals)

Overview 2008–2012

	2012	2011	2010	2009	2008
Total Community Hospitals					
in Census Division 5, East South Central . . .	433	440	441	446	449
Bed Size Category					
6-24	21	22	16	16	18
25-49	125	125	128	128	126
50-99	95	98	100	104	107
100-199	97	99	104	104	99
200-299	41	40	35	35	39
300-399	24	25	25	26	26
400-499	8	10	14	15	14
500 + ...	22	21	19	18	20
Location					
Hospitals Urban.	200	207	208	211	186
Hospitals Rural	233	233	233	235	263
Control					
State and Local Government.	111	112	112	115	119
Not for Profit	176	177	182	186	188
Investor owned	146	151	147	145	142
Physician Models					
Independent Practice Association	30	31	36	36	35
Group Practice without Walls.	7	7	7	10	10
Open Physician-Hospital Organization	45	43	43	41	49
Closed Physician-Hospital Organization	12	10	8	11	17
Management Service Organization	44	46	39	34	34
Integrated Salary Model	113	111	114	102	94
Equity Model	2	1	1	3	2
Foundation.	15	21	22	23	22
Insurance Products					
Health Maintenance Organization	26	25	32	26	39
Preferred Provider Organization.	65	80	75	70	83
Indemnity Fee for Service	19	18	21	15	28
Managed Care Contracts					
Health Maintenance Organization	159	165	165	164	176
Preferred Provider Organization.	194	204	215	211	233
Affiliations					
Hospitals in a System.	295	294	289	289	286
Hospitals in a Network	89	91	101	105	111
Hospitals in a Group Purchasing Organization. .	192	194	205	224	240

TABLE 5

U.S. CENSUS DIVISION 5: EAST SOUTH CENTRAL

U.S. Registered Community Hospitals
(Nonfederal, short-term general and other special hospitals)

Utilization, Personnel, Revenue and Expenses, Community Health Indicators 2008–2012

	2012	2011	2010	2009	2008
TOTAL FACILITY (Includes Hospital and Nursing Home Units)					
Utilization - Inpatient					
Beds	62,199	62,478	63,079	63,252	63,626
Admissions	2,430,269	2,424,397	2,486,454	2,535,115	2,587,919
Inpatient Days	13,150,314	13,300,397	13,614,893	13,973,205	14,460,015
Average Length of Stay	5.4	5.5	5.5	5.5	5.6
Inpatient Surgeries	728,421	732,580	728,125	746,929	736,745
Births	209,932	207,943	221,646	233,974	245,061
Utilization - Outpatient					
Emergency Outpatient Visits	9,782,661	9,526,218	9,527,974	9,630,514	9,557,382
Other Outpatient Visits	25,794,437	25,425,473	25,726,751	25,948,613	25,382,539
Total Outpatient Visits	35,577,098	34,951,691	35,254,725	35,579,127	34,939,921
Outpatient Surgeries	1,405,286	1,386,491	1,344,976	1,337,590	1,309,219
Personnel					
Full Time RNs	75,991	75,308	73,350	73,191	70,022
Full Time LPNs	6,263	6,748	7,457	8,025	8,614
Part Time RNs	25,437	24,560	25,319	24,568	25,507
Part Time LPNs	1,640	1,692	2,052	2,168	2,568
Total Full Time	266,388	265,560	262,113	265,884	263,757
Total Part Time	71,714	68,968	72,591	71,457	74,148
Revenue - Inpatient					
Gross Inpatient Revenue	$80,646,954,304	$75,686,751,272	$73,345,815,567	$70,177,022,070	$67,429,348,071
Revenue - Outpatient					
Gross Outpatient Revenue	$71,015,770,262	$61,846,614,466	$56,798,252,271	$52,231,598,393	$46,662,139,027
Revenue and Expenses - Totals					
(Includes Inpatient and Outpatient)					
Total Gross Revenue	$151,662,724,566	$137,533,365,738	$130,144,067,838	$122,408,620,463	$114,091,487,098
Deductions from Revenue	109,016,339,180	99,633,059,934	92,627,817,898	85,830,854,030	79,115,671,773
Net Patient Revenue	42,646,385,386	37,900,305,804	37,516,249,940	36,577,766,433	34,975,815,325
Other Operating Revenue	1,820,681,077	1,532,546,010	1,479,335,426	1,540,908,813	1,625,010,586
Other Nonoperating Revenue	407,005,231	481,348,514	696,071,058	193,864,288	-19,706,728
Total Net Revenue	44,874,071,694	39,914,200,328	39,691,656,424	38,312,539,534	36,581,119,183
Total Expenses	41,101,364,805	36,909,370,915	36,471,494,399	36,466,730,541	34,933,934,594
HOSPITAL UNIT (Excludes Separate Nursing Home Units)					
Utilization - Inpatient					
Beds	58,411	58,770	58,946	58,982	59,075
Admissions	2,413,202	2,407,693	2,471,184	2,518,083	2,569,243
Inpatient Days	11,963,248	12,159,845	12,327,182	12,606,657	12,982,972
Average Length of Stay	5.0	5.1	5.0	5.0	5.1
Personnel					
Total Full Time	263,124	262,518	258,805	262,043	259,932
Total Part Time	70,861	68,301	71,637	70,556	73,231
Revenue and Expenses - Totals					
(Includes Inpatient and Outpatient)					
Total Net Revenue	$44,641,587,474	$39,631,141,073	$39,425,199,072	$38,036,670,123	$36,298,364,734
Total Expenses	40,885,625,657	36,701,651,997	36,231,662,045	36,228,704,518	34,698,028,587
COMMUNITY HEALTH INDICATORS PER 1000 POPULATION					
Total Population (in thousands)	18,644	18,554	18,368	18,271	18,146
Inpatient					
Beds	3.3	3.4	3.4	3.5	3.5
Admissions	130.4	130.7	135.4	138.8	142.6
Inpatient Days	705.4	716.8	741.2	764.8	796.9
Inpatient Surgeries	39.1	39.5	39.6	40.9	40.6
Births	11.3	11.2	12.1	12.8	13.5
Outpatient					
Emergency Outpatient Visits	524.7	513.4	518.7	527.1	526.7
Other Outpatient Visits	1,383.6	1,370.4	1,400.7	1,420.2	1,398.8
Total Outpatient Visits	1,908.3	1,883.8	1,919.4	1,947.3	1,925.5
Outpatient Surgeries	75.4	74.7	73.2	73.2	72.1
Expense per Capita (per person)	$2,204.6	$1,989.3	$1,985.6	$1,995.9	$1,925.2

U.S. Census Divisions

TABLE **5**

U.S. CENSUS DIVISION 6: WEST NORTH CENTRAL

U.S. Registered Community Hospitals
(Nonfederal, short-term general and other special hospitals)

Overview 2008–2012

	2012	2011	2010	2009	2008
Total Community Hospitals					
in Census Division 6, West North Central . . .	692	682	685	689	683
Bed Size Category					
6-24	128	126	113	108	103
25-49	217	218	220	217	214
50-99	160	154	164	167	166
100-199	97	91	97	104	105
200-299	35	38	35	38	38
300-399	25	25	28	25	26
400-499	14	14	12	14	15
500 + ...	16	16	16	16	16
Location					
Hospitals Urban.	226	220	223	224	191
Hospitals Rural	466	462	462	465	492
Control					
State and Local Government.	233	236	235	237	236
Not for Profit	405	396	398	399	395
Investor owned	54	50	52	53	52
Physician Models					
Independent Practice Association	63	62	70	77	82
Group Practice without Walls.	16	12	11	14	13
Open Physician-Hospital Organization	70	68	70	84	89
Closed Physician-Hospital Organization	26	26	23	27	26
Management Service Organization	16	20	17	19	25
Integrated Salary Model.	336	330	317	339	315
Equity Model	7	6	2	5	6
Foundation.	17	22	17	14	21
Insurance Products					
Health Maintenance Organization	59	56	59	56	59
Preferred Provider Organization.	69	89	88	84	93
Indemnity Fee for Service	20	29	27	29	32
Managed Care Contracts					
Health Maintenance Organization	318	311	310	320	313
Preferred Provider Organization.	445	442	446	469	471
Affiliations					
Hospitals in a System.	372	352	348	347	339
Hospitals in a Network	288	287	277	282	280
Hospitals in a Group Purchasing Organization. .	562	557	552	573	570

TABLE 5

U.S. CENSUS DIVISION 6: WEST NORTH CENTRAL

U.S. Registered Community Hospitals
(Nonfederal, short-term general and other special hospitals)

Utilization, Personnel, Revenue and Expenses, Community Health Indicators 2008–2012

	2012	2011	2010	2009	2008
TOTAL FACILITY (Includes Hospital and Nursing Home Units)					
Utilization - Inpatient					
Beds	68,455	67,559	68,830	70,039	70,208
Admissions	2,421,698	2,453,988	2,464,267	2,523,626	2,589,852
Inpatient Days	14,638,214	14,718,938	14,928,227	15,492,237	15,912,612
Average Length of Stay	6.0	6.0	6.1	6.1	6.1
Inpatient Surgeries	667,171	674,685	683,170	705,862	722,817
Births	268,618	264,259	264,621	274,101	279,320
Utilization - Outpatient					
Emergency Outpatient Visits	8,725,139	8,573,615	8,260,672	8,272,930	8,056,684
Other Outpatient Visits	52,156,664	49,766,340	50,003,264	48,365,884	45,865,406
Total Outpatient Visits	60,881,803	58,339,955	58,263,936	56,638,814	53,922,090
Outpatient Surgeries	1,381,534	1,352,232	1,322,974	1,367,598	1,420,972
Personnel					
Full Time RNs	78,654	75,384	73,425	70,664	67,029
Full Time LPNs	7,145	7,158	7,282	7,481	7,692
Part Time RNs	54,342	51,864	52,648	54,581	55,475
Part Time LPNs	4,109	4,132	4,485	4,775	5,225
Total Full Time	311,613	301,105	297,067	289,975	285,576
Total Part Time	164,991	160,171	164,985	169,233	171,973
Revenue - Inpatient					
Gross Inpatient Revenue	$77,970,550,986	$74,583,373,377	$71,077,555,297	$68,351,872,323	$65,013,165,311
Revenue - Outpatient					
Gross Outpatient Revenue	$76,310,450,463	$68,953,101,651	$62,710,234,207	$58,193,971,919	$50,949,559,907
Revenue and Expenses - Totals					
(Includes Inpatient and Outpatient)					
Total Gross Revenue	$154,281,001,449	$143,536,475,028	$133,787,789,504	$126,545,844,242	$115,962,725,218
Deductions from Revenue	96,278,090,518	89,596,077,363	82,115,750,561	76,480,891,243	67,883,978,998
Net Patient Revenue	58,002,910,931	53,940,397,665	51,672,038,943	50,064,952,999	48,078,746,220
Other Operating Revenue	3,444,366,586	2,870,841,462	2,830,841,723	2,646,149,834	2,675,404,595
Other Nonoperating Revenue	1,330,357,727	1,096,847,381	1,318,194,215	557,107,759	-524,235,863
Total Net Revenue	62,777,635,244	57,908,086,508	55,821,074,881	53,268,210,592	50,229,914,952
Total Expenses	56,450,154,448	54,026,689,854	51,771,367,599	50,238,229,445	48,227,547,446
HOSPITAL UNIT (Excludes Separate Nursing Home Units)					
Utilization - Inpatient					
Beds	59,408	58,568	59,661	59,833	58,879
Admissions	2,400,701	2,432,961	2,443,671	2,498,928	2,561,317
Inpatient Days	11,768,543	11,849,105	12,018,243	12,233,218	12,328,044
Average Length of Stay	4.9	4.9	4.9	4.9	4.8
Personnel					
Total Full Time	305,819	295,954	291,819	283,837	279,159
Total Part Time	160,210	155,670	160,316	164,037	166,260
Revenue and Expenses - Totals					
(Includes Inpatient and Outpatient)					
Total Net Revenue	$62,194,053,711	$57,296,078,737	$55,268,629,929	$52,624,057,167	$49,501,040,808
Total Expenses	55,903,031,384	53,536,656,669	51,251,683,260	49,653,268,189	47,573,291,977
COMMUNITY HEALTH INDICATORS PER 1000 POPULATION					
Total Population (in thousands)	20,750	20,640	20,451	20,336	20,206
Inpatient					
Beds	3.3	3.3	3.4	3.4	3.5
Admissions	116.7	118.9	120.5	124.1	128.2
Inpatient Days	705.5	713.1	729.9	761.8	787.5
Inpatient Surgeries	32.2	32.7	33.4	34.7	35.8
Births	12.9	12.8	12.9	13.5	13.8
Outpatient					
Emergency Outpatient Visits	420.5	415.4	403.9	406.8	398.7
Other Outpatient Visits	2,513.6	2,411.2	2,445.0	2,378.3	2,269.9
Total Outpatient Visits	2,934.1	2,826.6	2,848.9	2,785.1	2,668.6
Outpatient Surgeries	66.6	65.5	64.7	67.2	70.3
Expense per Capita (per person)	$2,720.5	$2,617.6	$2,531.4	$2,470.4	$2,386.8

TABLE **5**

U.S. CENSUS DIVISION 7: WEST SOUTH CENTRAL

U.S. Registered Community Hospitals
(Nonfederal, short-term general and other special hospitals)

Overview 2008–2012

	2012	2011	2010	2009	2008
Total Community Hospitals					
in Census Division 7, West South Central...	749	746	750	758	757
Bed Size Category					
6-24	117	114	119	112	112
25-49	224	226	220	223	219
50-99	149	144	146	147	151
100-199	104	109	115	124	124
200-299	62	62	61	61	61
300-399	40	37	35	35	37
400-499	19	20	20	22	21
500 + ...	34	34	34	34	32
Location					
Hospitals Urban..........................	439	431	436	440	424
Hospitals Rural	310	315	314	318	333
Control					
State and Local Government................	206	210	221	230	225
Not for Profit	275	276	267	263	273
Investor owned	268	260	262	265	259
Physician Models					
Independent Practice Association	82	94	109	109	103
Group Practice without Walls................	28	31	33	41	28
Open Physician-Hospital Organization	128	126	128	137	143
Closed Physician-Hospital Organization	38	32	30	31	32
Management Service Organization	88	93	94	99	92
Integrated Salary Model....................	215	211	181	168	155
Equity Model	11	10	16	17	19
Foundation..............................	48	47	43	44	50
Insurance Products					
Health Maintenance Organization	93	101	96	90	78
Preferred Provider Organization..............	76	116	118	105	93
Indemnity Fee for Service	22	34	36	30	32
Managed Care Contracts					
Health Maintenance Organization	468	457	449	458	453
Preferred Provider Organization..............	542	554	540	544	551
Affiliations					
Hospitals in a System......................	451	436	434	457	454
Hospitals in a Network	193	193	184	175	177
Hospitals in a Group Purchasing Organization..	625	629	623	624	622

TABLE 5

U.S. CENSUS DIVISION 7: WEST SOUTH CENTRAL

U.S. Registered Community Hospitals
(Nonfederal, short-term general and other special hospitals)

Utilization, Personnel, Revenue and Expenses, Community Health Indicators 2008–2012

	2012	2011	2010	2009	2008
TOTAL FACILITY (Includes Hospital and Nursing Home Units)					
Utilization - Inpatient					
Beds	97,260	96,825	97,399	98,807	97,720
Admissions	3,908,065	3,929,807	4,005,387	4,083,758	4,061,559
Inpatient Days	20,396,936	20,460,393	20,922,699	21,466,556	21,234,945
Average Length of Stay	5.2	5.2	5.2	5.3	5.2
Inpatient Surgeries	1,080,738	1,118,349	1,150,547	1,181,045	1,169,284
Births	516,124	503,256	528,045	561,702	546,219
Utilization - Outpatient					
Emergency Outpatient Visits	16,269,062	15,575,261	15,392,542	14,987,499	14,148,116
Other Outpatient Visits	45,892,246	44,066,578	45,924,148	44,027,580	42,236,693
Total Outpatient Visits	62,161,308	59,641,839	61,316,690	59,015,079	56,384,809
Outpatient Surgeries	1,675,034	1,683,472	1,707,264	1,671,570	1,642,752
Personnel					
Full Time RNs	126,908	121,426	123,112	120,752	110,558
Full Time LPNs	13,783	14,606	15,573	16,584	17,702
Part Time RNs	36,330	35,553	33,058	33,815	33,899
Part Time LPNs	3,352	3,347	3,961	4,411	4,592
Total Full Time	435,758	428,649	434,296	436,301	419,150
Total Part Time	106,477	103,538	99,628	101,491	102,483
Revenue - Inpatient					
Gross Inpatient Revenue	$157,197,100,160	$146,271,380,775	$139,926,153,510	$132,565,357,014	$122,760,036,602
Revenue - Outpatient					
Gross Outpatient Revenue	$118,343,524,306	$104,883,587,404	$95,633,086,065	$84,978,216,080	$73,261,517,369
Revenue and Expenses - Totals					
(Includes Inpatient and Outpatient)					
Total Gross Revenue	$275,540,624,466	$251,154,968,179	$235,559,239,575	$217,543,573,094	$196,021,553,971
Deductions from Revenue	199,811,182,037	184,194,250,743	169,768,881,745	154,142,249,102	136,945,981,599
Net Patient Revenue	75,729,442,429	66,960,717,436	65,790,357,830	63,401,323,992	59,075,572,372
Other Operating Revenue	6,473,296,689	5,893,843,564	5,622,273,906	5,328,857,978	4,942,957,894
Other Nonoperating Revenue	1,074,127,947	1,909,520,980	1,791,442,768	267,367,879	412,762,180
Total Net Revenue	83,276,867,065	74,764,081,980	73,204,074,504	68,997,549,849	64,431,292,446
Total Expenses	74,523,034,451	67,280,680,393	65,549,933,822	64,399,048,894	60,693,798,710
HOSPITAL UNIT (Excludes Separate Nursing Home Units)					
Utilization - Inpatient					
Beds	95,188	94,783	95,427	96,504	95,219
Admissions	3,894,508	3,916,503	3,991,294	4,068,586	4,044,358
Inpatient Days	19,839,649	19,861,338	20,336,517	20,737,974	20,585,465
Average Length of Stay	5.1	5.1	5.1	5.1	5.1
Personnel					
Total Full Time	433,602	427,100	432,842	433,900	416,608
Total Part Time	106,091	103,146	99,156	100,856	101,661
Revenue and Expenses - Totals					
(Includes Inpatient and Outpatient)					
Total Net Revenue	$83,105,764,389	$74,607,353,353	$73,043,779,992	$68,839,731,724	$64,269,536,853
Total Expenses	74,387,874,023	67,137,888,126	65,399,265,396	64,241,260,529	60,516,951,798
COMMUNITY HEALTH INDICATORS PER 1000 POPULATION					
Total Population (in thousands)	37,425	36,979	36,378	35,851	35,268
Inpatient					
Beds	2.6	2.6	2.7	2.8	2.8
Admissions	104.4	106.3	110.1	113.9	115.2
Inpatient Days	545.0	553.3	575.2	598.8	602.1
Inpatient Surgeries	28.9	30.2	31.6	32.9	33.2
Births	13.8	13.6	14.5	15.7	15.5
Outpatient					
Emergency Outpatient Visits	434.7	421.2	423.1	418.1	401.2
Other Outpatient Visits	1,226.2	1,191.7	1,262.4	1,228.1	1,197.6
Total Outpatient Visits	1,661.0	1,612.9	1,685.6	1,646.1	1,598.8
Outpatient Surgeries	44.8	45.5	46.9	46.6	46.6
Expense per Capita (per person)	$1,991.3	$1,819.4	$1,801.9	$1,796.3	$1,721.0

U.S. Census Divisions

TABLE **5**

U.S. CENSUS DIVISION 8: MOUNTAIN

U.S. Registered Community Hospitals
(Nonfederal, short-term general and other special hospitals)

Overview 2008–2012

	2012	2011	2010	2009	2008
Total Community Hospitals					
in Census Division 8, Mountain..............	**388**	**384**	**382**	**382**	**374**
Bed Size Category					
6-24	57	55	53	50	48
25-49	102	99	98	96	94
50-99	84	87	88	96	92
100-199	65	63	66	61	66
200-299	34	35	32	35	34
300-399	20	20	21	21	17
400-499	14	13	11	8	9
500 + ...	12	12	13	15	14
Location					
Hospitals Urban...........................	193	191	189	189	166
Hospitals Rural	195	193	193	193	208
Control					
State and Local Government................	93	94	94	97	96
Not for Profit	196	197	195	191	189
Investor owned	99	93	93	94	89
Physician Models					
Independent Practice Association	40	41	42	48	46
Group Practice without Walls................	12	13	8	9	8
Open Physician-Hospital Organization	37	36	34	36	33
Closed Physician-Hospital Organization	13	15	14	16	16
Management Service Organization	21	24	27	26	22
Integrated Salary Model....................	148	140	125	130	122
Equity Model.............................	4	5	5	5	6
Foundation...............................	12	12	13	11	14
Insurance Products					
Health Maintenance Organization	55	57	54	53	53
Preferred Provider Organization..............	40	58	56	54	49
Indemnity Fee for Service	20	26	27	29	25
Managed Care Contracts					
Health Maintenance Organization	143	141	147	153	156
Preferred Provider Organization..............	190	184	185	198	199
Affiliations					
Hospitals in a System......................	234	229	230	232	225
Hospitals in a Network	99	110	112	111	110
Hospitals in a Group Purchasing Organization..	240	259	248	257	255

TABLE 5

U.S. CENSUS DIVISION 8: MOUNTAIN

U.S. Registered Community Hospitals
(Nonfederal, short-term general and other special hospitals)

Utilization, Personnel, Revenue and Expenses, Community Health Indicators 2008–2012

	2012	2011	2010	2009	2008
TOTAL FACILITY (Includes Hospital and Nursing Home Units)					
Utilization - Inpatient					
Beds	47,501	47,119	46,872	47,028	46,293
Admissions	2,060,596	2,064,195	2,091,454	2,089,087	2,098,239
Inpatient Days	10,231,226	10,303,057	10,379,491	10,509,716	10,533,261
Average Length of Stay.	5.0	5.0	5.0	5.0	5.0
Inpatient Surgeries.	614,124	646,125	662,412	673,176	638,455
Births.	269,841	268,969	278,694	300,722	314,340
Utilization - Outpatient					
Emergency Outpatient Visits	7,821,770	7,567,323	7,497,043	7,485,406	7,302,452
Other Outpatient Visits.	32,436,477	31,476,244	29,432,803	28,867,801	28,396,866
Total Outpatient Visits	40,258,247	39,043,567	36,929,846	36,353,207	35,699,318
Outpatient Surgeries	982,976	996,441	982,327	962,734	936,167
Personnel					
Full Time RNs	66,845	64,271	66,717	64,343	62,485
Full Time LPNs	3,085	3,129	3,511	4,372	4,011
Part Time RNs.	26,537	25,828	23,141	24,303	24,804
Part Time LPNs	1,204	1,197	1,170	1,401	1,594
Total Full Time.	234,035	228,851	233,880	229,182	224,101
Total Part Time	78,088	76,297	68,863	73,288	75,630
Revenue - Inpatient					
Gross Inpatient Revenue.	$83,441,071,276	$77,570,487,787	$74,568,371,912	$69,773,749,237	$65,876,774,754
Revenue - Outpatient					
Gross Outpatient Revenue	$65,655,835,782	$59,010,644,319	$53,530,101,037	$47,901,898,628	$41,380,379,213
Revenue and Expenses - Totals					
(Includes Inpatient and Outpatient)					
Total Gross Revenue.	$149,096,907,058	$136,581,132,106	$128,098,472,949	$117,675,647,865	$107,257,153,967
Deductions from Revenue.	102,954,441,992	94,240,727,395	86,894,343,376	78,561,440,721	70,987,810,766
Net Patient Revenue	46,142,465,066	42,340,404,711	41,204,129,573	39,114,207,144	36,269,343,201
Other Operating Revenue	1,890,523,158	1,885,009,958	1,804,886,179	1,641,533,021	1,612,417,661
Other Nonoperating Revenue	353,858,460	497,930,676	550,761,263	383,043,417	-20,098,533
Total Net Revenue.	48,386,846,684	44,723,345,345	43,559,777,015	41,138,783,582	37,861,662,329
Total Expenses.	43,346,401,522	40,362,478,873	38,771,182,258	37,489,628,683	35,816,821,042
HOSPITAL UNIT (Excludes Separate Nursing Home Units)					
Utilization - Inpatient					
Beds	44,388	43,922	43,563	43,572	42,780
Admissions	2,052,402	2,054,557	2,081,194	2,078,283	2,087,447
Inpatient Days	9,282,591	9,320,023	9,356,938	9,453,606	9,502,108
Average Length of Stay.	4.5	4.5	4.5	4.5	4.6
Personnel					
Total Full Time.	232,008	226,920	231,537	226,895	220,221
Total Part Time	76,862	75,224	67,617	72,075	74,179
Revenue and Expenses - Totals					
(Includes Inpatient and Outpatient)					
Total Net Revenue.	$48,172,247,901	$44,490,329,013	$43,323,260,876	$40,917,090,747	$37,657,242,332
Total Expenses.	43,160,567,568	40,156,890,139	38,565,221,584	37,287,396,355	35,628,245,086
COMMUNITY HEALTH INDICATORS PER 1000 POPULATION					
Total Population (in thousands)	22,618	22,373	22,379	22,123	21,793
Inpatient					
Beds	2.1	2.1	2.1	2.1	2.1
Admissions	91.1	92.3	93.5	94.4	96.3
Inpatient Days	452.4	460.5	463.8	475.1	483.3
Inpatient Surgeries.	27.2	28.9	29.6	30.4	29.3
Births.	11.9	12.0	12.5	13.6	14.4
Outpatient					
Emergency Outpatient Visits	345.8	338.2	335.0	338.4	335.1
Other Outpatient Visits.	1,434.1	1,406.9	1,315.2	1,304.9	1,303.0
Total Outpatient Visits	1,779.9	1,745.1	1,650.2	1,643.2	1,638.1
Outpatient Surgeries	43.5	44.5	43.9	43.5	43.0
Expense per Capita (per person).	$1,916.5	$1,804.0	$1,732.5	$1,694.6	$1,643.5

TABLE 5

U.S. CENSUS DIVISION 9: PACIFIC

U.S. Registered Community Hospitals
(Nonfederal, short-term general and other special hospitals)

Overview 2008–2012

	2012	2011	2010	2009	2008
Total Community Hospitals					
in Census Division 9, Pacific	541	535	535	535	543
Bed Size Category					
6-24	39	42	41	39	36
25-49	102	97	97	98	97
50-99	72	73	70	73	82
100-199	138	133	139	139	139
200-299	88	86	84	87	92
300-399	51	55	55	57	53
400-499	34	31	31	27	27
500 + ...	17	18	18	15	17
Location					
Hospitals Urban...........................	421	414	413	413	403
Hospitals Rural	120	121	122	122	140
Control					
State and Local Government................	132	133	135	135	141
Not for Profit	321	318	319	319	315
Investor owned	88	84	81	81	87
Physician Models					
Independent Practice Association	65	79	83	78	88
Group Practice without Walls................	21	24	24	24	22
Open Physician-Hospital Organization	16	22	20	19	22
Closed Physician-Hospital Organization	11	11	10	11	10
Management Service Organization	63	47	48	47	44
Integrated Salary Model.....................	112	115	113	110	107
Equity Model	6	6	7	5	2
Foundation................................	91	59	60	55	52
Insurance Products					
Health Maintenance Organization	66	64	55	64	64
Preferred Provider Organization..............	38	62	56	54	48
Indemnity Fee for Service	10	21	15	14	15
Managed Care Contracts					
Health Maintenance Organization	258	228	231	231	226
Preferred Provider Organization..............	268	252	259	270	263
Affiliations					
Hospitals in a System......................	339	336	330	324	328
Hospitals in a Network	110	121	110	111	107
Hospitals in a Group Purchasing Organization..	295	315	310	352	333

TABLE 5

U.S. CENSUS DIVISION 9: PACIFIC

U.S. Registered Community Hospitals
(Nonfederal, short-term general and other special hospitals)

Utilization, Personnel, Revenue and Expenses, Community Health Indicators 2008–2012

	2012	2011	2010	2009	2008
TOTAL FACILITY (Includes Hospital and Nursing Home Units)					
Utilization - Inpatient					
Beds	94,194	92,601	93,088	91,046	92,389
Admissions	4,403,646	4,471,783	4,501,591	4,514,874	4,557,658
Inpatient Days	22,168,393	22,232,780	22,640,225	22,791,572	23,454,079
Average Length of Stay	5.0	5.0	5.0	5.0	5.1
Inpatient Surgeries	1,195,847	1,192,531	1,241,853	1,252,243	1,260,249
Births	621,481	629,315	632,032	645,081	676,180
Utilization - Outpatient					
Emergency Outpatient Visits	16,342,076	15,480,506	15,128,224	15,055,923	14,473,721
Other Outpatient Visits	62,140,989	62,797,927	61,596,946	57,529,665	58,052,120
Total Outpatient Visits	78,483,065	78,278,433	76,725,170	72,585,588	72,525,841
Outpatient Surgeries	1,808,384	1,846,317	1,835,447	1,833,478	1,886,717
Personnel					
Full Time RNs	141,776	136,326	134,508	130,132	126,718
Full Time LPNs	7,614	7,594	8,301	8,642	9,011
Part Time RNs	77,206	72,866	71,284	70,581	72,526
Part Time LPNs	3,279	3,211	3,453	3,839	4,274
Total Full Time	508,241	493,680	487,053	477,901	477,563
Total Part Time	210,546	199,030	193,703	191,891	201,710
Revenue - Inpatient					
Gross Inpatient Revenue	$236,834,787,719	$219,593,141,460	$211,874,242,966	$193,636,178,785	$181,416,247,444
Revenue - Outpatient					
Gross Outpatient Revenue	$147,772,531,581	$138,274,865,366	$124,558,809,024	$109,199,995,898	$98,528,236,224
Revenue and Expenses - Totals					
(Includes Inpatient and Outpatient)					
Total Gross Revenue	$384,607,319,300	$357,868,006,826	$336,433,051,990	$302,836,174,683	$279,944,483,668
Deductions from Revenue	271,710,809,903	253,322,749,612	239,252,607,338	212,570,073,192	194,777,375,687
Net Patient Revenue	112,896,509,397	104,545,257,214	97,180,444,652	90,266,101,491	85,167,107,981
Other Operating Revenue	6,642,799,134	5,990,186,797	6,027,711,222	5,590,026,520	5,041,401,269
Other Nonoperating Revenue	1,979,204,632	2,259,696,906	1,866,228,283	1,090,362,535	23,014,193
Total Net Revenue	121,518,513,163	112,795,140,917	105,074,384,157	96,946,490,546	90,231,523,443
Total Expenses	113,537,965,473	105,001,431,937	98,998,692,542	93,038,063,591	88,037,635,750
HOSPITAL UNIT (Excludes Separate Nursing Home Units)					
Utilization - Inpatient					
Beds	88,926	88,926	88,925	86,836	87,253
Admissions	4,378,581	4,450,403	4,478,851	4,489,343	4,527,176
Inpatient Days	20,541,376	21,093,072	21,344,190	21,533,040	21,897,397
Average Length of Stay	4.7	4.7	4.8	4.8	4.8
Personnel					
Total Full Time	503,839	490,810	483,548	473,892	473,367
Total Part Time	208,555	197,584	192,111	189,876	199,475
Revenue and Expenses - Totals					
(Includes Inpatient and Outpatient)					
Total Net Revenue	$120,898,001,137	$112,319,758,152	$104,531,350,858	$96,415,616,765	$89,624,997,242
Total Expenses	112,990,603,410	104,639,691,795	98,595,961,703	92,611,409,620	87,584,896,173
COMMUNITY HEALTH INDICATORS PER 1000 POPULATION					
Total Population (in thousands)	50,962	50,491	49,877	49,445	48,905
Inpatient					
Beds	1.8	1.8	1.9	1.8	1.9
Admissions	86.4	88.6	90.3	91.3	93.2
Inpatient Days	435.0	440.3	453.9	460.9	479.6
Inpatient Surgeries	23.5	23.6	24.9	25.3	25.8
Births	12.2	12.5	12.7	13.0	13.8
Outpatient					
Emergency Outpatient Visits	320.7	306.6	303.3	304.5	296.0
Other Outpatient Visits	1,219.4	1,243.7	1,235.0	1,163.5	1,187.0
Total Outpatient Visits	1,540.0	1,550.3	1,538.3	1,468.0	1,483.0
Outpatient Surgeries	35.5	36.6	36.8	37.1	38.6
Expense per Capita (per person)	$2,227.9	$2,079.6	$1,984.8	$1,881.6	$1,800.2

U.S. Census Divisions

TABLE 6

Overview 2008–2012

	2012	2011	2010	2009	2008
Total Community Hospitals in Alabama	97	102	105	108	109
Bed Size Category					
6-24	7	9	7	7	8
25-49	23	23	27	27	25
50-99	21	21	22	24	27
100-199	23	24	28	28	25
200-299	10	12	9	9	11
300-399	6	6	6	7	7
400-499	2	3	3	3	3
500 + ...	5	4	3	3	3
Location					
Hospitals Urban	52	57	58	60	58
Hospitals Rural	45	45	47	48	51
Control					
State and Local Government	38	39	40	42	42
Not for Profit	24	24	24	26	27
Investor owned	35	39	41	40	40
Physician Models					
Independent Practice Association	3	4	7	8	8
Group Practice without Walls	0	0	1	2	2
Open Physician-Hospital Organization	6	7	7	3	3
Closed Physician-Hospital Organization	4	4	0	1	2
Management Service Organization	11	10	7	5	10
Integrated Salary Model	13	13	18	16	14
Equity Model	0	0	0	0	0
Foundation	4	5	7	5	5
Insurance Products					
Health Maintenance Organization	2	3	7	10	13
Preferred Provider Organization	9	12	8	9	10
Indemnity Fee for Service	0	1	1	1	3
Managed Care Contracts					
Health Maintenance Organization	34	35	37	36	35
Preferred Provider Organization	43	44	51	49	49
Affiliations					
Hospitals in a System	61	61	64	67	68
Hospitals in a Network	8	8	9	11	12
Hospitals in a Group Purchasing Organization . .	50	53	56	70	68

States

Table 6

ALABAMA

U.S. Registered Community Hospitals
(Nonfederal, short-term general and other special hospitals)

Utilization, Personnel, Revenue and Expenses, Community Health Indicators 2008–2012

	2012	2011	2010	2009	2008
TOTAL FACILITY (Includes Hospital and Nursing Home Units)					
Utilization - Inpatient					
Beds	14,983	15,387	15,086	15,290	15,250
Admissions	650,116	625,425	642,309	665,788	687,446
Inpatient Days	3,235,410	3,259,740	3,336,285	3,459,946	3,524,687
Average Length of Stay	5.0	5.2	5.2	5.2	5.1
Inpatient Surgeries	216,437	225,340	197,605	203,945	202,900
Births	54,169	56,038	58,287	62,819	62,436
Utilization - Outpatient					
Emergency Outpatient Visits	2,349,349	2,301,480	2,304,682	2,286,343	2,271,755
Other Outpatient Visits	5,787,211	6,428,214	6,496,039	6,905,010	6,746,766
Total Outpatient Visits	8,136,560	8,729,694	8,800,721	9,191,353	9,018,521
Outpatient Surgeries	416,822	410,937	372,359	380,226	364,648
Personnel					
Full Time RNs	18,971	19,179	19,033	18,906	17,930
Full Time LPNs	1,284	1,334	1,533	1,587	1,795
Part Time RNs	6,450	6,030	6,521	6,495	6,708
Part Time LPNs	423	407	544	584	755
Total Full Time	63,711	63,640	63,565	64,706	64,821
Total Part Time	17,393	16,258	17,485	17,181	18,103
Revenue - Inpatient					
Gross Inpatient Revenue	$21,905,302,437	$20,721,285,712	$20,382,077,101	$19,226,829,885	$18,436,910,861
Revenue - Outpatient					
Gross Outpatient Revenue	$18,451,159,730	$16,116,899,016	$15,107,168,189	$13,746,107,465	$11,949,849,370
Revenue and Expenses - Totals					
(Includes Inpatient and Outpatient)					
Total Gross Revenue	$40,356,462,167	$36,838,184,728	$35,489,245,290	$32,972,937,350	$30,386,760,231
Deductions from Revenue	30,849,527,537	28,275,034,462	26,885,327,851	24,887,051,667	22,550,588,921
Net Patient Revenue	9,506,934,630	8,563,150,266	8,603,917,439	8,085,885,683	7,836,171,310
Other Operating Revenue	530,660,281	419,270,245	398,593,891	476,168,844	499,586,864
Other Nonoperating Revenue	117,222,122	124,960,404	180,032,402	209,998,612	-56,405,573
Total Net Revenue	10,154,817,033	9,107,380,915	9,182,543,732	8,772,053,139	8,279,352,601
Total Expenses	9,009,790,217	8,285,877,588	8,334,444,846	8,276,604,492	8,288,702,647
HOSPITAL UNIT (Excludes Separate Nursing Home Units)					
Utilization - Inpatient					
Beds	14,684	14,953	14,569	14,861	14,824
Admissions	649,138	624,134	641,118	664,534	686,256
Inpatient Days	3,135,159	3,142,919	3,188,617	3,314,802	3,377,540
Average Length of Stay	4.8	5.0	5.0	5.0	4.9
Personnel					
Total Full Time	63,419	63,302	63,159	64,371	64,502
Total Part Time	17,324	16,224	17,373	17,120	18,073
Revenue and Expenses - Totals					
(Includes Inpatient and Outpatient)					
Total Net Revenue	$10,139,471,861	$9,085,772,314	$9,160,325,136	$8,749,089,004	$8,258,544,123
Total Expenses	8,994,674,312	8,272,890,643	8,308,793,595	8,249,699,883	8,268,150,713
COMMUNITY HEALTH INDICATORS PER 1000 POPULATION					
Total Population (in thousands)	4,822	4,803	4,730	4,709	4,677
Inpatient					
Beds	3.1	3.2	3.2	3.2	3.3
Admissions	134.8	130.2	135.8	141.4	147.0
Inpatient Days	671.0	678.7	705.4	734.8	753.5
Inpatient Surgeries	44.9	46.9	41.8	43.3	43.4
Births	11.2	11.7	12.3	13.3	13.3
Outpatient					
Emergency Outpatient Visits	487.2	479.2	487.3	485.6	485.7
Other Outpatient Visits	1,200.2	1,338.4	1,373.5	1,466.4	1,442.4
Total Outpatient Visits	1,687.4	1,817.6	1,860.8	1,952.0	1,928.1
Outpatient Surgeries	86.4	85.6	78.7	80.7	78.0
Expense per Capita (per person)	$1,868.5	$1,725.2	$1,762.2	$1,757.7	$1,772.1

States

TABLE 6

ALASKA

U.S. Registered Community Hospitals
(Nonfederal, short-term general and other special hospitals)

Overview 2008–2012

	2012	2011	2010	2009	2008
Total Community Hospitals in Alaska.........	23	23	22	22	22
Bed Size Category					
6-24	7	7	6	6	6
25-49	8	7	7	8	7
50-99	3	4	4	3	4
100-199	3	3	3	3	3
200-299	1	1	1	1	1
300-399	1	1	1	1	1
400-499	0	0	0	0	0
500 + ...	0	0	0	0	0
Location					
Hospitals Urban........................	6	6	5	5	3
Hospitals Rural	17	17	17	17	19
Control					
State and Local Government...............	7	7	7	6	7
Not for Profit............................	14	14	13	14	13
Investor owned	2	2	2	2	2
Physician Models					
Independent Practice Association	1	1	1	0	0
Group Practice without Walls................	0	0	0	0	0
Open Physician-Hospital Organization	2	2	2	2	2
Closed Physician-Hospital Organization	1	1	1	1	0
Management Service Organization	0	0	0	1	0
Integrated Salary Model....................	3	4	4	3	4
Equity Model	0	0	0	0	0
Foundation..............................	0	0	0	0	0
Insurance Products					
Health Maintenance Organization	0	0	0	0	0
Preferred Provider Organization..............	1	4	1	2	2
Indemnity Fee for Service	0	1	0	0	1
Managed Care Contracts					
Health Maintenance Organization	0	1	0	0	0
Preferred Provider Organization..............	5	7	5	7	8
Affiliations					
Hospitals in a System......................	8	9	9	8	8
Hospitals in a Network	2	1	3	5	3
Hospitals in a Group Purchasing Organization..	6	8	8	12	11

TABLE 6

ALASKA

U.S. Registered Community Hospitals
(Nonfederal, short-term general and other special hospitals)

Utilization, Personnel, Revenue and Expenses, Community Health Indicators 2008–2012

	2012	2011	2010	2009	2008
TOTAL FACILITY (Includes Hospital and Nursing Home Units)					
Utilization - Inpatient					
Beds............................	1,549	1,556	1,543	1,532	1,553
Admissions......................	56,131	54,715	57,005	57,227	58,204
Inpatient Days	341,987	340,060	342,960	338,547	346,837
Average Length of Stay............	6.1	6.2	6.0	5.9	6.0
Inpatient Surgeries...............	15,613	16,420	17,999	20,294	20,522
Births..........................	8,522	9,196	8,919	9,358	8,882
Utilization - Outpatient					
Emergency Outpatient Visits........	290,711	315,181	296,573	296,524	328,164
Other Outpatient Visits............	1,161,515	1,450,455	1,486,369	1,470,894	1,365,178
Total Outpatient Visits	1,452,226	1,765,636	1,782,942	1,767,418	1,693,342
Outpatient Surgeries	40,892	43,714	47,417	50,469	43,567
Personnel					
Full Time RNs	2,209	2,456	2,238	2,348	2,090
Full Time LPNs	145	177	178	163	163
Part Time RNs...................	893	820	906	816	848
Part Time LPNs..................	37	35	28	27	48
Total Full Time...................	8,723	10,064	9,608	9,421	8,809
Total Part Time	2,467	2,177	2,584	2,125	2,435
Revenue - Inpatient					
Gross Inpatient Revenue...........	$2,628,751,616	$2,510,713,374	$2,340,223,028	$1,920,419,380	$2,045,394,009
Revenue - Outpatient					
Gross Outpatient Revenue	$2,524,384,455	$2,540,116,099	$2,263,620,240	$1,956,296,065	$1,623,182,947
Revenue and Expenses - Totals					
(Includes Inpatient and Outpatient)					
Total Gross Revenue..............	$5,153,136,071	$5,050,829,473	$4,603,843,268	$3,876,715,445	$3,668,576,956
Deductions from Revenue..........	3,134,854,935	3,205,558,785	2,836,623,088	2,198,399,661	2,054,343,109
Net Patient Revenue	2,018,281,136	1,845,270,688	1,767,220,180	1,678,315,784	1,614,233,847
Other Operating Revenue	100,656,142	216,227,533	146,570,128	65,784,620	66,832,290
Other Nonoperating Revenue	33,745,177	19,647,439	21,027,327	18,948,295	16,635,452
Total Net Revenue................	2,152,682,455	2,081,145,660	1,934,817,635	1,763,048,699	1,697,701,589
Total Expenses...................	1,765,708,752	1,747,385,857	1,590,214,704	1,753,736,940	1,570,873,845
HOSPITAL UNIT (Excludes Separate Nursing Home Units)					
Utilization - Inpatient					
Beds............................	1,293	1,346	1,334	1,300	1,381
Admissions......................	55,667	54,498	56,797	56,918	58,081
Inpatient Days	257,797	270,835	275,518	263,515	293,939
Average Length of Stay............	4.6	5.0	4.9	4.6	5.1
Personnel					
Total Full Time...................	8,486	9,855	9,428	9,174	8,712
Total Part Time	2,371	2,080	2,443	1,990	2,350
Revenue and Expenses - Totals					
(Includes Inpatient and Outpatient)					
Total Net Revenue................	$2,105,900,495	$2,048,187,683	$1,900,578,038	$1,724,497,539	$1,678,203,874
Total Expenses...................	1,730,733,295	1,720,343,546	1,564,596,210	1,726,965,040	1,560,050,288
COMMUNITY HEALTH INDICATORS PER 1000 POPULATION					
Total Population (in thousands)	731	723	709	698	688
Inpatient					
Beds............................	2.1	2.2	2.2	2.2	2.3
Admissions......................	76.7	75.7	80.4	81.9	84.6
Inpatient Days	467.5	470.5	483.8	484.7	504.0
Inpatient Surgeries...............	21.3	22.7	25.4	29.1	29.8
Births..........................	11.7	12.7	12.6	13.4	12.9
Outpatient					
Emergency Outpatient Visits........	397.4	436.1	418.4	424.5	476.9
Other Outpatient Visits............	1,588.0	2,006.9	2,096.8	2,105.9	1,983.9
Total Outpatient Visits	1,985.4	2,443.0	2,515.2	2,530.4	2,460.8
Outpatient Surgeries	55.9	60.5	66.9	72.3	63.3
Expense per Capita (per person).....	$2,414.0	$2,417.8	$2,243.3	$2,510.8	$2,282.8

States

TABLE **6**

ARIZONA

U.S. Registered Community Hospitals
(Nonfederal, short-term general and other special hospitals)

Overview 2008–2012

	2012	2011	2010	2009	2008
Total Community Hospitals in Arizona	72	70	73	72	71
Bed Size Category					
6-24	5	5	5	4	4
25-49	12	12	10	10	10
50-99	15	14	18	18	18
100-199	13	12	13	11	12
200-299	10	11	11	12	11
300-399	6	4	5	8	7
400-499	5	7	6	4	4
500 + ...	6	5	5	5	5
Location					
Hospitals Urban.	58	56	58	58	54
Hospitals Rural	14	14	15	14	17
Control					
State and Local Government.	4	4	5	7	4
Not for Profit	46	47	46	43	44
Investor owned	22	19	22	22	23
Physician Models					
Independent Practice Association	9	7	8	9	10
Group Practice without Walls.	3	3	1	1	2
Open Physician-Hospital Organization	5	5	6	6	5
Closed Physician-Hospital Organization	3	2	3	4	4
Management Service Organization	7	9	8	4	3
Integrated Salary Model	16	19	15	16	12
Equity Model	0	0	0	0	0
Foundation.	1	2	2	2	3
Insurance Products					
Health Maintenance Organization	12	10	9	8	10
Preferred Provider Organization.	4	8	7	5	3
Indemnity Fee for Service	0	5	5	4	3
Managed Care Contracts					
Health Maintenance Organization	26	30	32	32	33
Preferred Provider Organization.	27	31	31	33	31
Affiliations					
Hospitals in a System.	49	46	48	49	48
Hospitals in a Network	17	17	19	14	14
Hospitals in a Group Purchasing Organization. .	37	40	45	41	43

States

TABLE 6

ARIZONA

U.S. Registered Community Hospitals
(Nonfederal, short-term general and other special hospitals)

Utilization, Personnel, Revenue and Expenses, Community Health Indicators 2008–2012

	2012	2011	2010	2009	2008
TOTAL FACILITY (Includes Hospital and Nursing Home Units)					
Utilization - Inpatient					
Beds	13,527	13,352	13,385	13,455	13,138
Admissions	674,808	700,855	711,901	705,371	716,136
Inpatient Days	2,977,605	3,106,331	3,160,244	3,203,551	3,235,063
Average Length of Stay	4.4	4.4	4.4	4.5	4.5
Inpatient Surgeries	216,991	239,277	247,886	249,404	225,735
Births	73,033	74,547	80,960	88,943	96,193
Utilization - Outpatient					
Emergency Outpatient Visits	2,309,621	2,189,955	2,240,946	2,137,007	2,172,149
Other Outpatient Visits	6,427,396	6,362,148	5,886,520	4,965,037	5,542,202
Total Outpatient Visits	8,737,017	8,552,103	8,127,466	7,102,044	7,714,351
Outpatient Surgeries	245,168	250,415	257,530	264,098	254,546
Personnel					
Full Time RNs	20,977	20,524	22,440	21,733	20,898
Full Time LPNs	590	649	807	1,428	957
Part Time RNs	6,167	5,929	5,419	6,207	6,462
Part Time LPNs	150	152	135	217	251
Total Full Time	66,940	67,996	71,092	68,218	65,568
Total Part Time	16,020	15,965	14,521	16,938	18,272
Revenue - Inpatient					
Gross Inpatient Revenue	$27,609,357,979	$26,796,619,071	$26,745,329,251	$25,403,304,711	$23,681,284,471
Revenue - Outpatient					
Gross Outpatient Revenue	$18,858,344,930	$16,955,905,216	$15,678,580,294	$14,088,508,773	$12,097,995,360
Revenue and Expenses - Totals					
(Includes Inpatient and Outpatient)					
Total Gross Revenue	$46,467,702,909	$43,752,524,287	$42,423,909,545	$39,491,813,484	$35,779,279,831
Deductions from Revenue	34,058,007,365	32,157,030,582	30,579,491,050	28,395,520,445	25,364,507,854
Net Patient Revenue	12,409,695,544	11,595,493,705	11,844,418,495	11,096,293,039	10,414,771,977
Other Operating Revenue	475,139,314	515,033,121	504,651,779	405,351,865	363,332,345
Other Nonoperating Revenue	86,412,468	82,344,006	65,552,870	146,545,191	-141,211,261
Total Net Revenue	12,971,247,326	12,192,870,832	12,414,623,144	11,648,190,095	10,636,893,061
Total Expenses	12,112,683,858	11,520,903,768	11,271,574,937	10,838,466,876	10,461,227,615
HOSPITAL UNIT (Excludes Separate Nursing Home Units)					
Utilization - Inpatient					
Beds	13,401	13,226	13,265	13,311	12,954
Admissions	672,834	698,689	709,606	703,074	713,487
Inpatient Days	2,944,802	3,063,786	3,120,611	3,154,344	3,189,855
Average Length of Stay	4.4	4.4	4.4	4.5	4.5
Personnel					
Total Full Time	66,850	67,911	70,791	68,133	63,940
Total Part Time	16,010	15,936	14,477	16,909	17,993
Revenue and Expenses - Totals					
(Includes Inpatient and Outpatient)					
Total Net Revenue	$12,943,620,235	$12,154,799,416	$12,377,572,952	$11,622,780,339	$10,627,564,240
Total Expenses	12,098,532,372	11,504,061,948	11,256,388,031	10,821,151,582	10,447,130,955
COMMUNITY HEALTH INDICATORS PER 1000 POPULATION					
Total Population (in thousands)	6,553	6,483	6,677	6,596	6,499
Inpatient					
Beds	2.1	2.1	2.0	2.0	2.0
Admissions	103.0	108.1	106.6	106.9	110.2
Inpatient Days	454.4	479.2	473.3	485.7	497.7
Inpatient Surgeries	33.1	36.9	37.1	37.8	34.7
Births	11.1	11.5	12.1	13.5	14.8
Outpatient					
Emergency Outpatient Visits	352.4	337.8	335.6	324.0	334.2
Other Outpatient Visits	980.8	981.4	881.7	752.8	852.7
Total Outpatient Visits	1,333.2	1,319.3	1,217.3	1,076.8	1,186.9
Outpatient Surgeries	37.4	38.6	38.6	40.0	39.2
Expense per Capita (per person)	$1,848.3	$1,777.2	$1,688.2	$1,643.2	$1,609.6

TABLE 6

ARKANSAS

U.S. Registered Community Hospitals
(Nonfederal, short-term general and other special hospitals)

Overview 2008–2012

	2012	2011	2010	2009	2008
Total Community Hospitals in Arkansas.......	**83**	**84**	**85**	**86**	**86**
Bed Size Category					
6-24	5	5	6	7	7
25-49	32	33	32	31	30
50-99	14	14	16	18	18
100-199	16	18	18	17	18
200-299	7	5	6	5	6
300-399	6	6	4	5	5
400-499	2	2	2	2	0
500 + ...	1	1	1	1	2
Location					
Hospitals Urban.......................	35	36	37	37	33
Hospitals Rural	48	48	48	49	53
Control					
State and Local Government................	11	11	14	15	13
Not for Profit	49	50	45	45	46
Investor owned	23	23	26	26	27
Physician Models					
Independent Practice Association	6	9	16	16	17
Group Practice without Walls...............	5	5	6	6	6
Open Physician-Hospital Organization	23	24	25	28	28
Closed Physician-Hospital Organization	4	5	6	6	4
Management Service Organization	9	10	10	10	10
Integrated Salary Model....................	20	18	21	20	18
Equity Model	1	0	1	2	2
Foundation..............................	5	6	7	8	11
Insurance Products					
Health Maintenance Organization	14	14	14	14	15
Preferred Provider Organization..............	7	10	14	14	13
Indemnity Fee for Service	1	2	4	3	4
Managed Care Contracts					
Health Maintenance Organization	40	46	46	50	47
Preferred Provider Organization..............	53	64	62	66	65
Affiliations					
Hospitals in a System.....................	46	44	46	47	46
Hospitals in a Network....................	22	26	26	28	29
Hospitals in a Group Purchasing Organization..	61	73	67	78	80

TABLE 6

ARKANSAS

U.S. Registered Community Hospitals
(Nonfederal, short-term general and other special hospitals)

Utilization, Personnel, Revenue and Expenses, Community Health Indicators 2008–2012

	2012	2011	2010	2009	2008
TOTAL FACILITY (Includes Hospital and Nursing Home Units)					
Utilization - Inpatient					
Beds	9,417	9,425	9,451	9,565	9,686
Admissions	352,752	363,516	370,401	380,478	376,158
Inpatient Days	1,845,443	1,882,912	1,908,843	1,957,556	1,989,969
Average Length of Stay	5.2	5.2	5.2	5.1	5.3
Inpatient Surgeries	101,156	102,964	104,912	101,681	102,681
Births	35,421	36,809	36,913	38,556	39,013
Utilization - Outpatient					
Emergency Outpatient Visits	1,382,183	1,391,537	1,376,649	1,355,032	1,301,330
Other Outpatient Visits	3,743,252	3,419,087	3,645,562	3,692,949	3,671,422
Total Outpatient Visits	5,125,435	4,810,624	5,022,211	5,047,981	4,972,752
Outpatient Surgeries	174,095	160,223	155,784	143,094	136,565
Personnel					
Full Time RNs	11,964	11,429	11,059	10,620	9,700
Full Time LPNs	1,587	1,897	1,890	2,080	2,455
Part Time RNs	3,576	3,700	4,068	4,030	3,596
Part Time LPNs	455	606	663	809	824
Total Full Time	40,286	39,108	38,553	38,571	38,483
Total Part Time	10,397	10,746	11,921	11,981	11,549
Revenue - Inpatient					
Gross Inpatient Revenue	$9,975,710,168	$9,587,181,461	$9,211,448,957	$8,800,185,973	$8,250,771,568
Revenue - Outpatient					
Gross Outpatient Revenue	$8,663,764,850	$7,800,635,792	$7,084,460,315	$6,421,124,915	$5,568,220,057
Revenue and Expenses - Totals					
(Includes Inpatient and Outpatient)					
Total Gross Revenue	$18,639,475,018	$17,387,817,253	$16,295,909,272	$15,221,310,888	$13,818,991,625
Deductions from Revenue	12,820,230,814	12,106,848,283	11,007,346,255	10,164,398,525	9,011,385,599
Net Patient Revenue	5,819,244,204	5,280,968,970	5,288,563,017	5,056,912,363	4,807,606,026
Other Operating Revenue	256,162,838	220,871,438	221,189,649	193,955,665	169,341,834
Other Nonoperating Revenue	85,908,563	52,395,249	69,605,801	73,678,302	31,674,701
Total Net Revenue	6,161,315,605	5,554,235,657	5,579,358,467	5,324,546,330	5,008,622,561
Total Expenses	5,759,240,612	5,236,539,234	5,246,234,974	5,161,176,256	4,921,858,438
HOSPITAL UNIT (Excludes Separate Nursing Home Units)					
Utilization - Inpatient					
Beds	9,200	9,041	9,228	9,132	9,250
Admissions	351,712	362,005	368,895	378,746	374,159
Inpatient Days	1,774,671	1,757,602	1,830,615	1,824,645	1,854,685
Average Length of Stay	5.0	4.9	5.0	4.8	5.0
Personnel					
Total Full Time	40,123	38,835	38,362	38,050	38,028
Total Part Time	10,347	10,639	11,881	11,767	11,398
Revenue and Expenses - Totals					
(Includes Inpatient and Outpatient)					
Total Net Revenue	$6,148,169,295	$5,526,988,517	$5,558,657,844	$5,301,946,109	$4,986,288,187
Total Expenses	5,749,516,565	5,219,018,613	5,234,362,445	5,141,870,990	4,902,909,300
COMMUNITY HEALTH INDICATORS PER 1000 POPULATION					
Total Population (in thousands)	2,949	2,938	2,910	2,889	2,868
Inpatient					
Beds	3.2	3.2	3.2	3.3	3.4
Admissions	119.6	123.7	127.3	131.7	131.2
Inpatient Days	625.8	640.9	655.9	677.5	693.9
Inpatient Surgeries	34.3	35.0	36.0	35.2	35.8
Births	12.0	12.5	12.7	13.3	13.6
Outpatient					
Emergency Outpatient Visits	468.7	473.6	473.0	469.0	453.8
Other Outpatient Visits	1,269.3	1,163.8	1,252.7	1,278.1	1,280.2
Total Outpatient Visits	1,737.9	1,637.4	1,725.7	1,747.0	1,734.0
Outpatient Surgeries	59.0	54.5	53.5	49.5	47.6
Expense per Capita (per person)	$1,952.9	$1,782.4	$1,802.7	$1,786.2	$1,716.3

States

TABLE **6**

CALIFORNIA

U.S. Registered Community Hospitals
(Nonfederal, short-term general and other special hospitals)

Overview 2008–2012

	2012	2011	2010	2009	2008
Total Community Hospitals in California	**349**	**345**	**343**	**343**	**352**
Bed Size Category					
6-24	11	13	13	13	14
25-49	44	39	38	37	36
50-99	40	43	42	42	50
100-199	105	101	104	106	107
200-299	67	65	61	64	66
300-399	44	47	47	50	44
400-499	25	23	24	20	22
500 + ...	13	14	14	11	13
Location					
Hospitals Urban.........................	318	314	312	313	315
Hospitals Rural	31	31	31	30	37
Control					
State and Local Government................	66	69	69	69	71
Not for Profit	206	202	202	202	202
Investor owned	77	74	72	72	79
Physician Models					
Independent Practice Association	51	64	66	62	72
Group Practice without Walls...............	10	11	11	12	12
Open Physician-Hospital Organization	4	6	5	5	6
Closed Physician-Hospital Organization	4	5	6	7	7
Management Service Organization	46	30	28	26	27
Integrated Salary Model....................	20	24	24	25	30
Equity Model	2	3	3	0	1
Foundation...............................	83	51	50	40	39
Insurance Products					
Health Maintenance Organization	47	40	35	42	46
Preferred Provider Organization..............	18	24	22	22	19
Indemnity Fee for Service	8	16	11	9	10
Managed Care Contracts					
Health Maintenance Organization	168	147	156	157	154
Preferred Provider Organization..............	160	146	157	159	158
Affiliations					
Hospitals in a System......................	231	230	226	225	231
Hospitals in a Network.....................	60	70	59	59	59
Hospitals in a Group Purchasing Organization..	174	185	182	210	206

TABLE 6

CALIFORNIA

U.S. Registered Community Hospitals
(Nonfederal, short-term general and other special hospitals)

Utilization, Personnel, Revenue and Expenses, Community Health Indicators 2008–2012

	2012	2011	2010	2009	2008
TOTAL FACILITY (Includes Hospital and Nursing Home Units)					
Utilization - Inpatient					
Beds	71,004	70,008	70,440	68,745	69,587
Admissions	3,304,230	3,393,166	3,423,820	3,433,319	3,460,688
Inpatient Days	16,919,921	17,090,593	17,443,427	17,582,055	18,044,888
Average Length of Stay	5.1	5.0	5.1	5.1	5.2
Inpatient Surgeries	867,839	858,118	907,650	899,439	904,722
Births	482,313	488,863	493,712	500,085	526,946
Utilization - Outpatient					
Emergency Outpatient Visits	11,859,123	11,073,272	10,945,256	10,554,310	10,068,613
Other Outpatient Visits	40,365,732	41,601,911	40,784,007	37,700,623	38,808,536
Total Outpatient Visits	52,224,855	52,675,183	51,729,263	48,254,933	48,877,149
Outpatient Surgeries	1,249,704	1,273,633	1,261,889	1,248,053	1,309,864
Personnel					
Full Time RNs	106,195	103,753	103,010	98,905	98,152
Full Time LPNs	6,108	6,227	6,817	7,145	7,531
Part Time RNs	55,861	50,209	48,553	48,356	49,205
Part Time LPNs	2,574	2,420	2,625	2,900	3,281
Total Full Time	370,238	365,577	358,559	353,440	356,834
Total Part Time	147,910	134,162	129,897	130,048	134,602
Revenue - Inpatient					
Gross Inpatient Revenue	$194,710,241,465	$183,080,834,445	$176,241,777,468	$160,482,118,425	$150,337,219,745
Revenue - Outpatient					
Gross Outpatient Revenue	$110,355,399,582	$105,412,786,768	$93,211,672,697	$81,537,158,136	$74,357,000,289
Revenue and Expenses - Totals					
(Includes Inpatient and Outpatient)					
Total Gross Revenue	$305,065,641,047	$288,493,621,213	$269,453,450,165	$242,019,276,561	$224,694,220,034
Deductions from Revenue	222,641,523,180	211,224,646,235	198,665,132,469	176,891,970,909	162,955,378,616
Net Patient Revenue	82,424,117,867	77,268,974,978	70,788,317,696	65,127,305,652	61,738,841,418
Other Operating Revenue	4,935,487,999	4,404,016,212	4,549,376,153	4,239,820,033	3,808,102,197
Other Nonoperating Revenue	1,579,522,303	1,779,948,031	1,405,680,400	900,886,474	139,168,261
Total Net Revenue	88,939,128,169	83,452,939,221	76,743,374,249	70,268,012,159	65,686,111,876
Total Expenses	83,074,054,310	77,265,358,490	72,279,546,582	67,532,620,386	64,441,142,995
HOSPITAL UNIT (Excludes Separate Nursing Home Units)					
Utilization - Inpatient					
Beds	66,826	67,306	67,288	65,699	65,773
Admissions	3,281,803	3,374,467	3,404,159	3,411,915	3,435,099
Inpatient Days	15,596,063	16,266,645	16,480,612	16,688,765	16,911,379
Average Length of Stay	4.8	4.8	4.8	4.9	4.9
Personnel					
Total Full Time	366,919	363,402	355,707	350,441	353,564
Total Part Time	146,283	133,098	128,661	128,548	132,907
Revenue and Expenses - Totals					
(Includes Inpatient and Outpatient)					
Total Net Revenue	$88,462,119,698	$83,072,725,098	$76,308,938,222	$69,852,937,155	$65,179,794,371
Total Expenses	82,671,685,266	77,001,174,879	71,979,685,381	67,204,581,934	64,094,102,118
COMMUNITY HEALTH INDICATORS PER 1000 POPULATION					
Total Population (in thousands)	38,041	37,692	37,267	36,962	36,580
Inpatient					
Beds	1.9	1.9	1.9	1.9	1.9
Admissions	86.9	90.0	91.9	92.9	94.6
Inpatient Days	444.8	453.4	468.1	475.7	493.3
Inpatient Surgeries	22.8	22.8	24.4	24.3	24.7
Births	12.7	13.0	13.2	13.5	14.4
Outpatient					
Emergency Outpatient Visits	311.7	293.8	293.7	285.5	275.2
Other Outpatient Visits	1,061.1	1,103.7	1,094.4	1,020.0	1,060.9
Total Outpatient Visits	1,372.8	1,397.5	1,388.1	1,305.5	1,336.2
Outpatient Surgeries	32.9	33.8	33.9	33.8	35.8
Expense per Capita (per person)	$2,183.8	$2,049.9	$1,939.5	$1,827.1	$1,761.6

States

TABLE **6**

COLORADO

U.S. Registered Community Hospitals
(Nonfederal, short-term general and other special hospitals)

Overview 2008–2012

	2012	2011	2010	2009	2008
Total Community Hospitals in Colorado.......	82	82	80	81	78
Bed Size Category					
6-24	12	11	11	13	10
25-49	22	23	21	19	21
50-99	17	17	16	18	16
100-199	12	12	14	11	13
200-299	7	7	6	10	9
300-399	6	8	8	5	4
400-499	6	3	2	3	3
500 + ...	0	1	2	2	2
Location					
Hospitals Urban..........................	44	44	43	43	40
Hospitals Rural	38	38	37	38	38
Control					
State and Local Government................	26	27	27	28	28
Not for Profit	39	38	37	37	37
Investor owned	17	17	16	16	13
Physician Models					
Independent Practice Association	10	11	10	9	9
Group Practice without Walls................	3	3	2	1	1
Open Physician-Hospital Organization	11	13	13	12	12
Closed Physician-Hospital Organization	3	4	3	3	2
Management Service Organization	4	4	4	3	3
Integrated Salary Model....................	40	37	34	33	32
Equity Model	1	2	2	1	2
Foundation..............................	3	2	4	1	2
Insurance Products					
Health Maintenance Organization	9	9	10	11	9
Preferred Provider Organization..............	3	9	10	10	9
Indemnity Fee for Service	1	1	2	3	3
Managed Care Contracts					
Health Maintenance Organization	44	40	46	47	48
Preferred Provider Organization..............	51	45	52	53	54
Affiliations					
Hospitals in a System.....................	47	46	46	46	44
Hospitals in a Network	19	27	27	24	25
Hospitals in a Group Purchasing Organization..	54	63	60	58	57

TABLE 6

COLORADO

U.S. Registered Community Hospitals
(Nonfederal, short-term general and other special hospitals)

Utilization, Personnel, Revenue and Expenses, Community Health Indicators 2008–2012

	2012	2011	2010	2009	2008
TOTAL FACILITY (Includes Hospital and Nursing Home Units)					
Utilization - Inpatient					
Beds	10,244	10,167	10,208	10,364	10,053
Admissions	444,430	432,887	449,369	445,291	442,161
Inpatient Days	2,253,793	2,170,349	2,234,925	2,237,893	2,210,340
Average Length of Stay	5.1	5.0	5.0	5.0	5.0
Inpatient Surgeries	134,849	137,218	141,751	143,822	141,724
Births	58,253	62,264	63,653	65,130	68,659
Utilization - Outpatient					
Emergency Outpatient Visits	1,818,858	1,730,788	1,677,353	1,725,417	1,621,056
Other Outpatient Visits	7,139,929	6,934,427	6,572,791	7,134,664	6,786,916
Total Outpatient Visits	8,958,787	8,665,215	8,250,144	8,860,081	8,407,972
Outpatient Surgeries	232,063	219,321	211,730	206,315	204,045
Personnel					
Full Time RNs	15,678	15,239	15,787	15,411	15,300
Full Time LPNs	479	472	551	684	775
Part Time RNs	6,456	6,449	5,235	5,377	5,123
Part Time LPNs	191	190	179	215	240
Total Full Time	54,125	53,370	55,072	54,311	53,002
Total Part Time	17,930	18,322	15,268	15,782	16,290
Revenue - Inpatient					
Gross Inpatient Revenue	$22,263,097,740	$19,860,096,681	$19,013,208,766	$17,525,068,092	$16,296,367,033
Revenue - Outpatient					
Gross Outpatient Revenue	$18,360,253,142	$16,603,620,063	$14,766,810,304	$13,322,614,754	$11,343,750,441
Revenue and Expenses - Totals					
(Includes Inpatient and Outpatient)					
Total Gross Revenue	$40,623,350,882	$36,463,716,744	$33,780,019,070	$30,847,682,846	$27,640,117,474
Deductions from Revenue	28,720,794,917	25,752,881,907	23,450,147,224	21,100,773,225	18,781,874,571
Net Patient Revenue	11,902,555,965	10,710,834,837	10,329,871,846	9,746,909,621	8,858,242,903
Other Operating Revenue	559,939,985	513,568,821	501,184,086	489,463,546	518,570,378
Other Nonoperating Revenue	156,458,722	143,185,607	196,854,806	146,646,198	-27,071,112
Total Net Revenue	12,618,954,672	11,367,589,265	11,027,910,738	10,383,019,365	9,349,742,169
Total Expenses	10,941,848,898	10,054,322,089	9,590,946,802	9,244,357,277	8,889,584,362
HOSPITAL UNIT (Excludes Separate Nursing Home Units)					
Utilization - Inpatient					
Beds	9,663	9,599	9,537	9,777	9,518
Admissions	442,623	430,676	447,782	443,718	441,061
Inpatient Days	2,067,062	1,995,737	2,026,168	2,056,115	2,076,120
Average Length of Stay	4.7	4.6	4.5	4.6	4.7
Personnel					
Total Full Time	53,774	52,935	54,554	53,795	52,602
Total Part Time	17,727	18,169	14,960	15,572	16,131
Revenue and Expenses - Totals					
(Includes Inpatient and Outpatient)					
Total Net Revenue	$12,577,500,290	$11,330,471,189	$10,984,832,365	$10,343,931,411	$9,321,879,151
Total Expenses	10,898,966,203	10,014,190,366	9,546,862,102	9,207,018,816	8,862,237,046
COMMUNITY HEALTH INDICATORS PER 1000 POPULATION					
Total Population (in thousands)	5,188	5,117	5,095	5,025	4,935
Inpatient					
Beds	2.0	2.0	2.0	2.1	2.0
Admissions	85.7	84.6	88.2	88.6	89.6
Inpatient Days	434.5	424.2	438.6	445.4	447.9
Inpatient Surgeries	26.0	26.8	27.8	28.6	28.7
Births	11.2	12.2	12.5	13.0	13.9
Outpatient					
Emergency Outpatient Visits	350.6	338.3	329.2	343.4	328.5
Other Outpatient Visits	1,376.4	1,355.2	1,290.0	1,419.9	1,375.2
Total Outpatient Visits	1,727.0	1,693.5	1,619.2	1,763.3	1,703.7
Outpatient Surgeries	44.7	42.9	41.6	41.1	41.3
Expense per Capita (per person)	$2,109.2	$1,965.0	$1,882.3	$1,839.8	$1,801.3

States

TABLE 6

CONNECTICUT

U.S. Registered Community Hospitals
(Nonfederal, short-term general and other special hospitals)

Overview 2008–2012

	2012	2011	2010	2009	2008
Total Community Hospitals in Connecticut	34	35	34	35	35
Bed Size Category					
6-24	0	0	0	0	0
25-49	2	2	1	1	1
50-99	9	8	8	8	8
100-199	10	12	10	12	12
200-299	4	4	5	3	4
300-399	5	5	5	6	5
400-499	1	1	2	2	2
500 + ...	3	3	3	3	3
Location					
Hospitals Urban..........................	29	30	29	30	29
Hospitals Rural	5	5	5	5	6
Control					
State and Local Government................	1	1	1	1	1
Not for Profit	32	33	32	33	32
Investor owned	1	1	1	1	2
Physician Models					
Independent Practice Association	7	6	7	8	8
Group Practice without Walls...............	0	0	2	0	1
Open Physician-Hospital Organization	5	4	5	6	3
Closed Physician-Hospital Organization	4	3	2	2	2
Management Service Organization	6	4	5	4	3
Integrated Salary Model....................	17	17	17	15	18
Equity Model	4	1	1	1	1
Foundation...............................	8	9	5	1	0
Insurance Products					
Health Maintenance Organization	0	0	2	2	3
Preferred Provider Organization..............	1	0	0	0	0
Indemnity Fee for Service	0	0	0	0	1
Managed Care Contracts					
Health Maintenance Organization	24	25	23	22	22
Preferred Provider Organization..............	24	25	22	23	22
Affiliations					
Hospitals in a System.....................	18	15	14	12	9
Hospitals in a Network	12	12	11	12	13
Hospitals in a Group Purchasing Organization..	25	27	28	28	28

TABLE 6

CONNECTICUT

U.S. Registered Community Hospitals
(Nonfederal, short-term general and other special hospitals)

Utilization, Personnel, Revenue and Expenses, Community Health Indicators 2008–2012

	2012	2011	2010	2009	2008
TOTAL FACILITY (Includes Hospital and Nursing Home Units)					
Utilization - Inpatient					
Beds............................	8,120	7,745	8,091	7,935	7,906
Admissions......................	378,130	402,838	406,718	407,710	400,632
Inpatient Days...................	2,053,559	2,110,564	2,290,323	2,345,878	2,296,558
Average Length of Stay............	5.4	5.2	5.6	5.8	5.7
Inpatient Surgeries................	99,309	103,828	108,070	109,334	107,611
Births...........................	35,891	37,565	37,483	38,932	40,963
Utilization - Outpatient					
Emergency Outpatient Visits........	1,643,476	1,643,282	1,661,088	1,607,670	1,524,545
Other Outpatient Visits............	7,342,754	6,884,506	6,605,714	6,567,848	6,550,089
Total Outpatient Visits............	8,986,230	8,527,788	8,266,802	8,175,518	8,074,634
Outpatient Surgeries	216,262	204,949	201,480	198,390	192,544
Personnel					
Full Time RNs...................	10,989	11,075	10,483	10,831	10,057
Full Time LPNs	261	258	264	311	348
Part Time RNs...................	7,221	7,107	6,609	6,512	6,883
Part Time LPNs.................	221	229	194	229	361
Total Full Time..................	44,994	44,784	43,689	44,091	42,558
Total Part Time	22,084	22,538	21,507	20,842	23,152
Revenue - Inpatient					
Gross Inpatient Revenue...........	$14,329,380,117	$14,148,582,803	$13,295,787,334	$12,736,578,199	$11,484,375,092
Revenue - Outpatient					
Gross Outpatient Revenue	$13,501,775,551	$11,773,260,720	$10,537,030,956	$9,767,664,004	$8,402,315,796
Revenue and Expenses - Totals					
(Includes Inpatient and Outpatient)					
Total Gross Revenue..............	$27,831,155,668	$25,921,843,523	$23,832,818,290	$22,504,242,203	$19,886,690,888
Deductions from Revenue..........	18,019,019,740	16,507,379,096	15,121,712,588	14,125,599,354	12,234,710,097
Net Patient Revenue	9,812,135,928	9,414,464,427	8,711,105,702	8,378,642,849	7,651,980,791
Other Operating Revenue	562,656,610	462,365,876	455,355,109	420,171,188	368,547,369
Other Nonoperating Revenue	123,095,744	57,595,778	115,215,987	-1,279,820	-125,823,897
Total Net Revenue................	10,497,888,282	9,934,426,081	9,281,676,798	8,797,534,217	7,894,704,263
Total Expenses..................	9,795,239,002	9,561,576,935	8,928,296,028	8,565,211,235	7,906,958,696
HOSPITAL UNIT (Excludes Separate Nursing Home Units)					
Utilization - Inpatient					
Beds............................	7,777	7,468	7,676	7,648	7,237
Admissions......................	377,468	402,394	405,842	407,207	399,384
Inpatient Days...................	1,973,687	2,109,561	2,146,637	2,245,293	2,060,023
Average Length of Stay............	5.2	5.2	5.3	5.5	5.2
Personnel					
Total Full Time..................	44,726	44,768	43,306	44,052	41,790
Total Part Time	21,876	22,521	21,256	20,826	22,313
Revenue and Expenses - Totals					
(Includes Inpatient and Outpatient)					
Total Net Revenue................	$10,439,662,013	$9,928,376,462	$9,235,623,435	$8,759,788,307	$7,822,208,146
Total Expenses..................	9,741,183,887	9,556,797,059	8,888,242,578	8,530,306,215	7,846,566,914
COMMUNITY HEALTH INDICATORS PER 1000 POPULATION					
Total Population (in thousands)	3,590	3,581	3,527	3,518	3,503
Inpatient					
Beds............................	2.3	2.2	2.3	2.3	2.3
Admissions......................	105.3	112.5	115.3	115.9	114.4
Inpatient Days...................	572.0	589.4	649.4	666.8	655.6
Inpatient Surgeries................	27.7	29.0	30.6	31.1	30.7
Births...........................	10.0	10.5	10.6	11.1	11.7
Outpatient					
Emergency Outpatient Visits........	457.7	458.9	471.0	456.9	435.2
Other Outpatient Visits............	2,045.1	1,922.7	1,872.9	1,866.8	1,869.9
Total Outpatient Visits............	2,502.9	2,381.6	2,343.9	2,323.7	2,305.1
Outpatient Surgeries	60.2	57.2	57.1	56.4	55.0
Expense per Capita (per person).....	$2,728.2	$2,670.3	$2,531.5	$2,434.5	$2,257.2

States

TABLE 6

DELAWARE

U.S. Registered Community Hospitals
(Nonfederal, short-term general and other special hospitals)

Overview 2008–2012

	2012	2011	2010	2009	2008
Total Community Hospitals in Delaware	7	7	7	7	7
Bed Size Category					
6-24	0	0	0	0	0
25-49	1	1	1	1	1
50-99	1	0	0	0	0
100-199	2	2	2	2	3
200-299	1	2	2	2	1
300-399	1	1	1	1	1
400-499	0	0	0	0	0
500 + ...	1	1	1	1	1
Location					
Hospitals Urban.........................	5	5	5	5	5
Hospitals Rural	2	2	2	2	2
Control					
State and Local Government................	0	0	0	0	0
Not for Profit	6	6	6	6	6
Investor owned	1	1	1	1	1
Physician Models					
Independent Practice Association	0	0	0	0	0
Group Practice without Walls...............	0	0	0	0	0
Open Physician-Hospital Organization	0	0	0	0	0
Closed Physician-Hospital Organization	0	0	0	0	0
Management Service Organization	0	0	0	0	0
Integrated Salary Model	1	2	3	3	2
Equity Model	0	0	0	0	0
Foundation..............................	1	1	1	1	1
Insurance Products					
Health Maintenance Organization	0	0	1	1	0
Preferred Provider Organization..............	0	0	1	1	0
Indemnity Fee for Service	0	0	1	1	0
Managed Care Contracts					
Health Maintenance Organization	3	3	4	5	5
Preferred Provider Organization..............	3	3	4	5	5
Affiliations					
Hospitals in a System......................	4	3	3	3	3
Hospitals in a Network	0	0	0	0	0
Hospitals in a Group Purchasing Organization..	5	5	6	6	6

TABLE 6

DELAWARE

U.S. Registered Community Hospitals
(Nonfederal, short-term general and other special hospitals)

Utilization, Personnel, Revenue and Expenses, Community Health Indicators 2008–2012

	2012	2011	2010	2009	2008
TOTAL FACILITY (Includes Hospital and Nursing Home Units)					
Utilization - Inpatient					
Beds	1,998	2,143	2,155	2,125	2,071
Admissions	104,803	100,288	101,735	102,153	103,726
Inpatient Days	526,678	578,466	580,261	597,993	613,049
Average Length of Stay.	5.0	5.8	5.7	5.9	5.9
Inpatient Surgeries.	32,163	31,852	28,828	29,930	30,845
Births.	11,358	11,496	11,486	12,158	12,536
Utilization - Outpatient					
Emergency Outpatient Visits	437,706	417,689	406,652	392,660	363,979
Other Outpatient Visits.	1,653,598	1,432,957	1,380,658	1,351,824	1,317,097
Total Outpatient Visits	2,091,304	1,850,646	1,787,310	1,744,484	1,681,076
Outpatient Surgeries	64,243	62,618	67,852	70,362	60,343
Personnel					
Full Time RNs	3,997	3,990	3,689	3,485	3,334
Full Time LPNs	142	171	126	135	164
Part Time RNs.	2,166	1,927	2,195	2,486	2,326
Part Time LPNs	118	136	125	133	156
Total Full Time.	15,421	14,456	13,885	13,707	13,954
Total Part Time	5,918	5,598	5,846	6,406	6,340
Revenue - Inpatient					
Gross Inpatient Revenue.	$3,097,560,492	$2,830,331,928	$2,671,560,601	$2,528,530,549	$2,385,974,140
Revenue - Outpatient					
Gross Outpatient Revenue	$2,677,941,719	$2,262,497,249	$2,026,156,087	$1,797,902,276	$1,569,559,056
Revenue and Expenses - Totals					
(Includes Inpatient and Outpatient)					
Total Gross Revenue.	$5,775,502,211	$5,092,829,177	$4,697,716,688	$4,326,432,825	$3,955,533,196
Deductions from Revenue.	3,063,219,162	2,640,575,715	2,394,621,807	2,111,070,905	1,865,226,783
Net Patient Revenue	2,712,283,049	2,452,253,462	2,303,094,881	2,215,361,920	2,090,306,413
Other Operating Revenue	118,067,679	178,700,023	165,608,644	159,598,810	121,047,453
Other Nonoperating Revenue	17,706,306	171,781,254	77,555,669	-156,561,766	81,948,435
Total Net Revenue.	2,848,057,034	2,802,734,739	2,546,259,194	2,218,398,964	2,293,302,301
Total Expenses.	2,662,272,646	2,408,075,977	2,344,087,243	2,264,467,218	2,119,860,075
HOSPITAL UNIT (Excludes Separate Nursing Home Units)					
Utilization - Inpatient					
Beds	1,998	2,033	1,941	1,911	1,967
Admissions	104,803	99,921	101,130	101,502	103,438
Inpatient Days	526,678	540,146	509,077	525,133	577,278
Average Length of Stay.	5.0	5.4	5.0	5.2	5.6
Personnel					
Total Full Time.	15,421	14,301	13,670	13,553	13,883
Total Part Time	5,918	5,582	5,705	6,246	6,316
Revenue and Expenses - Totals					
(Includes Inpatient and Outpatient)					
Total Net Revenue.	$2,848,057,034	$2,791,771,225	$2,525,583,028	$2,197,822,141	$2,283,604,301
Total Expenses.	2,662,272,646	2,396,081,133	2,323,082,005	2,243,045,075	2,110,993,075
COMMUNITY HEALTH INDICATORS PER 1000 POPULATION					
Total Population (in thousands)	917	907	891	885	876
Inpatient					
Beds	2.2	2.4	2.4	2.4	2.4
Admissions	114.3	110.6	114.1	115.4	118.4
Inpatient Days	574.3	637.7	650.9	675.6	699.7
Inpatient Surgeries.	35.1	35.1	32.3	33.8	35.2
Births.	12.4	12.7	12.9	13.7	14.3
Outpatient					
Emergency Outpatient Visits	477.3	460.4	456.2	443.6	415.4
Other Outpatient Visits.	1,803.1	1,579.7	1,548.8	1,527.3	1,503.2
Total Outpatient Visits	2,280.4	2,040.1	2,004.9	1,970.9	1,918.6
Outpatient Surgeries	70.1	69.0	76.1	79.5	68.9
Expense per Capita (per person).	$2,903.0	$2,654.6	$2,629.5	$2,558.4	$2,419.3

States

TABLE **6**

DISTRICT OF COLUMBIA

U.S. Registered Community Hospitals
(Nonfederal, short-term general and other special hospitals)

Overview 2008–2012

	2012	2011	2010	2009	2008
Total Community Hospitals in District of Columbia	11	11	11	10	10
Bed Size Category					
6-24	0	0	0	0	0
25-49	0	0	0	0	0
50-99	1	1	1	1	1
100-199	2	2	2	1	1
200-299	2	3	4	3	3
300-399	4	2	1	2	3
400-499	0	1	1	1	0
500 +	2	2	2	2	2
Location					
Hospitals Urban	11	11	11	10	10
Hospitals Rural	0	0	0	0	0
Control					
State and Local Government	1	1	1	0	0
Not for Profit	7	7	7	7	7
Investor owned	3	3	3	3	3
Physician Models					
Independent Practice Association	3	0	1	0	1
Group Practice without Walls	4	1	0	1	1
Open Physician-Hospital Organization	0	0	0	0	0
Closed Physician-Hospital Organization	3	1	1	1	1
Management Service Organization	3	1	1	1	1
Integrated Salary Model	5	4	5	5	4
Equity Model	0	0	0	0	0
Foundation	1	1	1	1	1
Insurance Products					
Health Maintenance Organization	5	4	2	3	3
Preferred Provider Organization	4	1	0	0	0
Indemnity Fee for Service	0	1	0	0	0
Managed Care Contracts					
Health Maintenance Organization	8	6	7	7	7
Preferred Provider Organization	7	6	6	7	7
Affiliations					
Hospitals in a System	8	8	9	7	7
Hospitals in a Network	1	4	5	4	2
Hospitals in a Group Purchasing Organization	9	7	8	8	8

TABLE 6

DISTRICT OF COLUMBIA

U.S. Registered Community Hospitals
(Nonfederal, short-term general and other special hospitals)

Utilization, Personnel, Revenue and Expenses, Community Health Indicators 2008–2012

	2012	2011	2010	2009	2008
TOTAL FACILITY (Includes Hospital and Nursing Home Units)					
Utilization - Inpatient					
Beds	3,617	3,635	3,458	3,452	3,358
Admissions	132,539	131,577	131,976	138,456	137,260
Inpatient Days	933,177	954,752	926,254	927,419	954,416
Average Length of Stay	7.0	7.3	7.0	6.7	7.0
Inpatient Surgeries	39,163	40,477	41,736	42,667	43,173
Births	13,783	13,792	13,814	14,507	14,901
Utilization - Outpatient					
Emergency Outpatient Visits	499,154	455,553	430,637	457,292	436,918
Other Outpatient Visits	1,961,067	1,994,547	1,888,245	1,954,514	1,919,145
Total Outpatient Visits	2,460,221	2,450,100	2,318,882	2,411,806	2,356,063
Outpatient Surgeries	66,622	62,767	58,907	62,497	65,742
Personnel					
Full Time RNs	5,647	5,435	5,458	5,222	4,447
Full Time LPNs	249	216	267	304	215
Part Time RNs	1,318	1,643	1,966	1,845	1,796
Part Time LPNs	38	32	46	35	38
Total Full Time	22,972	22,815	22,654	22,371	21,247
Total Part Time	3,313	4,525	5,259	4,666	4,463
Revenue - Inpatient					
Gross Inpatient Revenue	$6,515,832,670	$6,334,158,623	$6,016,677,081	$5,895,449,855	$5,686,127,872
Revenue - Outpatient					
Gross Outpatient Revenue	$3,968,228,093	$3,932,470,181	$3,476,432,807	$3,108,162,999	$2,835,491,356
Revenue and Expenses - Totals					
(Includes Inpatient and Outpatient)					
Total Gross Revenue	$10,484,060,763	$10,266,628,804	$9,493,109,888	$9,003,612,854	$8,521,619,228
Deductions from Revenue	6,640,686,593	6,617,584,769	5,971,324,649	5,592,219,614	5,300,645,413
Net Patient Revenue	3,843,374,170	3,649,044,035	3,521,785,239	3,411,393,240	3,220,973,815
Other Operating Revenue	299,523,683	277,637,308	205,891,415	214,814,678	192,446,948
Other Nonoperating Revenue	-15,527,022	95,995,539	33,913,566	32,415,954	-139,712,361
Total Net Revenue	4,127,370,831	4,022,676,882	3,761,590,220	3,658,623,872	3,273,708,402
Total Expenses	3,937,620,808	3,766,313,652	3,582,285,072	3,585,829,997	3,392,800,661
HOSPITAL UNIT (Excludes Separate Nursing Home Units)					
Utilization - Inpatient					
Beds	3,200	3,470	3,161	3,157	3,061
Admissions	130,696	130,232	130,125	136,578	135,521
Inpatient Days	791,242	909,564	822,314	822,965	850,769
Average Length of Stay	6.1	7.0	6.3	6.0	6.3
Personnel					
Total Full Time	22,602	22,710	22,327	22,067	21,151
Total Part Time	3,241	4,500	5,181	4,595	4,437
Revenue and Expenses - Totals					
(Includes Inpatient and Outpatient)					
Total Net Revenue	$4,074,614,436	$4,007,011,323	$3,726,836,744	$3,624,105,283	$3,244,092,304
Total Expenses	3,890,891,777	3,750,371,864	3,552,676,361	3,556,839,618	3,363,055,134
COMMUNITY HEALTH INDICATORS PER 1000 POPULATION					
Total Population (in thousands)	632	618	611	600	590
Inpatient					
Beds	5.7	5.9	5.7	5.8	5.7
Admissions	209.6	212.9	216.1	230.9	232.6
Inpatient Days	1,475.8	1,544.9	1,517.0	1,546.6	1,617.5
Inpatient Surgeries	61.9	65.5	68.4	71.2	73.2
Births	21.8	22.3	22.6	24.2	25.3
Outpatient					
Emergency Outpatient Visits	789.4	737.1	705.3	762.6	740.4
Other Outpatient Visits	3,101.4	3,227.4	3,092.5	3,259.4	3,252.4
Total Outpatient Visits	3,890.8	3,964.6	3,797.8	4,022.0	3,992.8
Outpatient Surgeries	105.4	101.6	96.5	104.2	111.4
Expense per Capita (per person)	$6,227.2	$6,094.4	$5,866.9	$5,979.8	$5,749.8

States

TABLE 6

FLORIDA

U.S. Registered Community Hospitals
(Nonfederal, short-term general and other special hospitals)

Overview 2008–2012

	2012	2011	2010	2009	2008
Total Community Hospitals in Florida.........	216	213	210	210	211
Bed Size Category					
6-24	4	3	2	2	3
25-49	23	21	21	21	23
50-99	39	38	39	39	35
100-199	55	55	50	51	55
200-299	37	37	38	37	37
300-399	25	27	27	25	25
400-499	10	9	9	12	11
500 + ...	23	23	24	23	22
Location					
Hospitals Urban...........................	186	184	181	181	177
Hospitals Rural	30	29	29	29	34
Control					
State and Local Government...............	24	26	27	25	25
Not for Profit	80	81	79	82	86
Investor owned	112	106	104	103	100
Physician Models					
Independent Practice Association	3	5	5	4	6
Group Practice without Walls................	6	9	7	9	3
Open Physician-Hospital Organization	19	24	19	19	12
Closed Physician-Hospital Organization	2	5	7	6	10
Management Service Organization	15	14	14	8	5
Integrated Salary Model....................	66	64	59	52	52
Equity Model	0	1	1	0	0
Foundation...............................	2	3	4	4	2
Insurance Products					
Health Maintenance Organization	14	15	11	13	8
Preferred Provider Organization..............	7	18	16	17	10
Indemnity Fee for Service	4	7	5	6	5
Managed Care Contracts					
Health Maintenance Organization	100	111	98	88	81
Preferred Provider Organization..............	100	113	101	91	82
Affiliations					
Hospitals in a System......................	176	167	160	160	159
Hospitals in a Network.....................	48	37	35	35	38
Hospitals in a Group Purchasing Organization..	113	101	106	116	118

TABLE 6

FLORIDA

U.S. Registered Community Hospitals
(Nonfederal, short-term general and other special hospitals)

Utilization, Personnel, Revenue and Expenses, Community Health Indicators 2008–2012

	2012	2011	2010	2009	2008
TOTAL FACILITY (Includes Hospital and Nursing Home Units)					
Utilization - Inpatient					
Beds	53,785	52,923	53,318	53,293	52,836
Admissions	2,472,181	2,508,311	2,452,089	2,452,546	2,396,691
Inpatient Days	12,372,261	12,365,513	12,191,209	12,261,161	12,192,327
Average Length of Stay	5.0	4.9	5.0	5.0	5.1
Inpatient Surgeries	610,533	614,726	650,557	655,203	659,237
Births	196,681	186,919	202,862	206,284	218,035
Utilization - Outpatient					
Emergency Outpatient Visits	8,126,914	7,580,718	7,559,853	7,477,209	7,161,108
Other Outpatient Visits	15,367,371	16,827,980	16,683,248	17,396,409	17,268,832
Total Outpatient Visits	23,494,285	24,408,698	24,243,101	24,873,618	24,429,940
Outpatient Surgeries	800,782	782,871	798,189	822,841	846,551
Personnel					
Full Time RNs	74,829	72,090	69,840	68,581	62,639
Full Time LPNs	3,495	3,595	4,111	4,470	4,563
Part Time RNs	18,183	16,461	16,844	17,495	20,188
Part Time LPNs	885	789	901	1,092	1,154
Total Full Time	239,356	234,893	232,349	229,515	220,165
Total Part Time	55,168	49,243	47,580	49,670	54,335
Revenue - Inpatient					
Gross Inpatient Revenue	$106,765,072,734	$100,263,145,301	$98,439,589,940	$90,412,617,613	$80,168,815,722
Revenue - Outpatient					
Gross Outpatient Revenue	$70,527,318,626	$63,221,928,643	$58,858,434,042	$52,572,001,561	$44,224,777,407
Revenue and Expenses - Totals					
(Includes Inpatient and Outpatient)					
Total Gross Revenue	$177,292,391,360	$163,485,073,944	$157,298,023,982	$142,984,619,174	$124,393,593,129
Deductions from Revenue	135,271,195,802	126,350,152,571	119,355,324,858	107,498,135,646	91,084,229,921
Net Patient Revenue	42,021,195,558	37,134,921,373	37,942,699,124	35,486,483,528	33,309,363,208
Other Operating Revenue	2,402,722,300	2,293,290,171	2,190,285,623	1,811,268,561	2,104,002,109
Other Nonoperating Revenue	498,972,173	613,632,452	562,284,781	483,113,737	64,179,556
Total Net Revenue	44,922,890,031	40,041,843,996	40,695,269,528	37,780,865,826	35,477,544,873
Total Expenses	40,816,430,398	36,908,772,722	36,318,160,204	34,922,141,446	33,117,894,364
HOSPITAL UNIT (Excludes Separate Nursing Home Units)					
Utilization - Inpatient					
Beds	52,723	52,055	52,415	52,361	51,863
Admissions	2,465,633	2,504,407	2,448,276	2,448,331	2,392,911
Inpatient Days	12,021,523	12,096,907	11,888,876	11,942,896	11,874,879
Average Length of Stay	4.9	4.8	4.9	4.9	5.0
Personnel					
Total Full Time	238,286	234,104	231,450	228,263	219,027
Total Part Time	54,951	49,111	47,423	49,227	54,203
Revenue and Expenses - Totals					
(Includes Inpatient and Outpatient)					
Total Net Revenue	$44,817,002,142	$39,961,735,021	$40,594,960,399	$37,709,543,480	$35,402,114,525
Total Expenses	40,697,886,032	36,803,286,544	36,197,864,998	34,839,959,163	33,027,271,463
COMMUNITY HEALTH INDICATORS PER 1000 POPULATION					
Total Population (in thousands)	19,318	19,058	18,678	18,538	18,424
Inpatient					
Beds	2.8	2.8	2.9	2.9	2.9
Admissions	128.0	131.6	131.3	132.3	130.1
Inpatient Days	640.5	648.9	652.7	661.4	661.8
Inpatient Surgeries	31.6	32.3	34.8	35.3	35.8
Births	10.2	9.8	10.9	11.1	11.8
Outpatient					
Emergency Outpatient Visits	420.7	397.8	404.7	403.3	388.7
Other Outpatient Visits	795.5	883.0	893.2	938.4	937.3
Total Outpatient Visits	1,216.2	1,280.8	1,297.9	1,341.8	1,326.0
Outpatient Surgeries	41.5	41.1	42.7	44.4	45.9
Expense per Capita (per person)	$2,112.9	$1,936.7	$1,944.4	$1,883.8	$1,797.6

States

TABLE 6

GEORGIA

U.S. Registered Community Hospitals
(Nonfederal, short-term general and other special hospitals)

Overview 2008–2012

	2012	2011	2010	2009	2008
Total Community Hospitals in Georgia	148	153	154	152	153
Bed Size Category					
6-24	4	6	6	6	4
25-49	38	38	39	38	41
50-99	25	26	24	24	22
100-199	39	41	42	42	44
200-299	18	17	17	16	15
300-399	6	6	7	8	9
400-499	10	8	10	10	9
500 + ...	8	11	9	8	9
Location					
Hospitals Urban............................	86	88	89	87	69
Hospitals Rural	62	65	65	65	84
Control					
State and Local Government................	49	49	52	53	56
Not for Profit	66	68	66	63	63
Investor owned	33	36	36	36	34
Physician Models					
Independent Practice Association	5	6	8	10	10
Group Practice without Walls................	0	0	0	1	2
Open Physician-Hospital Organization	12	14	18	15	19
Closed Physician-Hospital Organization	18	16	17	16	15
Management Service Organization	7	9	8	7	8
Integrated Salary Model....................	35	39	41	37	35
Equity Model	2	4	5	5	6
Foundation...............................	3	4	4	3	5
Insurance Products					
Health Maintenance Organization	6	8	9	12	10
Preferred Provider Organization..............	8	15	20	21	20
Indemnity Fee for Service	2	4	5	7	7
Managed Care Contracts					
Health Maintenance Organization	67	77	81	83	79
Preferred Provider Organization..............	72	83	94	95	89
Affiliations					
Hospitals in a System......................	78	80	81	79	81
Hospitals in a Network	36	41	40	39	42
Hospitals in a Group Purchasing Organization..	76	95	104	105	100

TABLE 6

GEORGIA

U.S. Registered Community Hospitals
(Nonfederal, short-term general and other special hospitals)

Utilization, Personnel, Revenue and Expenses, Community Health Indicators 2008–2012

	2012	2011	2010	2009	2008
TOTAL FACILITY (Includes Hospital and Nursing Home Units)					
Utilization - Inpatient					
Beds	24,657	25,282	25,513	25,419	25,583
Admissions	953,817	956,503	961,391	956,870	959,375
Inpatient Days	5,970,497	6,094,960	6,138,828	6,059,475	6,172,510
Average Length of Stay	6.3	6.4	6.4	6.3	6.4
Inpatient Surgeries	257,747	265,074	265,789	267,788	269,766
Births	119,564	123,546	128,531	135,505	142,382
Utilization - Outpatient					
Emergency Outpatient Visits	4,153,101	4,035,426	4,095,951	4,081,812	3,843,244
Other Outpatient Visits	10,881,116	10,740,295	10,195,629	10,308,523	10,340,848
Total Outpatient Visits	15,034,217	14,775,721	14,291,580	14,390,335	14,184,092
Outpatient Surgeries	474,453	494,889	497,929	511,272	487,070
Personnel					
Full Time RNs	31,786	30,458	30,393	29,719	27,823
Full Time LPNs	2,866	3,119	3,276	3,506	3,651
Part Time RNs	9,066	10,000	10,469	11,965	11,963
Part Time LPNs	591	740	857	977	1,035
Total Full Time	111,769	110,421	112,040	111,451	108,871
Total Part Time	26,565	29,260	29,110	32,522	32,169
Revenue - Inpatient					
Gross Inpatient Revenue	$32,638,245,514	$30,470,684,745	$28,768,523,466	$26,548,862,459	$25,139,478,750
Revenue - Outpatient					
Gross Outpatient Revenue	$26,952,133,432	$24,110,026,415	$22,700,713,568	$20,738,855,918	$18,392,697,423
Revenue and Expenses - Totals					
(Includes Inpatient and Outpatient)					
Total Gross Revenue	$59,590,378,946	$54,580,711,160	$51,469,237,034	$47,287,718,377	$43,532,176,173
Deductions from Revenue	41,286,051,494	38,089,080,759	35,169,736,402	31,401,538,356	28,602,816,610
Net Patient Revenue	18,304,327,452	16,491,630,401	16,299,500,632	15,886,180,021	14,929,359,563
Other Operating Revenue	896,928,314	811,702,301	773,260,104	755,206,277	788,733,742
Other Nonoperating Revenue	313,593,866	228,081,442	324,122,628	128,720,872	-102,237,534
Total Net Revenue	19,514,849,632	17,531,414,144	17,396,883,364	16,770,107,170	15,615,855,771
Total Expenses	17,663,914,623	16,450,926,776	16,079,597,038	15,616,820,380	15,098,639,746
HOSPITAL UNIT (Excludes Separate Nursing Home Units)					
Utilization - Inpatient					
Beds	21,695	21,581	21,605	21,868	22,332
Admissions	947,058	949,217	953,677	949,070	953,328
Inpatient Days	4,988,750	4,924,671	4,826,637	4,890,754	5,113,980
Average Length of Stay	5.3	5.2	5.1	5.2	5.4
Personnel					
Total Full Time	109,799	107,993	109,514	108,900	106,600
Total Part Time	26,140	28,663	28,416	31,885	31,471
Revenue and Expenses - Totals					
(Includes Inpatient and Outpatient)					
Total Net Revenue	$19,343,288,346	$17,334,774,424	$17,166,588,760	$16,591,803,789	$15,449,511,224
Total Expenses	17,517,267,271	16,266,797,779	15,896,591,116	15,452,332,194	14,947,753,769
COMMUNITY HEALTH INDICATORS PER 1000 POPULATION					
Total Population (in thousands)	9,920	9,815	9,908	9,829	9,698
Inpatient					
Beds	2.5	2.6	2.6	2.6	2.6
Admissions	96.2	97.5	97.0	97.3	98.9
Inpatient Days	601.9	621.0	619.6	616.5	636.5
Inpatient Surgeries	26.0	27.0	26.8	27.2	27.8
Births	12.1	12.6	13.0	13.8	14.7
Outpatient					
Emergency Outpatient Visits	418.7	411.1	413.4	415.3	396.3
Other Outpatient Visits	1,096.9	1,094.3	1,029.0	1,048.8	1,066.3
Total Outpatient Visits	1,515.6	1,505.4	1,442.4	1,464.0	1,462.6
Outpatient Surgeries	47.8	50.4	50.3	52.0	50.2
Expense per Capita (per person)	$1,780.6	$1,676.1	$1,622.8	$1,588.8	$1,556.9

States

TABLE **6**

HAWAII

U.S. Registered Community Hospitals
(Nonfederal, short-term general and other special hospitals)

Overview 2008–2012

	2012	2011	2010	2009	2008
Total Community Hospitals in Hawaii	24	23	26	25	25
Bed Size Category					
6-24	5	5	6	5	4
25-49	3	4	3	4	4
50-99	6	5	4	5	5
100-199	5	4	7	5	6
200-299	4	4	5	5	5
300-399	0	0	0	0	0
400-499	1	1	1	1	1
500 + ...	0	0	0	0	0
Location					
Hospitals Urban............................	12	11	14	13	14
Hospitals Rural	12	12	12	12	11
Control					
State and Local Government................	10	7	8	7	8
Not for Profit	14	16	18	18	17
Investor owned	0	0	0	0	0
Physician Models					
Independent Practice Association	2	2	2	1	1
Group Practice without Walls...............	0	0	0	0	0
Open Physician-Hospital Organization	2	2	2	2	3
Closed Physician-Hospital Organization	3	2	1	1	1
Management Service Organization	0	0	0	0	0
Integrated Salary Model....................	9	7	7	5	4
Equity Model	0	0	0	0	0
Foundation................................	0	0	0	2	1
Insurance Products					
Health Maintenance Organization	1	1	1	2	0
Preferred Provider Organization..............	0	3	3	3	1
Indemnity Fee for Service	0	0	1	1	0
Managed Care Contracts					
Health Maintenance Organization	14	10	7	9	9
Preferred Provider Organization..............	14	10	8	9	9
Affiliations					
Hospitals in a System......................	19	18	21	20	21
Hospitals in a Network	3	2	2	3	1
Hospitals in a Group Purchasing Organization..	15	13	15	14	13

TABLE 6

HAWAII

U.S. Registered Community Hospitals
(Nonfederal, short-term general and other special hospitals)

Utilization, Personnel, Revenue and Expenses, Community Health Indicators 2008–2012

	2012	2011	2010	2009	2008
TOTAL FACILITY (Includes Hospital and Nursing Home Units)					
Utilization - Inpatient					
Beds	2,803	2,562	3,148	2,966	3,087
Admissions	109,270	105,039	110,577	111,706	111,310
Inpatient Days	745,956	720,633	827,977	772,508	846,756
Average Length of Stay	6.8	6.9	7.5	6.9	7.6
Inpatient Surgeries	27,141	27,447	30,626	32,340	30,723
Births	11,085	10,756	9,271	11,031	10,522
Utilization - Outpatient					
Emergency Outpatient Visits	399,437	366,276	365,903	383,778	361,068
Other Outpatient Visits	1,635,223	1,639,876	1,828,179	1,773,550	1,658,064
Total Outpatient Visits	2,034,660	2,006,152	2,194,082	2,157,328	2,019,132
Outpatient Surgeries	48,246	55,968	58,602	61,508	59,191
Personnel					
Full Time RNs	3,863	3,637	3,858	3,860	3,776
Full Time LPNs	253	231	292	252	298
Part Time RNs	867	722	974	1,136	1,254
Part Time LPNs	46	42	53	82	78
Total Full Time	15,008	13,674	14,755	14,505	14,550
Total Part Time	3,143	2,369	3,083	3,514	3,712
Revenue - Inpatient					
Gross Inpatient Revenue	$4,003,578,286	$3,138,945,148	$3,433,349,265	$3,279,585,271	$3,209,458,842
Revenue - Outpatient					
Gross Outpatient Revenue	$3,523,042,969	$2,692,147,508	$2,820,300,482	$2,476,907,535	$2,484,934,032
Revenue and Expenses - Totals					
(Includes Inpatient and Outpatient)					
Total Gross Revenue	$7,526,621,255	$5,831,092,656	$6,253,649,747	$5,756,492,806	$5,694,392,874
Deductions from Revenue	4,871,561,656	3,693,272,779	3,827,427,740	3,433,368,063	3,484,200,407
Net Patient Revenue	2,655,059,599	2,137,819,877	2,426,222,007	2,323,124,743	2,210,192,467
Other Operating Revenue	202,568,356	170,282,864	171,665,631	174,637,723	150,555,239
Other Nonoperating Revenue	35,719,144	43,411,366	48,234,523	40,300,553	21,263,753
Total Net Revenue	2,893,347,099	2,351,514,107	2,646,122,161	2,538,063,019	2,382,011,459
Total Expenses	2,855,849,784	2,391,952,134	2,611,062,195	2,576,059,889	2,321,587,503
HOSPITAL UNIT (Excludes Separate Nursing Home Units)					
Utilization - Inpatient					
Beds	2,355	2,203	2,688	2,635	2,589
Admissions	107,534	103,143	108,956	109,467	108,918
Inpatient Days	644,358	598,213	660,450	657,887	667,147
Average Length of Stay	6.0	5.8	6.1	6.0	6.1
Personnel					
Total Full Time	14,408	13,399	14,428	14,178	14,172
Total Part Time	3,077	2,318	3,047	3,446	3,610
Revenue and Expenses - Totals					
(Includes Inpatient and Outpatient)					
Total Net Revenue	$2,828,961,559	$2,318,674,997	$2,601,754,091	$2,512,905,897	$2,353,764,329
Total Expenses	2,775,697,478	2,347,459,882	2,561,364,433	2,550,665,438	2,275,182,714
COMMUNITY HEALTH INDICATORS PER 1000 POPULATION					
Total Population (in thousands)	1,392	1,375	1,300	1,295	1,287
Inpatient					
Beds	2.0	1.9	2.4	2.3	2.4
Admissions	78.5	76.4	85.1	86.2	86.5
Inpatient Days	535.8	524.2	636.9	596.4	657.7
Inpatient Surgeries	19.5	20.0	23.6	25.0	23.9
Births	8.0	7.8	7.1	8.5	8.2
Outpatient					
Emergency Outpatient Visits	286.9	266.4	281.4	296.3	280.4
Other Outpatient Visits	1,174.5	1,192.8	1,406.2	1,369.3	1,287.8
Total Outpatient Visits	1,461.4	1,459.2	1,687.6	1,665.7	1,568.3
Outpatient Surgeries	34.7	40.7	45.1	47.5	46.0
Expense per Capita (per person)	$2,051.2	$1,739.8	$2,008.4	$1,989.0	$1,803.2

States

TABLE **6**

IDAHO

U.S. Registered Community Hospitals
(Nonfederal, short-term general and other special hospitals)

Overview 2008–2012

	2012	2011	2010	2009	2008
Total Community Hospitals in Idaho	40	40	41	41	39
Bed Size Category					
6-24	11	12	11	11	11
25-49	13	11	12	11	10
50-99	7	8	9	10	9
100-199	5	4	5	5	5
200-299	1	2	1	1	2
300-399	2	2	2	2	1
400-499	0	0	0	0	0
500 + ...	1	1	1	1	1
Location					
Hospitals Urban.	14	14	15	15	7
Hospitals Rural	26	26	26	26	32
Control					
State and Local Government.	19	19	20	20	22
Not for Profit	16	17	16	16	14
Investor owned	5	4	5	5	3
Physician Models					
Independent Practice Association	4	5	5	5	7
Group Practice without Walls.	0	1	1	2	2
Open Physician-Hospital Organization	10	7	4	4	3
Closed Physician-Hospital Organization	1	2	2	3	4
Management Service Organization	0	1	3	4	4
Integrated Salary Model	15	12	13	13	11
Equity Model	1	0	0	0	1
Foundation.	1	1	1	1	1
Insurance Products					
Health Maintenance Organization	0	1	2	2	2
Preferred Provider Organization.	2	2	2	4	4
Indemnity Fee for Service	1	1	0	1	1
Managed Care Contracts					
Health Maintenance Organization	14	13	14	15	16
Preferred Provider Organization.	17	17	19	22	21
Affiliations					
Hospitals in a System.	21	20	23	23	22
Hospitals in a Network	10	11	13	15	15
Hospitals in a Group Purchasing Organization. .	26	25	25	28	26

States

TABLE 6

IDAHO

U.S. Registered Community Hospitals
(Nonfederal, short-term general and other special hospitals)

Utilization, Personnel, Revenue and Expenses, Community Health Indicators 2008–2012

	2012	2011	2010	2009	2008
TOTAL FACILITY (Includes Hospital and Nursing Home Units)					
Utilization - Inpatient					
Beds	3,305	3,306	3,376	3,382	3,311
Admissions	123,794	128,742	131,375	129,645	135,697
Inpatient Days	611,785	605,718	628,840	627,077	643,039
Average Length of Stay.	4.9	4.7	4.8	4.8	4.7
Inpatient Surgeries.	40,313	39,858	39,614	40,358	41,234
Births.	20,117	19,487	18,941	20,126	23,014
Utilization - Outpatient					
Emergency Outpatient Visits	543,272	517,995	489,718	514,299	520,941
Other Outpatient Visits.	3,807,298	3,516,106	2,672,240	2,558,653	2,419,470
Total Outpatient Visits	4,350,570	4,034,101	3,161,958	3,072,952	2,940,411
Outpatient Surgeries	81,915	84,221	73,409	68,339	70,154
Personnel					
Full Time RNs	4,651	4,334	4,103	3,898	3,739
Full Time LPNs	443	458	403	399	421
Part Time RNs.	2,418	2,341	2,245	2,119	2,641
Part Time LPNs	193	209	166	169	215
Total Full Time.	20,340	19,181	18,010	16,594	16,336
Total Part Time	8,192	8,019	7,175	6,408	7,728
Revenue - Inpatient					
Gross Inpatient Revenue.	$3,543,382,140	$3,108,970,857	$2,899,758,710	$2,707,480,791	$2,561,301,943
Revenue - Outpatient					
Gross Outpatient Revenue	$4,029,848,296	$3,623,818,467	$3,113,164,805	$2,775,500,660	$2,451,235,258
Revenue and Expenses - Totals					
(Includes Inpatient and Outpatient)					
Total Gross Revenue.	$7,573,230,436	$6,732,789,324	$6,012,923,515	$5,482,981,451	$5,012,537,201
Deductions from Revenue.	4,057,678,208	3,621,413,551	3,190,452,073	2,796,704,816	2,484,822,454
Net Patient Revenue	3,515,552,228	3,111,375,773	2,822,471,442	2,686,276,635	2,527,714,747
Other Operating Revenue	116,996,412	103,709,342	96,182,670	83,202,052	90,838,094
Other Nonoperating Revenue	17,730,950	49,967,037	47,366,046	-11,931,355	15,092,420
Total Net Revenue.	3,650,279,590	3,265,052,152	2,966,020,158	2,757,547,332	2,633,645,261
Total Expenses.	3,127,967,915	2,791,035,799	2,546,624,205	2,563,109,938	2,406,259,158
HOSPITAL UNIT (Excludes Separate Nursing Home Units)					
Utilization - Inpatient					
Beds	3,041	2,950	3,027	3,013	3,004
Admissions	122,840	127,750	129,900	127,927	134,364
Inpatient Days	536,537	503,243	525,428	518,291	553,925
Average Length of Stay.	4.4	3.9	4.0	4.1	4.1
Personnel					
Total Full Time.	20,159	18,937	17,803	16,327	16,134
Total Part Time	8,074	7,878	7,040	6,227	7,599
Revenue and Expenses - Totals					
(Includes Inpatient and Outpatient)					
Total Net Revenue.	$3,630,538,385	$3,240,672,233	$2,934,932,796	$2,730,768,774	$2,607,116,770
Total Expenses.	3,117,054,550	2,775,730,301	2,524,919,767	2,541,756,270	2,389,059,009
COMMUNITY HEALTH INDICATORS PER 1000 POPULATION					
Total Population (in thousands)	1,596	1,585	1,560	1,546	1,528
Inpatient					
Beds	2.1	2.1	2.2	2.2	2.2
Admissions	77.6	81.2	84.2	83.9	88.8
Inpatient Days	383.4	382.2	403.2	405.7	421.0
Inpatient Surgeries.	25.3	25.1	25.4	26.1	27.0
Births.	12.6	12.3	12.1	13.0	15.1
Outpatient					
Emergency Outpatient Visits	340.5	326.8	314.0	332.7	341.0
Other Outpatient Visits.	2,385.9	2,218.4	1,713.2	1,655.2	1,583.9
Total Outpatient Visits	2,726.4	2,545.2	2,027.2	1,987.9	1,925.0
Outpatient Surgeries	51.3	53.1	47.1	44.2	45.9
Expense per Capita (per person).	$1,960.2	$1,760.9	$1,632.7	$1,658.1	$1,575.3

States

TABLE 6

ILLINOIS

U.S. Registered Community Hospitals
(Nonfederal, short-term general and other special hospitals)

Overview 2008–2012

	2012	2011	2010	2009	2008
Total Community Hospitals in Illinois	188	188	189	189	191
Bed Size Category					
6-24	12	11	10	8	6
25-49	38	36	32	31	33
50-99	27	31	36	37	34
100-199	53	51	50	49	50
200-299	22	24	25	29	30
300-399	20	18	19	17	21
400-499	9	9	9	10	9
500 + ...	7	8	8	8	8
Location					
Hospitals Urban.	124	124	125	125	120
Hospitals Rural	64	64	64	64	71
Control					
State and Local Government.	24	24	26	26	26
Not for Profit	144	145	143	147	149
Investor owned	20	19	20	16	16
Physician Models					
Independent Practice Association	26	22	28	30	29
Group Practice without Walls.	8	8	4	5	8
Open Physician-Hospital Organization	46	43	43	47	41
Closed Physician-Hospital Organization	9	11	13	11	8
Management Service Organization	21	21	22	27	24
Integrated Salary Model.	63	59	62	64	61
Equity Model	3	3	2	4	3
Foundation.	8	8	13	6	7
Insurance Products					
Health Maintenance Organization	21	16	19	18	20
Preferred Provider Organization.	13	17	17	16	18
Indemnity Fee for Service	4	7	7	7	10
Managed Care Contracts					
Health Maintenance Organization	122	114	123	127	120
Preferred Provider Organization.	137	127	134	142	133
Affiliations					
Hospitals in a System.	114	113	108	104	105
Hospitals in a Network	52	43	47	47	45
Hospitals in a Group Purchasing Organization. .	145	142	157	158	149

TABLE 6

ILLINOIS

U.S. Registered Community Hospitals
(Nonfederal, short-term general and other special hospitals)

Utilization, Personnel, Revenue and Expenses, Community Health Indicators 2008–2012

	2012	2011	2010	2009	2008
TOTAL FACILITY (Includes Hospital and Nursing Home Units)					
Utilization - Inpatient					
Beds	32,662	32,775	33,310	33,856	34,506
Admissions	1,484,155	1,511,770	1,542,958	1,557,816	1,610,844
Inpatient Days	7,190,230	7,398,797	7,552,956	7,769,059	8,069,859
Average Length of Stay.	4.8	4.9	4.9	5.0	5.0
Inpatient Surgeries.	376,684	386,166	403,226	399,042	406,437
Births.	150,234	152,929	159,563	166,005	176,458
Utilization - Outpatient					
Emergency Outpatient Visits	5,422,193	5,414,964	5,366,010	5,312,763	5,123,091
Other Outpatient Visits.	27,694,668	26,277,834	27,192,086	26,780,252	25,863,666
Total Outpatient Visits	33,116,861	31,692,798	32,558,096	32,093,015	30,986,757
Outpatient Surgeries	728,808	731,909	738,783	723,461	728,072
Personnel					
Full Time RNs	44,894	42,707	41,948	39,989	39,613
Full Time LPNs	1,684	1,730	1,769	1,882	2,142
Part Time RNs.	23,656	23,563	23,493	24,237	23,785
Part Time LPNs	690	769	808	827	1,051
Total Full Time.	168,745	163,470	163,519	162,002	164,936
Total Part Time	72,684	74,154	74,448	76,241	73,769
Revenue - Inpatient					
Gross Inpatient Revenue.	$54,040,034,827	$51,831,662,656	$50,630,716,983	$48,011,580,288	$45,587,537,606
Revenue - Outpatient					
Gross Outpatient Revenue	$51,085,072,799	$45,237,976,561	$41,884,636,238	$38,198,138,940	$34,572,195,642
Revenue and Expenses - Totals					
(Includes Inpatient and Outpatient)					
Total Gross Revenue.	$105,125,107,626	$97,069,639,217	$92,515,353,221	$86,209,719,228	$80,159,733,248
Deductions from Revenue.	73,249,630,932	67,477,849,736	63,248,692,053	58,012,296,593	53,322,130,324
Net Patient Revenue	31,875,476,694	29,591,789,481	29,266,661,168	28,197,422,635	26,837,602,924
Other Operating Revenue	1,930,010,171	1,900,816,882	1,918,358,653	1,923,701,500	1,822,911,841
Other Nonoperating Revenue	597,357,110	1,093,755,704	712,723,108	-244,005,396	38,822,875
Total Net Revenue.	34,402,843,975	32,586,362,067	31,897,742,929	29,877,118,739	28,699,337,640
Total Expenses.	31,914,764,033	29,831,858,047	29,193,599,201	28,870,203,691	27,982,801,609
HOSPITAL UNIT (Excludes Separate Nursing Home Units)					
Utilization - Inpatient					
Beds	31,431	31,305	31,615	32,096	32,847
Admissions	1,471,741	1,497,436	1,526,371	1,540,936	1,597,722
Inpatient Days	6,891,159	7,012,553	7,117,426	7,294,792	7,595,924
Average Length of Stay.	4.7	4.7	4.7	4.7	4.8
Personnel					
Total Full Time.	168,056	162,704	162,567	160,793	163,669
Total Part Time	72,171	73,555	73,868	75,623	73,011
Revenue and Expenses - Totals					
(Includes Inpatient and Outpatient)					
Total Net Revenue.	$34,307,140,177	$32,474,980,131	$31,785,482,525	$29,750,884,315	$28,605,435,197
Total Expenses.	31,835,376,910	29,734,524,075	29,102,876,687	28,774,155,633	27,899,476,892
COMMUNITY HEALTH INDICATORS PER 1000 POPULATION					
Total Population (in thousands)	12,875	12,869	12,944	12,910	12,843
Inpatient					
Beds	2.5	2.5	2.6	2.6	2.7
Admissions	115.3	117.5	119.2	120.7	125.4
Inpatient Days	558.5	574.9	583.5	601.8	628.3
Inpatient Surgeries.	29.3	30.0	31.2	30.9	31.6
Births.	11.7	11.9	12.3	12.9	13.7
Outpatient					
Emergency Outpatient Visits	421.1	420.8	414.5	411.5	398.9
Other Outpatient Visits.	2,151.0	2,041.9	2,100.7	2,074.3	2,013.8
Total Outpatient Visits	2,572.1	2,462.7	2,515.2	2,485.8	2,412.7
Outpatient Surgeries	56.6	56.9	57.1	56.0	56.7
Expense per Capita (per person).	$2,478.8	$2,318.1	$2,255.3	$2,236.2	$2,178.8

TABLE 6

INDIANA

U.S. Registered Community Hospitals
(Nonfederal, short-term general and other special hospitals)

Overview 2008–2012

	2012	2011	2010	2009	2008
Total Community Hospitals in Indiana	**124**	**125**	**125**	**123**	**123**
Bed Size Category					
6-24	6	5	5	5	6
25-49	40	40	41	41	40
50-99	28	30	28	27	28
100-199	24	23	21	23	20
200-299	11	13	16	14	16
300-399	5	5	5	4	4
400-499	4	3	3	2	2
500 + ...	6	6	6	7	7
Location					
Hospitals Urban..........................	84	85	85	83	79
Hospitals Rural	40	40	40	40	44
Control					
State and Local Government................	30	30	33	34	39
Not for Profit	69	71	67	64	59
Investor owned	25	24	25	25	25
Physician Models					
Independent Practice Association	7	3	6	9	8
Group Practice without Walls...............	5	4	2	2	4
Open Physician-Hospital Organization	21	21	26	26	25
Closed Physician-Hospital Organization	8	7	8	9	9
Management Service Organization	7	8	9	9	9
Integrated Salary Model....................	58	53	55	53	49
Equity Model	3	3	2	3	2
Foundation...............................	4	2	5	7	6
Insurance Products					
Health Maintenance Organization	28	27	29	26	26
Preferred Provider Organization..............	29	30	33	27	25
Indemnity Fee for Service	9	4	6	4	5
Managed Care Contracts					
Health Maintenance Organization	64	62	65	69	64
Preferred Provider Organization..............	76	71	77	84	80
Affiliations					
Hospitals in a System.....................	85	87	85	82	79
Hospitals in a Network....................	42	45	46	44	42
Hospitals in a Group Purchasing Organization..	92	87	97	98	103

TABLE 6

INDIANA

U.S. Registered Community Hospitals
(Nonfederal, short-term general and other special hospitals)

Utilization, Personnel, Revenue and Expenses, Community Health Indicators 2008–2012

	2012	2011	2010	2009	2008
TOTAL FACILITY (Includes Hospital and Nursing Home Units)					
Utilization - Inpatient					
Beds	17,556	17,467	17,759	17,298	17,612
Admissions	731,046	737,438	718,348	713,456	732,627
Inpatient Days	3,739,056	3,724,041	3,756,021	3,687,549	3,829,835
Average Length of Stay	5.1	5.0	5.2	5.2	5.2
Inpatient Surgeries	200,708	200,907	206,124	206,101	217,917
Births	73,460	76,049	77,124	78,371	82,040
Utilization - Outpatient					
Emergency Outpatient Visits	3,207,214	3,144,973	3,185,166	3,004,721	3,041,160
Other Outpatient Visits	14,711,090	15,367,982	15,543,606	14,446,277	13,981,154
Total Outpatient Visits	17,918,304	18,512,955	18,728,772	17,450,998	17,022,314
Outpatient Surgeries	441,917	429,164	423,827	430,435	433,467
Personnel					
Full Time RNs	23,611	23,243	22,345	21,653	20,417
Full Time LPNs	1,536	1,697	1,664	1,742	2,092
Part Time RNs	14,379	13,697	14,136	13,502	14,045
Part Time LPNs	722	768	874	995	1,275
Total Full Time	88,265	87,241	86,266	86,530	83,800
Total Part Time	41,617	39,619	41,019	40,675	43,202
Revenue - Inpatient					
Gross Inpatient Revenue	$26,099,729,709	$23,724,867,721	$21,889,172,836	$19,297,952,821	$18,735,608,044
Revenue - Outpatient					
Gross Outpatient Revenue	$26,487,465,316	$23,279,155,929	$20,791,179,952	$18,451,255,529	$16,228,904,838
Revenue and Expenses - Totals					
(Includes Inpatient and Outpatient)					
Total Gross Revenue	$52,587,195,025	$47,004,023,650	$42,680,352,788	$37,749,208,350	$34,964,512,882
Deductions from Revenue	33,296,640,742	30,555,814,094	26,936,969,969	22,765,297,520	20,658,195,492
Net Patient Revenue	19,290,554,283	16,448,209,556	15,743,382,819	14,983,910,830	14,306,317,390
Other Operating Revenue	1,104,200,980	1,117,137,691	881,745,072	769,461,090	837,647,729
Other Nonoperating Revenue	439,930,085	405,284,123	434,805,381	282,345,047	-665,292,556
Total Net Revenue	20,834,685,348	17,970,631,370	17,059,933,272	16,035,716,967	14,478,672,563
Total Expenses	17,926,526,564	16,082,098,784	15,349,922,777	14,724,925,283	14,654,457,324
HOSPITAL UNIT (Excludes Separate Nursing Home Units)					
Utilization - Inpatient					
Beds	16,911	16,942	17,208	16,879	16,911
Admissions	726,693	732,496	713,224	707,886	724,499
Inpatient Days	3,569,377	3,562,156	3,584,106	3,567,515	3,612,957
Average Length of Stay	4.9	4.9	5.0	5.0	5.0
Personnel					
Total Full Time	87,873	86,943	85,948	85,900	82,933
Total Part Time	41,296	39,255	40,630	40,280	42,676
Revenue and Expenses - Totals					
(Includes Inpatient and Outpatient)					
Total Net Revenue	$20,781,574,841	$17,906,999,370	$17,017,380,655	$15,997,778,555	$14,424,793,981
Total Expenses	17,894,880,475	16,032,853,104	15,311,258,669	14,696,533,580	14,603,238,942
COMMUNITY HEALTH INDICATORS PER 1000 POPULATION					
Total Population (in thousands)	6,537	6,517	6,445	6,423	6,388
Inpatient					
Beds	2.7	2.7	2.8	2.7	2.8
Admissions	111.8	113.2	111.5	111.1	114.7
Inpatient Days	572.0	571.4	582.8	574.1	599.5
Inpatient Surgeries	30.7	30.8	32.0	32.1	34.1
Births	11.2	11.7	12.0	12.2	12.8
Outpatient					
Emergency Outpatient Visits	490.6	482.6	494.2	467.8	476.1
Other Outpatient Visits	2,250.3	2,358.2	2,411.6	2,249.1	2,188.6
Total Outpatient Visits	2,740.9	2,840.8	2,905.8	2,716.9	2,664.6
Outpatient Surgeries	67.6	65.9	65.8	67.0	67.9
Expense per Capita (per person)	$2,742.2	$2,467.7	$2,381.6	$2,292.5	$2,293.9

States

TABLE 6

IOWA

U.S. Registered Community Hospitals
(Nonfederal, short-term general and other special hospitals)

Overview 2008–2012

	2012	2011	2010	2009	2008
Total Community Hospitals in Iowa............	**118**	**118**	**118**	**118**	**118**
Bed Size Category					
6-24	19	19	18	15	13
25-49	48	48	49	51	53
50-99	26	27	27	26	26
100-199	11	10	10	12	11
200-299	6	6	6	6	6
300-399	5	5	5	5	5
400-499	1	1	1	1	2
500 + ...	2	2	2	2	2
Location					
Hospitals Urban...........................	34	34	34	34	23
Hospitals Rural	84	84	84	84	95
Control					
State and Local Government...............	59	59	59	59	59
Not for Profit	57	57	57	58	58
Investor owned	2	2	2	1	1
Physician Models					
Independent Practice Association	14	12	13	13	15
Group Practice without Walls...............	5	5	4	3	3
Open Physician-Hospital Organization	19	18	20	24	27
Closed Physician-Hospital Organization	11	11	10	10	10
Management Service Organization	8	9	8	9	12
Integrated Salary Model....................	76	74	72	70	65
Equity Model	1	1	0	0	0
Foundation...............................	3	5	4	4	6
Insurance Products					
Health Maintenance Organization	10	8	8	9	9
Preferred Provider Organization..............	12	20	23	22	20
Indemnity Fee for Service	4	5	5	6	4
Managed Care Contracts					
Health Maintenance Organization	75	74	73	71	70
Preferred Provider Organization..............	95	94	99	98	97
Affiliations					
Hospitals in a System......................	69	64	66	64	64
Hospitals in a Network	79	77	73	72	70
Hospitals in a Group Purchasing Organization..	116	115	115	112	112

TABLE 6

IOWA

U.S. Registered Community Hospitals
(Nonfederal, short-term general and other special hospitals)

Utilization, Personnel, Revenue and Expenses, Community Health Indicators 2008–2012

	2012	2011	2010	2009	2008
TOTAL FACILITY (Includes Hospital and Nursing Home Units)					
Utilization - Inpatient					
Beds	9,962	9,981	10,075	10,276	10,531
Admissions	336,765	340,412	341,744	354,534	373,330
Inpatient Days	2,022,552	2,058,730	2,058,304	2,185,446	2,248,874
Average Length of Stay	6.0	6.0	6.0	6.2	6.0
Inpatient Surgeries	84,008	83,333	87,343	92,154	101,343
Births	37,967	37,284	38,193	39,522	39,060
Utilization - Outpatient					
Emergency Outpatient Visits	1,297,129	1,273,985	1,223,271	1,230,737	1,226,568
Other Outpatient Visits	9,318,536	9,053,438	9,805,308	9,724,268	9,154,060
Total Outpatient Visits	10,615,665	10,327,423	11,028,579	10,955,005	10,380,628
Outpatient Surgeries	253,460	256,117	253,148	265,368	337,632
Personnel					
Full Time RNs	11,208	11,084	10,516	10,657	10,589
Full Time LPNs	761	788	775	814	902
Part Time RNs	6,913	6,843	6,988	7,147	7,573
Part Time LPNs	563	412	548	587	734
Total Full Time	44,797	44,535	43,589	43,659	45,177
Total Part Time	23,460	23,019	23,392	24,045	26,052
Revenue - Inpatient					
Gross Inpatient Revenue	$8,408,565,148	$7,955,026,036	$7,478,207,382	$7,402,854,971	$7,173,320,596
Revenue - Outpatient					
Gross Outpatient Revenue	$10,161,337,605	$9,276,348,064	$8,615,345,555	$7,932,610,080	$7,008,785,229
Revenue and Expenses - Totals					
(Includes Inpatient and Outpatient)					
Total Gross Revenue	$18,569,902,753	$17,231,374,100	$16,093,552,937	$15,335,465,051	$14,182,105,825
Deductions from Revenue	11,074,628,171	10,246,167,955	9,374,915,563	8,788,605,112	7,919,893,373
Net Patient Revenue	7,495,274,582	6,985,206,145	6,718,637,374	6,546,859,939	6,262,212,452
Other Operating Revenue	591,931,420	502,660,629	483,246,348	490,608,985	479,246,797
Other Nonoperating Revenue	149,767,795	223,831,009	236,093,511	9,177,812	-17,782,222
Total Net Revenue	8,236,973,797	7,711,697,783	7,437,977,233	7,046,646,736	6,723,677,027
Total Expenses	7,709,621,525	7,174,090,504	6,934,527,799	6,824,533,485	6,518,050,247
HOSPITAL UNIT (Excludes Separate Nursing Home Units)					
Utilization - Inpatient					
Beds	8,275	8,287	8,341	8,385	8,524
Admissions	332,949	336,335	337,483	348,765	365,727
Inpatient Days	1,501,406	1,533,884	1,521,829	1,602,497	1,616,630
Average Length of Stay	4.5	4.6	4.5	4.6	4.4
Personnel					
Total Full Time	44,073	43,792	42,836	42,865	44,290
Total Part Time	22,722	22,278	22,670	23,241	25,160
Revenue and Expenses - Totals					
(Includes Inpatient and Outpatient)					
Total Net Revenue	$8,147,277,912	$7,624,566,231	$7,354,382,506	$6,945,244,251	$6,614,103,911
Total Expenses	7,631,417,462	7,096,506,924	6,860,708,589	6,739,111,985	6,429,352,282
COMMUNITY HEALTH INDICATORS PER 1000 POPULATION					
Total Population (in thousands)	3,074	3,062	3,023	3,008	2,994
Inpatient					
Beds	3.2	3.3	3.3	3.4	3.5
Admissions	109.5	111.2	113.0	117.9	124.7
Inpatient Days	657.9	672.3	680.9	726.6	751.1
Inpatient Surgeries	27.3	27.2	28.9	30.6	33.8
Births	12.4	12.2	12.6	13.1	13.0
Outpatient					
Emergency Outpatient Visits	421.9	416.0	404.6	409.2	409.7
Other Outpatient Visits	3,031.2	2,956.4	3,243.5	3,233.0	3,057.5
Total Outpatient Visits	3,453.2	3,372.4	3,648.1	3,642.1	3,467.2
Outpatient Surgeries	82.4	83.6	83.7	88.2	112.8
Expense per Capita (per person)	$2,507.9	$2,342.7	$2,293.9	$2,268.9	$2,177.0

States

TABLE **6**

KANSAS

U.S. Registered Community Hospitals
(Nonfederal, short-term general and other special hospitals)

Overview 2008–2012

	2012	2011	2010	2009	2008
Total Community Hospitals in Kansas	131	132	130	133	132
Bed Size Category					
6-24	20	20	19	18	15
25-49	49	50	49	50	51
50-99	37	38	37	40	39
100-199	16	14	16	15	17
200-299	4	5	4	5	5
300-399	2	2	2	2	2
400-499	0	0	0	0	0
500 + ...	3	3	3	3	3
Location					
Hospitals Urban..........................	34	33	33	33	28
Hospitals Rural	97	99	97	100	104
Control					
State and Local Government................	61	63	62	62	62
Not for Profit	53	53	51	54	53
Investor owned	17	16	17	17	17
Physician Models					
Independent Practice Association	13	15	13	14	14
Group Practice without Walls...............	4	3	2	2	3
Open Physician-Hospital Organization	12	12	11	14	15
Closed Physician-Hospital Organization	2	1	0	2	2
Management Service Organization	2	5	3	4	4
Integrated Salary Model....................	79	77	69	71	65
Equity Model.............................	2	1	0	0	1
Foundation...............................	5	8	5	3	3
Insurance Products					
Health Maintenance Organization	2	1	1	2	5
Preferred Provider Organization..............	7	9	9	8	11
Indemnity Fee for Service	3	0	1	2	3
Managed Care Contracts					
Health Maintenance Organization	56	55	56	52	51
Preferred Provider Organization..............	112	110	109	111	112
Affiliations					
Hospitals in a System.....................	56	55	53	54	52
Hospitals in a Network....................	79	82	83	83	82
Hospitals in a Group Purchasing Organization..	128	129	128	126	126

TABLE 6

KANSAS

U.S. Registered Community Hospitals
(Nonfederal, short-term general and other special hospitals)

Utilization, Personnel, Revenue and Expenses, Community Health Indicators 2008–2012

	2012	2011	2010	2009	2008
TOTAL FACILITY (Includes Hospital and Nursing Home Units)					
Utilization - Inpatient					
Beds	10,127	10,023	9,965	10,127	10,269
Admissions	296,267	302,351	304,769	315,820	328,279
Inpatient Days	1,915,826	1,923,661	1,960,261	2,014,165	2,079,667
Average Length of Stay.	6.5	6.4	6.4	6.4	6.3
Inpatient Surgeries.	73,240	76,828	79,305	79,857	82,907
Births.	38,623	38,707	39,777	41,092	41,592
Utilization - Outpatient					
Emergency Outpatient Visits	1,114,026	1,041,234	1,019,521	1,042,407	1,028,706
Other Outpatient Visits.	6,179,011	5,955,302	5,660,293	5,687,308	5,497,497
Total Outpatient Visits	7,293,037	6,996,536	6,679,814	6,729,715	6,526,203
Outpatient Surgeries	166,253	161,889	157,746	160,653	162,784
Personnel					
Full Time RNs	11,619	10,968	10,852	10,517	9,924
Full Time LPNs	1,009	1,014	1,056	1,132	1,104
Part Time RNs.	4,917	4,533	4,535	4,550	4,448
Part Time LPNs	405	409	441	495	502
Total Full Time.	40,129	39,286	38,881	38,833	38,038
Total Part Time	14,838	14,111	14,183	14,585	14,394
Revenue - Inpatient					
Gross Inpatient Revenue.	$10,396,751,854	$9,707,362,014	$9,158,840,266	$8,857,616,660	$8,347,025,856
Revenue - Outpatient					
Gross Outpatient Revenue	$10,046,165,626	$8,606,191,704	$7,804,133,580	$7,296,946,111	$6,341,227,760
Revenue and Expenses - Totals					
(Includes Inpatient and Outpatient)					
Total Gross Revenue.	$20,442,917,480	$18,313,553,718	$16,962,973,846	$16,154,562,771	$14,688,253,616
Deductions from Revenue.	13,766,315,018	12,295,093,634	11,147,817,611	10,508,920,047	9,366,195,974
Net Patient Revenue	6,676,602,462	6,018,460,084	5,815,156,235	5,645,642,724	5,322,057,642
Other Operating Revenue	284,943,541	215,888,633	203,257,460	212,360,609	194,026,086
Other Nonoperating Revenue	160,005,906	66,106,732	128,773,371	25,755,861	33,604,548
Total Net Revenue.	7,121,551,909	6,300,455,449	6,147,187,066	5,883,759,194	5,549,688,276
Total Expenses.	6,513,729,367	5,963,380,431	5,759,373,331	5,603,169,760	5,330,135,811
HOSPITAL UNIT (Excludes Separate Nursing Home Units)					
Utilization - Inpatient					
Beds	8,568	8,495	8,338	8,418	8,435
Admissions	293,835	299,829	302,003	313,046	325,383
Inpatient Days	1,440,628	1,449,789	1,447,040	1,507,027	1,551,696
Average Length of Stay.	4.9	4.8	4.8	4.8	4.8
Personnel					
Total Full Time.	39,007	38,237	37,806	37,721	36,923
Total Part Time	14,268	13,543	13,660	13,972	13,775
Revenue and Expenses - Totals					
(Includes Inpatient and Outpatient)					
Total Net Revenue.	$7,040,162,578	$6,224,061,786	$6,068,771,082	$5,807,209,303	$5,472,326,781
Total Expenses.	6,440,417,821	5,897,756,162	5,694,269,627	5,536,264,786	5,262,852,507
COMMUNITY HEALTH INDICATORS PER 1000 POPULATION					
Total Population (in thousands)	2,886	2,871	2,841	2,819	2,797
Inpatient					
Beds	3.5	3.5	3.5	3.6	3.7
Admissions	102.7	105.3	107.3	112.0	117.4
Inpatient Days	663.9	670.0	690.0	714.6	743.4
Inpatient Surgeries.	25.4	26.8	27.9	28.3	29.6
Births.	13.4	13.5	14.0	14.6	14.9
Outpatient					
Emergency Outpatient Visits	386.0	362.6	358.8	369.8	367.7
Other Outpatient Visits.	2,141.1	2,074.1	1,992.3	2,017.7	1,965.2
Total Outpatient Visits	2,527.1	2,436.8	2,351.1	2,387.5	2,333.0
Outpatient Surgeries	57.6	56.4	55.5	57.0	58.2
Expense per Capita (per person).	$2,257.1	$2,076.9	$2,027.1	$1,987.8	$1,905.4

States

TABLE 6

KENTUCKY

U.S. Registered Community Hospitals
(Nonfederal, short-term general and other special hospitals)

Overview 2008–2012

	2012	2011	2010	2009	2008
Total Community Hospitals in Kentucky.......	106	106	106	104	105
Bed Size Category					
6-24	3	3	1	1	1
25-49	36	34	34	33	34
50-99	19	22	24	24	23
100-199	25	25	24	23	22
200-299	10	7	8	8	10
300-399	9	10	10	9	9
400-499	0	1	3	3	3
500 + ...	4	4	2	3	3
Location					
Hospitals Urban........................	43	43	43	42	35
Hospitals Rural	63	63	63	62	70
Control					
State and Local Government................	12	12	11	11	14
Not for Profit	74	74	75	73	71
Investor owned	20	20	20	20	20
Physician Models					
Independent Practice Association	6	5	5	6	7
Group Practice without Walls...............	1	0	0	2	2
Open Physician-Hospital Organization	6	7	9	12	11
Closed Physician-Hospital Organization	1	2	3	4	5
Management Service Organization	10	8	8	3	2
Integrated Salary Model...................	44	42	43	38	39
Equity Model	0	0	0	1	1
Foundation.............................	2	3	4	3	3
Insurance Products					
Health Maintenance Organization	7	7	10	5	4
Preferred Provider Organization.............	7	14	15	9	9
Indemnity Fee for Service	3	5	8	2	3
Managed Care Contracts					
Health Maintenance Organization	43	44	48	46	41
Preferred Provider Organization.............	44	53	59	57	60
Affiliations					
Hospitals in a System.....................	80	80	79	76	72
Hospitals in a Network	24	17	22	23	24
Hospitals in a Group Purchasing Organization..	74	71	80	77	82

Utilization, Personnel, Revenue and Expenses, Community Health Indicators 2008–2012

	2012	2011	2010	2009	2008
TOTAL FACILITY (Includes Hospital and Nursing Home Units)					
Utilization - Inpatient					
Beds	14,180	14,182	14,238	14,124	14,180
Admissions	572,294	599,601	608,644	597,224	610,449
Inpatient Days	2,908,461	3,061,415	3,141,502	3,113,326	3,216,149
Average Length of Stay.	5.1	5.1	5.2	5.2	5.3
Inpatient Surgeries.	166,885	170,702	173,656	173,196	176,178
Births.	53,538	49,657	53,630	50,085	54,872
Utilization - Outpatient					
Emergency Outpatient Visits	2,404,826	2,350,367	2,386,673	2,321,519	2,339,390
Other Outpatient Visits.	8,166,103	8,182,293	8,050,866	7,798,087	7,319,408
Total Outpatient Visits	10,570,929	10,532,660	10,437,539	10,119,606	9,658,798
Outpatient Surgeries	371,089	400,593	385,960	372,057	385,428
Personnel					
Full Time RNs	18,672	17,989	17,666	16,592	16,222
Full Time LPNs	1,290	1,436	1,648	1,849	1,807
Part Time RNs.	6,093	6,060	6,087	6,016	6,151
Part Time LPNs	268	343	397	419	445
Total Full Time.	64,131	64,035	63,493	61,699	61,610
Total Part Time	17,391	18,453	18,309	18,144	18,576
Revenue - Inpatient					
Gross Inpatient Revenue.	$16,779,961,324	$16,313,648,119	$15,503,184,961	$14,536,872,535	$13,943,782,950
Revenue - Outpatient					
Gross Outpatient Revenue	$16,724,256,215	$15,995,475,627	$14,305,855,765	$12,460,315,729	$11,459,995,978
Revenue and Expenses - Totals					
(Includes Inpatient and Outpatient)					
Total Gross Revenue.	$33,504,217,539	$32,309,123,746	$29,809,040,726	$26,997,188,264	$25,403,778,928
Deductions from Revenue.	22,702,995,327	22,051,533,008	19,784,508,926	17,477,244,235	16,462,600,038
Net Patient Revenue	10,801,222,212	10,257,590,738	10,024,531,800	9,519,944,029	8,941,178,890
Other Operating Revenue	406,456,390	383,110,150	338,831,936	353,366,856	309,734,161
Other Nonoperating Revenue	56,938,657	135,433,381	145,526,221	-11,001,226	-81,140,239
Total Net Revenue.	11,264,617,259	10,776,134,269	10,508,889,957	9,862,309,659	9,169,772,812
Total Expenses.	10,400,750,170	10,049,280,333	9,801,870,954	9,424,000,735	8,831,617,722
HOSPITAL UNIT (Excludes Separate Nursing Home Units)					
Utilization - Inpatient					
Beds	13,573	13,595	13,367	13,243	13,383
Admissions	564,937	592,962	602,635	591,112	603,967
Inpatient Days	2,743,755	2,886,190	2,889,658	2,843,189	2,975,158
Average Length of Stay.	4.9	4.9	4.8	4.8	4.9
Personnel					
Total Full Time.	63,588	63,514	62,730	60,717	60,776
Total Part Time	17,221	18,315	17,998	17,826	18,322
Revenue and Expenses - Totals					
(Includes Inpatient and Outpatient)					
Total Net Revenue.	$11,207,210,342	$10,690,507,752	$10,416,730,891	$9,778,913,020	$9,092,827,775
Total Expenses.	10,337,675,256	9,975,988,671	9,715,872,866	9,348,520,481	8,766,577,356
COMMUNITY HEALTH INDICATORS PER 1000 POPULATION					
Total Population (in thousands)	4,380	4,369	4,339	4,314	4,288
Inpatient					
Beds	3.2	3.2	3.3	3.3	3.3
Admissions	130.6	137.2	140.3	138.4	142.4
Inpatient Days	664.0	700.7	723.9	721.7	750.0
Inpatient Surgeries.	38.1	39.1	40.0	40.1	41.1
Births.	12.2	11.4	12.4	11.6	12.8
Outpatient					
Emergency Outpatient Visits	549.0	537.9	550.0	538.1	545.6
Other Outpatient Visits.	1,864.2	1,872.7	1,855.3	1,807.6	1,707.0
Total Outpatient Visits	2,413.2	2,410.6	2,405.3	2,345.7	2,252.6
Outpatient Surgeries	84.7	91.7	88.9	86.2	89.9
Expense per Capita (per person).	$2,374.4	$2,299.9	$2,258.8	$2,184.5	$2,059.6

States

TABLE 6

LOUISIANA

U.S. Registered Community Hospitals
(Nonfederal, short-term general and other special hospitals)

Overview 2008–2012

	2012	2011	2010	2009	2008
Total Community Hospitals in Louisiana	**124**	**127**	**126**	**128**	**130**
Bed Size Category					
6-24	17	18	18	16	19
25-49	38	40	40	39	37
50-99	25	24	22	24	22
100-199	20	19	21	26	28
200-299	10	12	12	10	9
300-399	7	8	6	5	7
400-499	4	2	3	3	5
500 + ...	3	4	4	5	3
Location					
Hospitals Urban.........................	77	77	76	77	80
Hospitals Rural	47	50	50	51	50
Control					
State and Local Government................	49	48	50	54	50
Not for Profit	38	39	38	35	38
Investor owned	37	40	38	39	42
Physician Models					
Independent Practice Association	5	7	7	9	8
Group Practice without Walls..............	3	7	6	5	4
Open Physician-Hospital Organization	10	12	12	14	14
Closed Physician-Hospital Organization	5	6	5	7	8
Management Service Organization	8	5	4	4	8
Integrated Salary Model....................	28	30	29	27	24
Equity Model	1	0	2	2	4
Foundation..............................	4	3	1	2	4
Insurance Products					
Health Maintenance Organization	6	9	8	7	9
Preferred Provider Organization..............	7	11	10	8	6
Indemnity Fee for Service	3	2	2	1	2
Managed Care Contracts					
Health Maintenance Organization	45	45	47	47	51
Preferred Provider Organization..............	51	57	57	55	61
Affiliations					
Hospitals in a System.....................	57	60	57	64	70
Hospitals in a Network....................	22	22	22	22	24
Hospitals in a Group Purchasing Organization..	62	66	71	71	72

TABLE 6

LOUISIANA

U.S. Registered Community Hospitals
(Nonfederal, short-term general and other special hospitals)

Utilization, Personnel, Revenue and Expenses, Community Health Indicators 2008–2012

	2012	2011	2010	2009	2008
TOTAL FACILITY (Includes Hospital and Nursing Home Units)					
Utilization - Inpatient					
Beds	15,204	15,342	15,421	15,857	16,007
Admissions	582,425	607,413	625,489	639,450	636,767
Inpatient Days	3,138,473	3,257,484	3,341,419	3,517,185	3,378,368
Average Length of Stay	5.4	5.4	5.3	5.5	5.3
Inpatient Surgeries	142,744	171,534	174,853	180,909	184,754
Births	60,736	54,963	61,525	71,711	67,081
Utilization - Outpatient					
Emergency Outpatient Visits	2,539,449	2,446,704	2,514,006	2,450,514	2,381,889
Other Outpatient Visits	7,011,868	7,096,563	9,840,934	9,922,624	8,779,479
Total Outpatient Visits	9,551,317	9,543,267	12,354,940	12,373,138	11,161,368
Outpatient Surgeries	253,503	277,370	283,987	279,065	278,141
Personnel					
Full Time RNs	18,885	18,529	18,458	18,666	17,187
Full Time LPNs	2,829	2,819	2,884	2,803	3,034
Part Time RNs	5,624	5,250	4,899	5,230	5,039
Part Time LPNs	728	594	628	686	773
Total Full Time	70,723	70,360	71,458	73,220	70,862
Total Part Time	17,577	15,769	15,447	16,165	15,367
Revenue - Inpatient					
Gross Inpatient Revenue	$18,651,353,386	$17,640,121,981	$17,480,238,475	$16,516,892,572	$15,609,477,577
Revenue - Outpatient					
Gross Outpatient Revenue	$15,579,961,189	$14,296,885,978	$13,195,535,770	$11,720,385,666	$10,443,222,809
Revenue and Expenses - Totals					
(Includes Inpatient and Outpatient)					
Total Gross Revenue	$34,231,314,575	$31,937,007,959	$30,675,774,245	$28,237,278,238	$26,052,700,386
Deductions from Revenue	24,308,385,152	22,487,315,530	21,158,064,386	19,280,756,846	17,411,142,732
Net Patient Revenue	9,922,929,423	9,449,692,429	9,517,709,859	8,956,521,392	8,641,557,654
Other Operating Revenue	650,768,859	727,155,809	672,891,456	549,360,404	521,425,542
Other Nonoperating Revenue	118,810,348	297,471,661	498,721,170	-74,290,469	33,327,586
Total Net Revenue	10,692,508,630	10,474,319,899	10,689,322,485	9,431,591,327	9,196,310,782
Total Expenses	10,146,975,702	9,705,109,556	9,593,366,678	9,451,348,220	9,014,212,755
HOSPITAL UNIT (Excludes Separate Nursing Home Units)					
Utilization - Inpatient					
Beds	14,552	14,874	14,721	15,199	15,323
Admissions	580,792	606,108	623,661	638,013	634,313
Inpatient Days	3,001,522	3,126,298	3,134,514	3,306,229	3,273,703
Average Length of Stay	5.2	5.2	5.0	5.2	5.2
Personnel					
Total Full Time	69,836	69,994	70,950	72,664	70,017
Total Part Time	17,416	15,644	15,241	15,946	15,147
Revenue and Expenses - Totals					
(Includes Inpatient and Outpatient)					
Total Net Revenue	$10,660,949,288	$10,452,759,116	$10,655,165,063	$9,395,699,394	$9,161,979,219
Total Expenses	10,112,917,995	9,680,765,455	9,556,204,131	9,410,102,839	8,973,038,466
COMMUNITY HEALTH INDICATORS PER 1000 POPULATION					
Total Population (in thousands)	4,602	4,575	4,529	4,492	4,452
Inpatient					
Beds	3.3	3.4	3.4	3.5	3.6
Admissions	126.6	132.8	138.1	142.4	143.0
Inpatient Days	682.0	712.0	737.7	783.0	758.9
Inpatient Surgeries	31.0	37.5	38.6	40.3	41.5
Births	13.2	12.0	13.6	16.0	15.1
Outpatient					
Emergency Outpatient Visits	551.8	534.8	555.0	545.5	535.1
Other Outpatient Visits	1,523.7	1,551.2	2,172.7	2,208.9	1,972.2
Total Outpatient Visits	2,075.5	2,086.0	2,727.7	2,754.4	2,507.3
Outpatient Surgeries	55.1	60.6	62.7	62.1	62.5
Expense per Capita (per person)	$2,205.0	$2,121.4	$2,118.0	$2,104.0	$2,025.0

States

TABLE **6**

MAINE

U.S. Registered Community Hospitals
(Nonfederal, short-term general and other special hospitals)

Overview 2008–2012

	2012	2011	2010	2009	2008
Total Community Hospitals in Maine..........	37	37	37	37	37
Bed Size Category					
6-24	2	2	2	2	2
25-49	17	16	15	16	16
50-99	8	9	10	9	9
100-199	7	7	7	7	7
200-299	1	1	1	1	1
300-399	1	1	1	1	1
400-499	0	0	0	0	0
500 + ...	1	1	1	1	1
Location					
Hospitals Urban..........................	15	15	15	15	8
Hospitals Rural	22	22	22	22	29
Control					
State and Local Government................	2	2	2	2	2
Not for Profit	34	34	34	34	34
Investor owned	1	1	1	1	1
Physician Models					
Independent Practice Association	2	3	4	4	3
Group Practice without Walls................	2	4	4	4	2
Open Physician-Hospital Organization	9	10	10	10	12
Closed Physician-Hospital Organization	3	3	4	1	0
Management Service Organization	3	4	5	5	5
Integrated Salary Model....................	22	24	24	23	20
Equity Model	1	1	1	1	1
Foundation...............................	1	1	1	1	0
Insurance Products					
Health Maintenance Organization	3	4	5	3	5
Preferred Provider Organization..............	3	4	4	3	4
Indemnity Fee for Service	0	2	3	2	2
Managed Care Contracts					
Health Maintenance Organization	21	25	23	20	21
Preferred Provider Organization..............	23	26	26	22	20
Affiliations					
Hospitals in a System.....................	20	20	20	12	14
Hospitals in a Network....................	18	19	18	18	17
Hospitals in a Group Purchasing Organization..	32	33	33	32	31

TABLE 6

MAINE

U.S. Registered Community Hospitals
(Nonfederal, short-term general and other special hospitals)

Utilization, Personnel, Revenue and Expenses, Community Health Indicators 2008–2012

	2012	2011	2010	2009	2008
TOTAL FACILITY (Includes Hospital and Nursing Home Units)					
Utilization - Inpatient					
Beds	3,523	3,557	3,571	3,583	3,504
Admissions	142,159	144,718	145,806	150,199	148,635
Inpatient Days	783,992	814,216	808,166	822,849	845,428
Average Length of Stay	5.5	5.6	5.5	5.5	5.7
Inpatient Surgeries	42,816	39,585	42,190	43,395	44,812
Births	11,224	12,434	12,874	13,146	13,489
Utilization - Outpatient					
Emergency Outpatient Visits	790,258	765,481	790,243	792,592	780,874
Other Outpatient Visits	5,387,237	5,388,213	5,174,906	4,967,837	4,312,504
Total Outpatient Visits	6,177,495	6,153,694	5,965,149	5,760,429	5,093,378
Outpatient Surgeries	117,491	123,494	137,762	115,503	130,708
Personnel					
Full Time RNs	5,229	4,999	4,813	4,909	4,707
Full Time LPNs	190	204	248	262	234
Part Time RNs	3,884	3,429	3,658	3,232	3,384
Part Time LPNs	149	132	116	153	159
Total Full Time	23,343	23,480	22,775	23,628	23,172
Total Part Time	12,446	12,998	12,597	10,590	11,058
Revenue - Inpatient					
Gross Inpatient Revenue	$3,743,957,102	$3,332,670,956	$3,184,130,431	$3,177,081,239	$3,043,869,279
Revenue - Outpatient					
Gross Outpatient Revenue	$5,068,158,029	$4,713,427,286	$4,265,543,968	$3,904,796,010	$3,446,970,975
Revenue and Expenses - Totals					
(Includes Inpatient and Outpatient)					
Total Gross Revenue	$8,812,115,131	$8,046,098,242	$7,449,674,399	$7,081,877,249	$6,490,840,254
Deductions from Revenue	4,477,604,537	3,940,954,482	3,559,422,414	3,352,561,094	2,989,235,436
Net Patient Revenue	4,334,510,594	4,105,143,760	3,890,251,985	3,729,316,155	3,501,604,818
Other Operating Revenue	257,362,641	195,118,835	106,225,360	98,806,755	93,262,738
Other Nonoperating Revenue	52,339,735	40,642,341	36,578,921	24,828,817	13,684,134
Total Net Revenue	4,644,212,970	4,340,904,936	4,033,056,266	3,852,951,727	3,608,551,690
Total Expenses	4,421,717,517	4,160,648,639	4,238,756,324	3,725,426,220	3,516,496,379
HOSPITAL UNIT (Excludes Separate Nursing Home Units)					
Utilization - Inpatient					
Beds	3,109	3,135	3,185	3,189	3,108
Admissions	141,049	143,500	144,564	148,985	147,524
Inpatient Days	645,365	669,361	673,425	685,582	712,754
Average Length of Stay	4.6	4.7	4.7	4.6	4.8
Personnel					
Total Full Time	22,538	23,121	22,465	23,103	22,480
Total Part Time	11,898	12,682	12,310	10,299	10,596
Revenue and Expenses - Totals					
(Includes Inpatient and Outpatient)					
Total Net Revenue	$4,608,434,715	$4,305,024,694	$4,000,528,653	$3,820,585,488	$3,580,910,825
Total Expenses	4,389,756,790	4,127,705,413	4,208,922,953	3,694,875,984	3,486,675,727
COMMUNITY HEALTH INDICATORS PER 1000 POPULATION					
Total Population (in thousands)	1,329	1,328	1,313	1,318	1,320
Inpatient					
Beds	2.7	2.7	2.7	2.7	2.7
Admissions	107.0	109.0	111.1	113.9	112.6
Inpatient Days	589.8	613.0	615.5	624.2	640.6
Inpatient Surgeries	32.2	29.8	32.1	32.9	34.0
Births	8.4	9.4	9.8	10.0	10.2
Outpatient					
Emergency Outpatient Visits	594.5	576.3	601.9	601.2	591.7
Other Outpatient Visits	4,053.0	4,056.8	3,941.5	3,768.4	3,267.8
Total Outpatient Visits	4,647.6	4,633.1	4,543.4	4,369.6	3,859.5
Outpatient Surgeries	88.4	93.0	104.9	87.6	99.0
Expense per Capita (per person)	$3,326.6	$3,132.6	$3,228.4	$2,825.9	$2,664.6

TABLE 6

MARYLAND

U.S. Registered Community Hospitals
(Nonfederal, short-term general and other special hospitals)

Overview 2008–2012

	2012	2011	2010	2009	2008
Total Community Hospitals in Maryland.......	50	48	47	49	50
Bed Size Category					
6-24.....................................	0	0	0	0	0
25-49...................................	3	3	2	2	2
50-99...................................	8	6	6	6	6
100-199.................................	11	14	13	13	13
200-299.................................	11	9	11	15	15
300-399.................................	9	8	9	6	8
400-499.................................	6	5	4	5	3
500 +..................................	2	3	2	2	3
Location					
Hospitals Urban.........................	44	42	41	43	41
Hospitals Rural.........................	6	6	6	6	9
Control					
State and Local Government................	0	0	0	0	0
Not for Profit.............................	48	46	45	47	48
Investor owned..........................	2	2	2	2	2
Physician Models					
Independent Practice Association............	12	8	7	5	3
Group Practice without Walls...............	8	2	3	3	3
Open Physician-Hospital Organization........	6	5	6	4	4
Closed Physician-Hospital Organization.......	9	4	1	2	2
Management Service Organization...........	14	11	10	7	6
Integrated Salary Model....................	32	29	30	29	27
Equity Model............................	4	4	3	3	4
Foundation..............................	6	6	6	4	5
Insurance Products					
Health Maintenance Organization............	16	16	16	14	12
Preferred Provider Organization.............	13	6	5	5	5
Indemnity Fee for Service..................	5	2	2	2	2
Managed Care Contracts					
Health Maintenance Organization............	31	30	32	34	36
Preferred Provider Organization.............	30	29	29	32	33
Affiliations					
Hospitals in a System.....................	35	32	30	33	32
Hospitals in a Network....................	16	16	17	17	15
Hospitals in a Group Purchasing Organization..	42	43	42	42	44

TABLE 6

MARYLAND

U.S. Registered Community Hospitals
(Nonfederal, short-term general and other special hospitals)

Utilization, Personnel, Revenue and Expenses, Community Health Indicators 2008–2012

	2012	2011	2010	2009	2008
TOTAL FACILITY (Includes Hospital and Nursing Home Units)					
Utilization - Inpatient					
Beds	12,271	11,887	11,682	11,887	12,018
Admissions	659,128	683,678	707,549	715,496	711,267
Inpatient Days	3,230,567	3,147,613	3,160,045	3,252,959	3,298,930
Average Length of Stay.	4.9	4.6	4.5	4.5	4.6
Inpatient Surgeries.	193,816	195,892	195,577	201,144	196,641
Births.	67,554	68,727	69,042	70,210	73,595
Utilization - Outpatient					
Emergency Outpatient Visits	2,552,154	2,469,637	2,460,678	2,429,724	2,282,417
Other Outpatient Visits.	7,244,174	6,301,934	5,912,927	5,864,175	5,800,698
Total Outpatient Visits	9,796,328	8,771,571	8,373,605	8,293,899	8,083,115
Outpatient Surgeries	348,264	363,469	352,770	354,443	355,489
Personnel					
Full Time RNs	19,382	18,228	17,338	16,670	16,216
Full Time LPNs	502	453	429	472	554
Part Time RNs	8,776	8,618	8,448	9,291	8,857
Part Time LPNs	241	188	185	236	271
Total Full Time.	75,558	72,370	68,011	66,942	66,471
Total Part Time	28,069	27,470	26,604	28,595	27,048
Revenue - Inpatient					
Gross Inpatient Revenue.	$11,340,693,112	$10,026,767,506	$9,444,745,728	$9,330,184,751	$8,955,048,928
Revenue - Outpatient					
Gross Outpatient Revenue	$8,221,461,005	$6,952,785,584	$5,942,458,212	$5,482,610,364	$4,920,676,123
Revenue and Expenses - Totals					
(Includes Inpatient and Outpatient)					
Total Gross Revenue.	$19,562,154,117	$16,979,553,090	$15,387,203,940	$14,812,795,115	$13,875,725,051
Deductions from Revenue	5,814,859,991	4,223,063,054	3,358,927,214	3,011,679,371	2,596,608,560
Net Patient Revenue	13,747,294,126	12,756,490,036	12,028,276,726	11,801,115,744	11,279,116,491
Other Operating Revenue	587,505,820	520,917,847	481,101,758	477,892,272	462,807,673
Other Nonoperating Revenue	16,735,289	289,518,580	134,850,598	-253,477,709	-106,798,785
Total Net Revenue.	14,351,535,235	13,566,926,463	12,644,229,082	12,025,530,307	11,635,125,379
Total Expenses.	13,808,394,036	12,730,746,066	12,132,497,694	11,898,147,143	11,389,973,159
HOSPITAL UNIT (Excludes Separate Nursing Home Units)					
Utilization - Inpatient					
Beds	11,503	11,310	11,113	11,318	11,272
Admissions	653,062	677,236	700,707	708,844	704,669
Inpatient Days	3,003,853	2,995,832	2,998,068	3,079,527	3,104,039
Average Length of Stay.	4.6	4.4	4.3	4.3	4.4
Personnel					
Total Full Time.	74,873	71,903	67,425	66,271	65,813
Total Part Time	27,724	27,194	26,242	28,247	26,682
Revenue and Expenses - Totals					
(Includes Inpatient and Outpatient)					
Total Net Revenue.	$14,246,938,190	$13,476,477,632	$12,543,530,248	$11,912,050,531	$11,517,892,326
Total Expenses.	13,710,327,354	12,629,434,037	12,026,632,893	11,787,009,932	11,280,192,702
COMMUNITY HEALTH INDICATORS PER 1000 POPULATION					
Total Population (in thousands)	5,885	5,828	5,737	5,699	5,659
Inpatient					
Beds	2.1	2.0	2.0	2.1	2.1
Admissions	112.0	117.3	123.3	125.5	125.7
Inpatient Days	549.0	540.1	550.8	570.7	583.0
Inpatient Surgeries.	32.9	33.6	34.1	35.3	34.8
Births.	11.5	11.8	12.0	12.3	13.0
Outpatient					
Emergency Outpatient Visits	433.7	423.7	428.9	426.3	403.3
Other Outpatient Visits.	1,231.0	1,081.3	1,030.6	1,028.9	1,025.1
Total Outpatient Visits	1,664.8	1,505.0	1,459.5	1,455.2	1,428.5
Outpatient Surgeries	59.2	62.4	61.5	62.2	62.8
Expense per Capita (per person).	$2,346.5	$2,184.3	$2,114.7	$2,087.6	$2,012.8

States

TABLE 6

MASSACHUSETTS

U.S. Registered Community Hospitals
(Nonfederal, short-term general and other special hospitals)

Overview 2008–2012

	2012	2011	2010	2009	2008
Total Community Hospitals in Massachusetts..	83	79	79	78	75
Bed Size Category					
6-24	5	5	6	6	6
25-49	8	8	8	8	7
50-99	19	13	10	12	11
100-199	22	24	29	25	22
200-299	14	15	12	11	11
300-399	7	7	6	8	9
400-499	2	1	1	1	2
500 +...................................	6	6	7	7	7
Location					
Hospitals Urban...........................	81	77	77	76	63
Hospitals Rural	2	2	2	2	12
Control					
State and Local Government................	3	1	1	2	2
Not for Profit	61	65	67	68	65
Investor owned	19	13	11	8	8
Physician Models					
Independent Practice Association	17	20	26	22	21
Group Practice without Walls................	2	2	3	2	2
Open Physician-Hospital Organization	18	20	19	17	15
Closed Physician-Hospital Organization	5	5	7	7	6
Management Service Organization	9	11	12	9	10
Integrated Salary Model....................	31	32	35	32	30
Equity Model	1	2	2	4	4
Foundation...............................	3	4	5	6	4
Insurance Products					
Health Maintenance Organization	9	11	9	8	6
Preferred Provider Organization..............	4	8	5	5	3
Indemnity Fee for Service	2	5	3	2	1
Managed Care Contracts					
Health Maintenance Organization	47	56	59	52	48
Preferred Provider Organization..............	45	51	55	51	45
Affiliations					
Hospitals in a System......................	51	46	43	41	39
Hospitals in a Network.....................	24	27	25	20	22
Hospitals in a Group Purchasing Organization..	50	55	62	55	58

TABLE 6

MASSACHUSETTS

U.S. Registered Community Hospitals
(Nonfederal, short-term general and other special hospitals)

Utilization, Personnel, Revenue and Expenses, Community Health Indicators 2008–2012

	2012	2011	2010	2009	2008
TOTAL FACILITY (Includes Hospital and Nursing Home Units)					
Utilization - Inpatient					
Beds	16,233	15,865	15,694	15,483	15,710
Admissions	802,312	838,080	823,246	819,625	808,489
Inpatient Days	4,130,110	4,168,038	4,164,008	4,187,076	4,190,441
Average Length of Stay.	5.1	5.0	5.1	5.1	5.2
Inpatient Surgeries.	197,450	205,653	209,277	213,059	216,569
Births.	70,702	72,707	72,306	73,363	77,002
Utilization - Outpatient					
Emergency Outpatient Visits	3,164,871	3,092,821	3,153,290	3,116,535	3,119,580
Other Outpatient Visits.	19,349,547	19,206,984	18,597,755	18,237,800	17,340,178
Total Outpatient Visits	22,514,418	22,299,805	21,751,045	21,354,335	20,459,758
Outpatient Surgeries	421,694	418,519	471,811	446,779	451,925
Personnel					
Full Time RNs	21,137	21,636	20,665	20,920	20,635
Full Time LPNs	868	827	797	825	857
Part Time RNs.	22,948	23,007	22,332	21,508	21,666
Part Time LPNs	708	686	707	745	814
Total Full Time.	113,291	114,923	112,453	112,122	108,893
Total Part Time	69,520	69,916	67,465	64,882	64,047
Revenue - Inpatient					
Gross Inpatient Revenue.	$25,212,735,967	$23,543,488,752	$22,838,917,130	$22,083,175,335	$21,768,649,075
Revenue - Outpatient					
Gross Outpatient Revenue	$28,198,949,623	$26,601,731,821	$26,120,785,816	$24,897,792,185	$22,264,309,254
Revenue and Expenses - Totals					
(Includes Inpatient and Outpatient)					
Total Gross Revenue.	$53,411,685,590	$50,145,220,573	$48,959,702,946	$46,980,967,520	$44,032,958,329
Deductions from Revenue.	31,738,657,662	29,585,822,724	28,469,292,992	27,289,257,271	25,449,205,856
Net Patient Revenue	21,673,027,928	20,559,397,849	20,490,409,954	19,691,710,249	18,583,752,473
Other Operating Revenue	3,570,796,587	3,539,011,217	3,161,300,000	3,056,380,254	2,794,111,079
Other Nonoperating Revenue	158,781,349	59,227,576	180,218,312	-134,832,543	-71,544,749
Total Net Revenue.	25,402,605,864	24,157,636,642	23,831,928,266	22,613,257,960	21,306,318,803
Total Expenses.	24,080,576,139	23,068,835,920	22,819,002,547	22,049,297,978	20,772,347,640
HOSPITAL UNIT (Excludes Separate Nursing Home Units)					
Utilization - Inpatient					
Beds	16,204	15,836	15,569	15,374	15,586
Admissions	801,583	837,325	820,368	817,254	805,960
Inpatient Days	4,121,270	4,158,948	4,125,806	4,153,746	4,156,756
Average Length of Stay.	5.1	5.0	5.0	5.1	5.2
Personnel					
Total Full Time.	113,273	114,916	112,401	112,051	108,805
Total Part Time	69,452	69,898	67,389	64,777	63,855
Revenue and Expenses - Totals					
(Includes Inpatient and Outpatient)					
Total Net Revenue.	$25,397,992,218	$24,152,583,333	$23,814,188,986	$22,595,437,262	$21,279,253,160
Total Expenses.	24,075,430,900	23,064,002,066	22,805,667,399	22,031,539,336	20,753,005,237
COMMUNITY HEALTH INDICATORS PER 1000 POPULATION					
Total Population (in thousands)	6,646	6,588	6,631	6,594	6,544
Inpatient					
Beds	2.4	2.4	2.4	2.3	2.4
Admissions	120.7	127.2	124.1	124.3	123.6
Inpatient Days	621.4	632.7	627.9	635.0	640.4
Inpatient Surgeries.	29.7	31.2	31.6	32.3	33.1
Births.	10.6	11.0	10.9	11.1	11.8
Outpatient					
Emergency Outpatient Visits	476.2	469.5	475.5	472.7	476.7
Other Outpatient Visits.	2,911.4	2,915.7	2,804.5	2,766.0	2,649.9
Total Outpatient Visits	3,387.6	3,385.2	3,280.1	3,238.7	3,126.7
Outpatient Surgeries	63.4	63.5	71.1	67.8	69.1
Expense per Capita (per person).	$3,623.2	$3,501.9	$3,441.1	$3,344.1	$3,174.5

States

TABLE **6**

MICHIGAN

U.S. Registered Community Hospitals
(Nonfederal, short-term general and other special hospitals)

Overview 2008–2012

	2012	2011	2010	2009	2008
Total Community Hospitals in Michigan.......	151	153	156	158	153
Bed Size Category					
6-24	12	12	12	11	9
25-49	46	45	44	42	40
50-99	29	30	35	38	39
100-199	20	19	18	21	20
200-299	15	18	18	17	15
300-399	11	14	15	14	14
400-499	7	5	3	4	6
500 + ...	11	10	11	11	10
Location					
Hospitals Urban...........................	93	95	97	99	95
Hospitals Rural	58	58	59	59	58
Control					
State and Local Government................	15	14	14	15	15
Not for Profit	114	119	125	126	123
Investor owned	22	20	17	17	15
Physician Models					
Independent Practice Association	14	18	15	15	13
Group Practice without Walls................	8	9	9	5	5
Open Physician-Hospital Organization	45	45	39	41	41
Closed Physician-Hospital Organization	11	15	17	13	14
Management Service Organization	16	18	19	15	12
Integrated Salary Model....................	85	83	86	88	85
Equity Model............................	1	1	0	0	0
Foundation.............................	6	8	8	9	7
Insurance Products					
Health Maintenance Organization	38	39	41	44	40
Preferred Provider Organization..............	27	39	41	45	42
Indemnity Fee for Service	10	14	13	17	16
Managed Care Contracts					
Health Maintenance Organization	102	106	114	120	117
Preferred Provider Organization..............	104	110	119	124	123
Affiliations					
Hospitals in a System.....................	96	96	96	96	89
Hospitals in a Network	62	65	70	72	71
Hospitals in a Group Purchasing Organization..	119	121	127	130	132

TABLE 6

MICHIGAN

U.S. Registered Community Hospitals
(Nonfederal, short-term general and other special hospitals)

Utilization, Personnel, Revenue and Expenses, Community Health Indicators 2008–2012

	2012	2011	2010	2009	2008
TOTAL FACILITY (Includes Hospital and Nursing Home Units)					
Utilization - Inpatient					
Beds	25,100	25,351	25,623	25,863	25,272
Admissions	1,182,541	1,191,236	1,207,546	1,219,893	1,221,970
Inpatient Days	6,037,474	6,173,528	6,214,588	6,332,816	6,350,025
Average Length of Stay............	5.1	5.2	5.1	5.2	5.2
Inpatient Surgeries...............	325,219	342,090	355,358	359,169	370,118
Births..........................	106,525	107,031	111,192	113,883	118,965
Utilization - Outpatient					
Emergency Outpatient Visits........	4,781,685	4,675,863	4,550,617	4,538,588	4,428,070
Other Outpatient Visits.............	28,037,761	26,307,833	25,699,720	24,759,189	23,570,226
Total Outpatient Visits	32,819,446	30,983,696	30,250,337	29,297,777	27,998,296
Outpatient Surgeries	678,329	656,318	704,866	694,079	707,236
Personnel					
Full Time RNs	38,759	37,356	36,166	34,530	33,536
Full Time LPNs	1,270	1,255	1,377	1,591	1,770
Part Time RNs...................	19,313	18,736	18,803	18,878	18,989
Part Time LPNs	748	810	916	949	1,156
Total Full Time...................	146,597	143,186	144,577	141,897	139,918
Total Part Time	63,422	63,510	64,909	65,113	65,331
Revenue - Inpatient					
Gross Inpatient Revenue...........	$34,248,317,962	$33,127,653,060	$32,307,141,469	$31,376,243,717	$29,869,338,749
Revenue - Outpatient					
Gross Outpatient Revenue	$34,632,987,398	$31,983,063,304	$30,177,541,390	$28,205,271,055	$26,487,242,565
Revenue and Expenses - Totals					
(Includes Inpatient and Outpatient)					
Total Gross Revenue..............	$68,881,305,360	$65,110,716,364	$62,484,682,859	$59,581,514,772	$56,356,581,314
Deductions from Revenue..........	41,938,126,634	40,060,740,730	38,000,334,594	35,829,939,127	33,607,413,797
Net Patient Revenue	26,943,178,726	25,049,975,634	24,484,348,265	23,751,575,645	22,749,167,517
Other Operating Revenue	1,306,714,292	1,133,933,341	1,105,518,315	1,092,750,061	1,094,570,561
Other Nonoperating Revenue	242,121,301	626,908,309	555,064,648	-550,883,455	-268,360,656
Total Net Revenue................	28,492,014,319	26,810,817,284	26,144,931,228	24,293,442,251	23,575,377,422
Total Expenses..................	27,293,081,777	25,328,136,970	24,872,817,460	24,366,675,781	23,392,920,738
HOSPITAL UNIT (Excludes Separate Nursing Home Units)					
Utilization - Inpatient					
Beds	23,759	24,256	24,243	24,499	23,838
Admissions	1,177,789	1,187,933	1,203,343	1,215,211	1,217,600
Inpatient Days	5,600,603	5,802,388	5,761,918	5,877,775	5,868,107
Average Length of Stay............	4.8	4.9	4.8	4.8	4.8
Personnel					
Total Full Time...................	145,517	142,322	143,514	140,743	138,950
Total Part Time	62,504	62,695	64,019	64,048	64,550
Revenue and Expenses - Totals					
(Includes Inpatient and Outpatient)					
Total Net Revenue................	$28,374,005,103	$26,702,789,590	$26,022,486,264	$24,172,162,834	$23,455,611,994
Total Expenses..................	27,190,001,432	25,261,120,163	24,753,757,439	24,287,466,409	23,316,518,420
COMMUNITY HEALTH INDICATORS PER 1000 POPULATION					
Total Population (in thousands)	9,883	9,876	9,931	9,970	10,002
Inpatient					
Beds	2.5	2.6	2.6	2.6	2.5
Admissions	119.6	120.6	121.6	122.4	122.2
Inpatient Days	610.9	625.1	625.8	635.2	634.8
Inpatient Surgeries...............	32.9	34.6	35.8	36.0	37.0
Births..........................	10.8	10.8	11.2	11.4	11.9
Outpatient					
Emergency Outpatient Visits........	483.8	473.4	458.2	455.2	442.7
Other Outpatient Visits.............	2,836.9	2,663.8	2,587.8	2,483.4	2,356.4
Total Outpatient Visits	3,320.7	3,137.2	3,046.0	2,938.7	2,799.1
Outpatient Surgeries	68.6	66.5	71.0	69.6	70.7
Expense per Capita (per person).....	$2,761.5	$2,564.6	$2,504.5	$2,444.1	$2,338.7

States

TABLE 6

MINNESOTA

U.S. Registered Community Hospitals
(Nonfederal, short-term general and other special hospitals)

Overview 2008–2012

	2012	2011	2010	2009	2008
Total Community Hospitals in Minnesota......	133	132	133	132	130
Bed Size Category					
6-24	21	23	19	19	17
25-49	32	29	29	26	25
50-99	37	34	38	37	37
100-199	26	29	30	34	35
200-299	4	4	5	4	4
300-399	7	6	5	4	4
400-499	3	4	4	5	5
500 + ...	3	3	3	3	3
Location					
Hospitals Urban..........................	51	51	51	50	46
Hospitals Rural	82	81	82	82	84
Control					
State and Local Government................	37	38	36	38	37
Not for Profit	95	93	96	93	93
Investor owned	1	1	1	1	0
Physician Models					
Independent Practice Association	10	10	18	20	20
Group Practice without Walls................	2	2	3	4	2
Open Physician-Hospital Organization	8	8	9	10	11
Closed Physician-Hospital Organization	2	3	3	3	3
Management Service Organization	2	1	1	1	2
Integrated Salary Model....................	56	52	49	52	47
Equity Model.............................	0	1	0	1	1
Foundation...............................	1	2	1	1	2
Insurance Products					
Health Maintenance Organization	19	15	14	11	9
Preferred Provider Organization..............	19	16	15	13	14
Indemnity Fee for Service	5	6	6	3	4
Managed Care Contracts					
Health Maintenance Organization	44	47	46	54	51
Preferred Provider Organization..............	49	53	52	57	55
Affiliations					
Hospitals in a System.....................	82	78	77	73	69
Hospitals in a Network.....................	30	29	27	22	24
Hospitals in a Group Purchasing Organization..	90	90	90	93	91

TABLE **6**

MINNESOTA

U.S. Registered Community Hospitals
(Nonfederal, short-term general and other special hospitals)

Utilization, Personnel, Revenue and Expenses, Community Health Indicators 2008–2012

	2012	2011	2010	2009	2008
TOTAL FACILITY (Includes Hospital and Nursing Home Units)					
Utilization - Inpatient					
Beds	14,895	14,985	15,346	15,589	15,621
Admissions	583,142	596,199	591,919	623,504	640,976
Inpatient Days	3,479,304	3,592,914	3,596,879	3,726,573	3,873,690
Average Length of Stay	6.0	6.0	6.1	6.0	6.0
Inpatient Surgeries	166,285	178,802	177,600	186,593	186,775
Births	64,001	64,004	62,885	67,064	69,360
Utilization - Outpatient					
Emergency Outpatient Visits	1,898,093	1,928,364	1,832,257	1,873,419	1,772,982
Other Outpatient Visits	9,532,070	8,863,642	9,232,626	8,906,635	8,233,087
Total Outpatient Visits	11,430,163	10,792,006	11,064,883	10,780,054	10,006,069
Outpatient Surgeries	302,985	315,819	303,839	311,336	294,628
Personnel					
Full Time RNs	11,693	11,275	11,163	9,976	9,744
Full Time LPNs	1,538	1,491	1,467	1,361	1,365
Part Time RNs	20,586	20,434	21,198	22,208	22,355
Part Time LPNs	1,524	1,716	1,767	1,862	2,031
Total Full Time	62,967	58,426	56,863	51,952	51,432
Total Part Time	57,938	58,167	62,186	64,411	64,764
Revenue - Inpatient					
Gross Inpatient Revenue	$19,494,970,283	$19,485,000,173	$18,410,175,974	$17,936,453,916	$17,008,252,322
Revenue - Outpatient					
Gross Outpatient Revenue	$17,426,213,830	$16,843,850,432	$15,401,043,442	$13,869,730,845	$12,005,677,625
Revenue and Expenses - Totals					
(Includes Inpatient and Outpatient)					
Total Gross Revenue	$36,921,184,113	$36,328,850,605	$33,811,219,416	$31,806,184,761	$29,013,929,947
Deductions from Revenue	21,566,323,331	21,780,756,415	20,208,906,364	18,729,750,687	16,742,727,027
Net Patient Revenue	15,354,860,782	14,548,094,190	13,602,313,052	13,076,434,074	12,271,202,920
Other Operating Revenue	736,968,011	673,017,078	627,863,165	654,722,103	615,406,723
Other Nonoperating Revenue	105,178,701	265,096,109	222,331,201	35,427,093	-172,569,600
Total Net Revenue	16,197,007,494	15,486,207,377	14,452,507,418	13,766,583,270	12,714,040,043
Total Expenses	15,069,347,845	14,474,689,902	13,507,569,053	12,894,812,345	12,401,406,555
HOSPITAL UNIT (Excludes Separate Nursing Home Units)					
Utilization - Inpatient					
Beds	12,798	12,651	13,128	13,443	12,837
Admissions	579,267	592,372	588,566	620,484	637,183
Inpatient Days	2,790,444	2,813,323	2,835,161	2,987,272	2,943,441
Average Length of Stay	4.8	4.7	4.8	4.8	4.6
Personnel					
Total Full Time	61,780	57,414	55,794	51,026	50,078
Total Part Time	56,197	56,546	60,461	62,837	62,661
Revenue and Expenses - Totals					
(Includes Inpatient and Outpatient)					
Total Net Revenue	$16,055,142,778	$15,260,507,840	$14,309,968,863	$13,627,368,247	$12,531,828,490
Total Expenses	14,927,729,599	14,318,110,391	13,362,374,519	12,751,881,151	12,221,469,706
COMMUNITY HEALTH INDICATORS PER 1000 POPULATION					
Total Population (in thousands)	5,379	5,345	5,290	5,266	5,231
Inpatient					
Beds	2.8	2.8	2.9	3.0	3.0
Admissions	108.4	111.5	111.9	118.4	122.5
Inpatient Days	646.8	672.2	679.9	707.6	740.6
Inpatient Surgeries	30.9	33.5	33.6	35.4	35.7
Births	11.9	12.0	11.9	12.7	13.3
Outpatient					
Emergency Outpatient Visits	352.9	360.8	346.3	355.7	339.0
Other Outpatient Visits	1,772.0	1,658.3	1,745.2	1,691.3	1,574.0
Total Outpatient Visits	2,124.9	2,019.1	2,091.5	2,047.0	1,913.0
Outpatient Surgeries	56.3	59.1	57.4	59.1	56.3
Expense per Capita (per person)	$2,801.4	$2,708.2	$2,553.2	$2,448.6	$2,370.9

States

TABLE 6

MISSISSIPPI

U.S. Registered Community Hospitals
(Nonfederal, short-term general and other special hospitals)

Overview 2008–2012

	2012	2011	2010	2009	2008
Total Community Hospitals in Mississippi	98	99	96	97	98
Bed Size Category					
6-24	2	3	2	2	2
25-49	32	32	32	32	31
50-99	24	23	22	24	25
100-199	23	24	23	23	23
200-299	8	8	6	5	6
300-399	2	2	3	3	3
400-499	3	3	3	3	3
500 + ...	4	4	5	5	5
Location					
Hospitals Urban	28	29	29	28	22
Hospitals Rural	70	70	67	69	76
Control					
State and Local Government	40	40	41	40	41
Not for Profit	29	29	27	28	30
Investor owned	29	30	28	29	27
Physician Models					
Independent Practice Association	5	5	5	5	6
Group Practice without Walls	2	2	2	3	2
Open Physician-Hospital Organization	16	18	16	15	16
Closed Physician-Hospital Organization	3	1	2	3	5
Management Service Organization	9	11	8	8	7
Integrated Salary Model	26	27	22	22	22
Equity Model	2	1	1	2	1
Foundation	7	10	7	8	6
Insurance Products					
Health Maintenance Organization	8	7	7	6	8
Preferred Provider Organization	36	37	35	36	38
Indemnity Fee for Service	9	9	9	10	12
Managed Care Contracts					
Health Maintenance Organization	26	18	14	15	14
Preferred Provider Organization	45	38	33	30	37
Affiliations					
Hospitals in a System	47	48	45	43	42
Hospitals in a Network	26	28	29	30	30
Hospitals in a Group Purchasing Organization . .	0	0	0	0	1

States

TABLE **6**

MISSISSIPPI

U.S. Registered Community Hospitals
(Nonfederal, short-term general and other special hospitals)

Utilization, Personnel, Revenue and Expenses, Community Health Indicators 2008–2012

	2012	2011	2010	2009	2008
TOTAL FACILITY (Includes Hospital and Nursing Home Units)					
Utilization - Inpatient					
Beds	12,882	12,867	12,925	12,879	13,094
Admissions	384,078	393,566	402,947	412,912	430,680
Inpatient Days	2,505,846	2,513,957	2,557,704	2,600,075	2,807,964
Average Length of Stay.	6.5	6.4	6.3	6.3	6.5
Inpatient Surgeries.	104,043	102,170	107,497	114,231	113,847
Births.	37,565	38,046	39,044	41,266	43,775
Utilization - Outpatient					
Emergency Outpatient Visits	1,767,684	1,761,207	1,705,959	1,720,780	1,694,645
Other Outpatient Visits.	3,321,143	3,015,093	2,880,177	2,964,042	3,320,962
Total Outpatient Visits	5,088,827	4,776,300	4,586,136	4,684,822	5,015,607
Outpatient Surgeries	169,096	169,856	174,969	172,105	173,799
Personnel					
Full Time RNs	12,179	12,842	12,176	11,847	11,143
Full Time LPNs	1,437	1,475	1,570	1,651	1,726
Part Time RNs	3,784	3,346	3,489	3,543	3,757
Part Time LPNs	339	290	344	423	487
Total Full Time.	46,695	48,461	46,910	46,451	46,424
Total Part Time	11,755	10,875	11,258	11,656	12,158
Revenue - Inpatient					
Gross Inpatient Revenue.	$12,982,460,621	$10,947,704,087	$10,614,195,531	$11,045,652,557	$11,036,455,713
Revenue - Outpatient					
Gross Outpatient Revenue	$11,618,451,746	$9,159,843,292	$8,108,639,171	$8,571,533,053	$7,520,162,560
Revenue and Expenses - Totals					
(Includes Inpatient and Outpatient)					
Total Gross Revenue.	$24,600,912,367	$20,107,547,379	$18,722,834,702	$19,617,185,610	$18,556,618,273
Deductions from Revenue.	17,485,118,401	14,441,074,648	13,026,769,588	13,518,559,893	12,632,981,913
Net Patient Revenue	7,115,793,966	5,666,472,731	5,696,065,114	6,098,625,717	5,923,636,360
Other Operating Revenue	336,578,667	284,527,695	332,166,296	279,046,585	319,430,782
Other Nonoperating Revenue	124,396,684	62,903,487	101,837,598	76,839,630	36,224,687
Total Net Revenue.	7,576,769,317	6,013,903,913	6,130,069,008	6,454,511,932	6,279,291,829
Total Expenses.	6,982,689,683	5,804,948,349	5,635,912,981	6,071,620,664	5,817,368,267
HOSPITAL UNIT (Excludes Separate Nursing Home Units)					
Utilization - Inpatient					
Beds	11,102	11,142	11,260	11,196	11,401
Admissions	383,020	392,650	402,148	412,159	429,960
Inpatient Days	1,906,203	1,948,010	2,004,002	2,048,068	2,233,999
Average Length of Stay.	5.0	5.0	5.0	5.0	5.2
Personnel					
Total Full Time.	45,222	47,168	45,658	45,069	45,125
Total Part Time	11,330	10,502	10,899	11,336	11,832
Revenue and Expenses - Totals					
(Includes Inpatient and Outpatient)					
Total Net Revenue.	$7,501,877,310	$5,924,570,004	$6,056,564,286	$6,377,178,448	$6,211,348,322
Total Expenses.	6,920,499,818	5,744,275,169	5,576,805,214	6,011,102,605	5,767,228,058
COMMUNITY HEALTH INDICATORS PER 1000 POPULATION					
Total Population (in thousands)	2,985	2,979	2,960	2,952	2,940
Inpatient					
Beds	4.3	4.3	4.4	4.4	4.5
Admissions	128.7	132.1	136.1	139.9	146.5
Inpatient Days	839.5	844.0	864.0	880.8	955.0
Inpatient Surgeries.	34.9	34.3	36.3	38.7	38.7
Births.	12.6	12.8	13.2	14.0	14.9
Outpatient					
Emergency Outpatient Visits	592.2	591.3	576.2	582.9	576.4
Other Outpatient Visits.	1,112.6	1,012.3	972.9	1,004.1	1,129.5
Total Outpatient Visits	1,704.8	1,603.6	1,549.1	1,587.0	1,705.9
Outpatient Surgeries	56.6	57.0	59.1	58.3	59.1
Expense per Capita (per person).	$2,339.3	$1,948.9	$1,903.7	$2,056.8	$1,978.6

TABLE **6**

MISSOURI

U.S. Registered Community Hospitals
(Nonfederal, short-term general and other special hospitals)

Overview 2008–2012

	2012	2011	2010	2009	2008
Total Community Hospitals in Missouri	**123**	**120**	**122**	**125**	**123**
Bed Size Category					
6-24	9	8	7	8	8
25-49	39	40	41	39	38
50-99	20	19	21	22	19
100-199	25	21	22	24	26
200-299	11	12	11	12	12
300-399	7	9	11	9	9
400-499	6	5	3	5	5
500 + ...	6	6	6	6	6
Location					
Hospitals Urban..........................	70	67	69	72	64
Hospitals Rural	53	53	53	53	59
Control					
State and Local Government................	34	35	35	35	35
Not for Profit	64	63	64	64	62
Investor owned	25	22	23	26	26
Physician Models					
Independent Practice Association	8	6	8	8	10
Group Practice without Walls...............	0	0	0	0	0
Open Physician-Hospital Organization	15	15	14	15	14
Closed Physician-Hospital Organization	6	7	8	8	8
Management Service Organization	0	0	1	1	2
Integrated Salary Model....................	66	66	67	69	66
Equity Model	1	1	1	1	1
Foundation...............................	2	2	4	2	3
Insurance Products					
Health Maintenance Organization	11	16	16	15	16
Preferred Provider Organization..............	10	14	14	13	14
Indemnity Fee for Service	2	5	4	4	5
Managed Care Contracts					
Health Maintenance Organization	99	93	95	99	97
Preferred Provider Organization..............	105	101	103	107	106
Affiliations					
Hospitals in a System.....................	77	70	72	73	72
Hospitals in a Network....................	38	36	37	38	38
Hospitals in a Group Purchasing Organization..	121	116	114	115	115

TABLE 6

MISSOURI

U.S. Registered Community Hospitals
(Nonfederal, short-term general and other special hospitals)

Utilization, Personnel, Revenue and Expenses, Community Health Indicators 2008–2012

	2012	2011	2010	2009	2008
TOTAL FACILITY (Includes Hospital and Nursing Home Units)					
Utilization - Inpatient					
Beds	19,032	18,749	18,745	19,101	18,968
Admissions	799,256	815,640	821,322	825,090	841,118
Inpatient Days	4,120,318	4,172,415	4,196,865	4,256,929	4,396,779
Average Length of Stay.	5.2	5.1	5.1	5.2	5.2
Inpatient Surgeries.	206,215	210,625	213,685	219,835	222,378
Births.	75,301	73,779	74,903	77,799	80,282
Utilization - Outpatient					
Emergency Outpatient Visits.	3,042,008	2,952,675	2,871,884	2,894,040	2,860,410
Other Outpatient Visits.	18,024,433	17,251,450	16,929,041	16,319,944	15,968,175
Total Outpatient Visits	21,066,441	20,204,125	19,800,925	19,213,984	18,828,585
Outpatient Surgeries	382,699	370,574	374,120	382,232	377,592
Personnel					
Full Time RNs	27,597	27,023	26,334	25,768	24,084
Full Time LPNs	2,375	2,407	2,398	2,508	2,711
Part Time RNs.	12,913	11,436	11,453	12,399	12,367
Part Time LPNs	664	654	719	826	837
Total Full Time.	102,089	101,030	100,265	98,635	96,722
Total Part Time	38,730	35,841	36,219	37,004	36,336
Revenue - Inpatient					
Gross Inpatient Revenue.	$27,122,625,962	$25,816,258,642	$24,578,843,364	$23,360,022,165	$22,713,673,771
Revenue - Outpatient					
Gross Outpatient Revenue	$26,031,861,914	$23,228,488,113	$20,597,557,308	$19,480,819,585	$17,415,385,697
Revenue and Expenses - Totals					
(Includes Inpatient and Outpatient)					
Total Gross Revenue.	$53,154,487,876	$49,044,746,755	$45,176,400,672	$42,840,841,750	$40,129,059,468
Deductions from Revenue	35,362,416,605	32,241,337,674	28,944,744,487	27,014,970,190	24,102,018,264
Net Patient Revenue	17,792,071,271	16,803,409,081	16,231,656,185	15,825,871,560	16,027,041,204
Other Operating Revenue	1,281,736,177	999,246,088	1,085,534,981	875,169,162	985,155,809
Other Nonoperating Revenue	794,602,472	214,485,919	529,984,875	522,159,166	-360,477,386
Total Net Revenue.	19,868,409,920	18,017,141,088	17,847,176,041	17,223,199,888	16,651,719,627
Total Expenses.	17,024,103,374	17,172,219,045	16,521,828,978	16,235,293,324	15,824,162,545
HOSPITAL UNIT (Excludes Separate Nursing Home Units)					
Utilization - Inpatient					
Beds	18,035	17,772	17,754	18,188	17,970
Admissions	793,155	809,450	816,764	818,739	834,653
Inpatient Days	3,822,166	3,892,314	3,946,461	3,999,089	4,109,631
Average Length of Stay.	4.8	4.8	4.8	4.9	4.9
Personnel					
Total Full Time.	101,135	100,248	99,631	97,598	96,023
Total Part Time	38,172	35,394	35,866	36,601	35,963
Revenue and Expenses - Totals					
(Includes Inpatient and Outpatient)					
Total Net Revenue.	$19,777,379,107	$17,938,622,213	$17,771,368,041	$17,122,754,301	$16,539,007,342
Total Expenses.	16,948,096,420	17,109,487,583	16,444,776,729	16,149,196,359	15,727,570,466
COMMUNITY HEALTH INDICATORS PER 1000 POPULATION					
Total Population (in thousands)	6,022	6,011	6,012	5,988	5,956
Inpatient					
Beds	3.2	3.1	3.1	3.2	3.2
Admissions	132.7	135.7	136.6	137.8	141.2
Inpatient Days	684.2	694.2	698.1	711.0	738.2
Inpatient Surgeries.	34.2	35.0	35.5	36.7	37.3
Births.	12.5	12.3	12.5	13.0	13.5
Outpatient					
Emergency Outpatient Visits	505.2	491.2	477.7	483.3	480.2
Other Outpatient Visits.	2,993.1	2,870.1	2,816.0	2,725.6	2,680.9
Total Outpatient Visits	3,498.3	3,361.4	3,293.7	3,209.0	3,161.1
Outpatient Surgeries	63.6	61.7	62.2	63.8	63.4
Expense per Capita (per person).	$2,827.0	$2,856.9	$2,748.3	$2,711.5	$2,656.7

States

TABLE 6

MONTANA

U.S. Registered Community Hospitals
(Nonfederal, short-term general and other special hospitals)

Overview 2008–2012

	2012	2011	2010	2009	2008
Total Community Hospitals in Montana	48	48	48	48	48
Bed Size Category					
6-24	10	11	10	8	9
25-49	13	12	15	16	14
50-99	15	14	12	13	15
100-199	7	8	8	8	7
200-299	1	1	1	1	1
300-399	1	1	1	1	1
400-499	1	1	1	0	1
500 + ...	0	0	0	1	0
Location					
Hospitals Urban.........................	6	6	6	6	3
Hospitals Rural	42	42	42	42	45
Control					
State and Local Government...............	10	10	8	7	8
Not for Profit	37	37	39	40	39
Investor owned	1	1	1	1	1
Physician Models					
Independent Practice Association	4	5	7	9	9
Group Practice without Walls................	4	4	3	3	3
Open Physician-Hospital Organization	4	4	5	5	6
Closed Physician-Hospital Organization	1	1	1	1	2
Management Service Organization	5	5	6	7	6
Integrated Salary Model....................	28	29	27	28	29
Equity Model	1	1	2	2	2
Foundation...............................	6	6	4	3	5
Insurance Products					
Health Maintenance Organization	2	4	4	4	4
Preferred Provider Organization..............	9	7	8	8	9
Indemnity Fee for Service	4	5	6	6	4
Managed Care Contracts					
Health Maintenance Organization	8	9	11	11	13
Preferred Provider Organization..............	27	25	22	25	27
Affiliations					
Hospitals in a System.....................	11	12	12	12	11
Hospitals in a Network	23	23	22	22	24
Hospitals in a Group Purchasing Organization..	40	41	39	44	47

TABLE 6

MONTANA

U.S. Registered Community Hospitals
(Nonfederal, short-term general and other special hospitals)

Utilization, Personnel, Revenue and Expenses, Community Health Indicators 2008–2012

	2012	2011	2010	2009	2008
TOTAL FACILITY (Includes Hospital and Nursing Home Units)					
Utilization - Inpatient					
Beds	3,710	3,626	3,692	3,820	3,765
Admissions	93,423	94,966	97,453	101,327	103,840
Inpatient Days	809,199	828,778	848,356	869,897	903,981
Average Length of Stay	8.7	8.7	8.7	8.6	8.7
Inpatient Surgeries	27,627	28,395	29,136	30,167	30,697
Births	10,191	10,254	10,217	10,432	10,708
Utilization - Outpatient					
Emergency Outpatient Visits	366,756	369,610	357,543	357,066	346,670
Other Outpatient Visits	3,218,282	3,173,110	3,146,841	2,973,218	2,807,604
Total Outpatient Visits	3,585,038	3,542,720	3,504,384	3,330,284	3,154,274
Outpatient Surgeries	48,788	47,582	48,043	45,364	45,012
Personnel					
Full Time RNs	3,191	2,860	2,946	2,843	2,496
Full Time LPNs	486	454	478	508	497
Part Time RNs	2,047	2,088	1,930	2,067	1,936
Part Time LPNs	280	256	257	283	328
Total Full Time	15,720	14,304	14,816	14,621	13,974
Total Part Time	7,743	7,502	7,138	7,470	7,358
Revenue - Inpatient					
Gross Inpatient Revenue	$2,279,133,191	$2,102,143,134	$2,049,917,318	$2,001,422,796	$1,868,192,302
Revenue - Outpatient					
Gross Outpatient Revenue	$2,990,024,968	$2,622,907,633	$2,452,151,901	$2,187,645,447	$1,879,526,779
Revenue and Expenses - Totals					
(Includes Inpatient and Outpatient)					
Total Gross Revenue	$5,269,158,159	$4,725,050,767	$4,502,069,219	$4,189,068,243	$3,747,719,081
Deductions from Revenue	2,595,587,712	2,261,961,105	2,145,913,313	1,939,387,748	1,670,030,190
Net Patient Revenue	2,673,570,447	2,463,089,662	2,356,155,906	2,249,680,495	2,077,688,891
Other Operating Revenue	110,280,462	98,796,127	93,587,995	90,423,031	80,597,184
Other Nonoperating Revenue	22,151,981	56,310,483	64,235,515	-5,428,277	16,554,468
Total Net Revenue	2,806,002,890	2,618,196,272	2,513,970,416	2,334,675,249	2,174,840,543
Total Expenses	2,660,995,740	2,485,931,042	2,379,151,295	2,263,313,965	2,077,753,777
HOSPITAL UNIT (Excludes Separate Nursing Home Units)					
Utilization - Inpatient					
Beds	2,403	2,347	2,398	2,421	2,292
Admissions	91,325	92,852	95,238	99,163	101,233
Inpatient Days	410,312	430,418	442,106	435,087	440,713
Average Length of Stay	4.5	4.6	4.6	4.4	4.4
Personnel					
Total Full Time	14,970	13,628	14,038	13,813	12,999
Total Part Time	7,213	7,007	6,602	6,946	6,770
Revenue and Expenses - Totals					
(Includes Inpatient and Outpatient)					
Total Net Revenue	$2,733,592,548	$2,538,770,978	$2,441,209,709	$2,259,366,824	$2,092,696,080
Total Expenses	2,591,928,424	2,403,184,670	2,306,425,879	2,191,842,514	2,002,337,963
COMMUNITY HEALTH INDICATORS PER 1000 POPULATION					
Total Population (in thousands)	1,005	998	980	975	968
Inpatient					
Beds	3.7	3.6	3.8	3.9	3.9
Admissions	92.9	95.1	99.4	103.9	107.3
Inpatient Days	805.1	830.3	865.5	892.2	933.8
Inpatient Surgeries	27.5	28.4	29.7	30.9	31.7
Births	10.1	10.3	10.4	10.7	11.1
Outpatient					
Emergency Outpatient Visits	364.9	370.3	364.8	366.2	358.1
Other Outpatient Visits	3,201.8	3,178.8	3,210.6	3,049.5	2,900.3
Total Outpatient Visits	3,566.7	3,549.1	3,575.3	3,415.7	3,258.4
Outpatient Surgeries	48.5	47.7	49.0	46.5	46.5
Expense per Capita (per person)	$2,647.4	$2,490.4	$2,427.3	$2,321.4	$2,146.4

TABLE **6**

NEBRASKA

U.S. Registered Community Hospitals
(Nonfederal, short-term general and other special hospitals)

Overview 2008–2012

	2012	2011	2010	2009	2008
Total Community Hospitals in Nebraska.......	**89**	**86**	**88**	**87**	**86**
Bed Size Category					
6-24	26	24	23	22	21
25-49	21	25	23	22	23
50-99	22	19	23	22	23
100-199	10	8	9	10	7
200-299	5	6	4	6	7
300-399	3	2	4	4	4
400-499	2	1	1	0	0
500 + ...	0	1	1	1	1
Location					
Hospitals Urban........................	18	16	17	16	14
Hospitals Rural	71	70	71	71	72
Control					
State and Local Government................	38	37	39	40	38
Not for Profit	49	46	46	45	46
Investor owned	2	3	3	2	2
Physician Models					
Independent Practice Association	6	6	6	6	8
Group Practice without Walls...............	2	0	1	2	2
Open Physician-Hospital Organization	11	10	12	13	13
Closed Physician-Hospital Organization	2	1	0	1	0
Management Service Organization	2	2	3	2	3
Integrated Salary Model....................	24	26	27	33	32
Equity Model	0	0	0	0	0
Foundation.............................	2	1	0	1	2
Insurance Products					
Health Maintenance Organization	2	3	3	2	3
Preferred Provider Organization..............	7	12	11	13	14
Indemnity Fee for Service	1	4	3	3	4
Managed Care Contracts					
Health Maintenance Organization	16	15	16	17	19
Preferred Provider Organization..............	43	43	43	50	53
Affiliations					
Hospitals in a System......................	29	29	26	28	29
Hospitals in a Network	30	32	28	33	36
Hospitals in a Group Purchasing Organization..	42	44	47	54	56

States

TABLE 6

NEBRASKA

U.S. Registered Community Hospitals
(Nonfederal, short-term general and other special hospitals)

Utilization, Personnel, Revenue and Expenses, Community Health Indicators 2008–2012

	2012	2011	2010	2009	2008
TOTAL FACILITY (Includes Hospital and Nursing Home Units)					
Utilization - Inpatient					
Beds	6,997	6,592	7,246	7,442	7,264
Admissions	205,065	203,394	208,949	209,750	214,808
Inpatient Days	1,411,707	1,313,451	1,461,558	1,552,206	1,562,960
Average Length of Stay	6.9	6.5	7.0	7.4	7.3
Inpatient Surgeries	81,170	65,592	65,316	67,275	71,248
Births	25,859	25,778	24,575	26,224	26,802
Utilization - Outpatient					
Emergency Outpatient Visits	671,332	716,718	700,818	688,519	639,756
Other Outpatient Visits	4,556,326	4,239,738	3,870,823	3,969,589	3,987,333
Total Outpatient Visits	5,227,658	4,956,456	4,571,641	4,658,108	4,627,089
Outpatient Surgeries	130,932	118,596	112,213	120,310	130,440
Personnel					
Full Time RNs	8,429	7,863	8,038	7,653	7,104
Full Time LPNs	681	687	856	876	913
Part Time RNs	4,274	4,182	4,286	4,111	4,477
Part Time LPNs	388	393	489	512	530
Total Full Time	29,039	27,779	29,024	28,451	27,407
Total Part Time	13,789	13,543	14,502	13,922	15,212
Revenue - Inpatient					
Gross Inpatient Revenue	$6,600,070,735	$6,329,607,253	$6,579,976,131	$6,240,788,042	$5,994,545,329
Revenue - Outpatient					
Gross Outpatient Revenue	$6,127,521,502	$5,571,277,484	$5,335,861,059	$4,923,545,533	$4,349,628,655
Revenue and Expenses - Totals					
(Includes Inpatient and Outpatient)					
Total Gross Revenue	$12,727,592,237	$11,900,884,737	$11,915,837,190	$11,164,333,575	$10,344,173,984
Deductions from Revenue	7,443,134,120	7,094,550,376	7,060,882,109	6,451,826,044	5,885,164,745
Net Patient Revenue	5,284,458,117	4,806,334,361	4,854,955,081	4,712,507,531	4,459,009,239
Other Operating Revenue	276,960,199	243,522,454	211,231,348	209,020,415	210,752,208
Other Nonoperating Revenue	61,823,105	203,146,705	132,518,504	-28,338,616	-24,908,037
Total Net Revenue	5,623,241,421	5,253,003,520	5,198,704,933	4,893,189,330	4,644,853,410
Total Expenses	4,972,245,644	4,659,397,050	4,710,906,183	4,471,302,656	4,380,337,731
HOSPITAL UNIT (Excludes Separate Nursing Home Units)					
Utilization - Inpatient					
Beds	5,979	5,817	6,168	6,102	5,793
Admissions	202,588	201,622	206,235	206,131	211,021
Inpatient Days	1,097,274	1,082,517	1,128,398	1,144,790	1,117,877
Average Length of Stay	5.4	5.4	5.5	5.6	5.3
Personnel					
Total Full Time	28,349	27,230	28,177	27,569	26,467
Total Part Time	13,362	13,178	13,927	13,239	14,524
Revenue and Expenses - Totals					
(Includes Inpatient and Outpatient)					
Total Net Revenue	$5,554,405,718	$5,207,994,214	$5,123,202,118	$4,790,650,335	$4,527,469,170
Total Expenses	4,897,073,033	4,613,479,154	4,634,581,746	4,379,557,407	4,274,392,152
COMMUNITY HEALTH INDICATORS PER 1000 POPULATION					
Total Population (in thousands)	1,856	1,843	1,811	1,797	1,782
Inpatient					
Beds	3.8	3.6	4.0	4.1	4.1
Admissions	110.5	110.4	115.4	116.7	120.5
Inpatient Days	760.8	712.8	807.0	864.0	877.1
Inpatient Surgeries	43.7	35.6	36.1	37.4	40.0
Births	13.9	14.0	13.6	14.6	15.0
Outpatient					
Emergency Outpatient Visits	361.8	389.0	387.0	383.2	359.0
Other Outpatient Visits	2,455.5	2,300.9	2,137.3	2,209.5	2,237.6
Total Outpatient Visits	2,817.3	2,689.9	2,524.3	2,592.7	2,596.6
Outpatient Surgeries	70.6	64.4	62.0	67.0	73.2
Expense per Capita (per person)	$2,679.7	$2,528.7	$2,601.2	$2,488.7	$2,458.2

States

TABLE 6

NEVADA

U.S. Registered Community Hospitals
(Nonfederal, short-term general and other special hospitals)

Overview 2008–2012

	2012	2011	2010	2009	2008
Total Community Hospitals in Nevada	38	38	36	35	35
Bed Size Category					
6-24	5	4	4	4	4
25-49	6	6	6	6	6
50-99	11	12	12	11	11
100-199	7	7	6	6	6
200-299	4	4	3	3	3
300-399	2	2	2	2	2
400-499	0	0	0	0	0
500 + ...	3	3	3	3	3
Location					
Hospitals Urban...........................	27	27	25	24	25
Hospitals Rural	11	11	11	11	10
Control					
State and Local Government................	6	6	6	6	6
Not for Profit	12	13	13	13	13
Investor owned	20	19	17	16	16
Physician Models					
Independent Practice Association	4	4	2	3	3
Group Practice without Walls...............	0	0	0	0	0
Open Physician-Hospital Organization	1	1	1	1	0
Closed Physician-Hospital Organization	2	2	2	2	1
Management Service Organization	1	2	2	4	3
Integrated Salary Model....................	9	7	2	3	4
Equity Model	0	1	0	0	0
Foundation.............................	0	0	0	0	0
Insurance Products					
Health Maintenance Organization	6	7	7	5	4
Preferred Provider Organization..............	6	7	7	6	5
Indemnity Fee for Service	6	3	4	3	3
Managed Care Contracts					
Health Maintenance Organization	17	20	13	12	11
Preferred Provider Organization..............	17	21	15	15	14
Affiliations					
Hospitals in a System.....................	27	27	25	24	24
Hospitals in a Network....................	6	6	5	5	5
Hospitals in a Group Purchasing Organization..	18	22	16	18	18

TABLE **6**

NEVADA

U.S. Registered Community Hospitals
(Nonfederal, short-term general and other special hospitals)

Utilization, Personnel, Revenue and Expenses, Community Health Indicators 2008–2012

	2012	2011	2010	2009	2008
TOTAL FACILITY (Includes Hospital and Nursing Home Units)					
Utilization - Inpatient					
Beds	5,504	5,507	5,192	5,119	5,144
Admissions	260,781	249,805	241,296	245,866	247,232
Inpatient Days	1,361,402	1,359,447	1,296,929	1,311,084	1,300,514
Average Length of Stay............	5.2	5.4	5.4	5.3	5.3
Inpatient Surgeries...............	63,184	63,902	69,928	72,737	68,365
Births...........................	26,384	21,822	24,844	30,373	29,248
Utilization - Outpatient					
Emergency Outpatient Visits........	865,371	820,812	820,675	820,980	780,500
Other Outpatient Visits.............	2,045,456	1,859,971	1,849,263	1,988,669	2,135,809
Total Outpatient Visits	2,910,827	2,680,783	2,669,938	2,809,649	2,916,309
Outpatient Surgeries	88,694	98,155	103,406	104,340	100,526
Personnel					
Full Time RNs	6,951	6,582	6,436	6,357	6,457
Full Time LPNs	322	351	406	404	452
Part Time RNs	1,816	2,011	1,439	1,340	1,521
Part Time LPNs	69	85	68	74	83
Total Full Time..................	21,297	20,545	20,948	20,386	21,672
Total Part Time	4,899	5,339	3,779	3,636	3,766
Revenue - Inpatient					
Gross Inpatient Revenue...........	$12,294,975,694	$11,616,603,674	$10,608,864,288	$10,439,117,032	$10,133,945,714
Revenue - Outpatient					
Gross Outpatient Revenue	$6,990,158,850	$6,466,989,068	$5,826,489,194	$5,312,533,278	$4,647,890,751
Revenue and Expenses - Totals					
(Includes Inpatient and Outpatient)					
Total Gross Revenue..............	$19,285,134,544	$18,083,592,742	$16,435,353,482	$15,751,650,310	$14,781,836,465
Deductions from Revenue..........	15,017,726,173	14,019,540,936	12,559,876,799	11,866,367,378	10,926,597,214
Net Patient Revenue..............	4,267,408,371	4,064,051,806	3,875,476,683	3,885,282,932	3,855,239,251
Other Operating Revenue	102,905,260	107,770,969	97,417,940	98,119,383	94,718,637
Other Nonoperating Revenue	35,498,438	75,853,300	93,314,155	73,065,405	49,631,516
Total Net Revenue...............	4,405,812,069	4,247,676,075	4,066,208,778	4,056,467,720	3,999,589,404
Total Expenses..................	4,199,882,893	4,070,512,098	3,940,182,337	3,957,622,058	3,912,575,991
HOSPITAL UNIT (Excludes Separate Nursing Home Units)					
Utilization - Inpatient					
Beds	5,479	5,443	5,174	5,076	5,119
Admissions	260,768	249,708	241,287	245,844	247,208
Inpatient Days	1,354,258	1,341,532	1,291,351	1,298,643	1,293,475
Average Length of Stay............	5.2	5.4	5.4	5.3	5.2
Personnel					
Total Full Time..................	21,284	20,517	20,939	20,368	21,651
Total Part Time	4,899	5,312	3,779	3,630	3,763
Revenue and Expenses - Totals					
(Includes Inpatient and Outpatient)					
Total Net Revenue...............	$4,403,869,456	$4,243,197,676	$4,065,636,650	$4,053,142,416	$3,997,480,744
Total Expenses..................	4,198,988,696	4,067,942,062	3,939,711,041	3,956,074,612	3,911,278,159
COMMUNITY HEALTH INDICATORS PER 1000 POPULATION					
Total Population (in thousands)	2,759	2,723	2,655	2,643	2,616
Inpatient					
Beds	2.0	2.0	2.0	1.9	2.0
Admissions	94.5	91.7	90.9	93.0	94.5
Inpatient Days	493.5	499.2	488.5	496.0	497.2
Inpatient Surgeries...............	22.9	23.5	26.3	27.5	26.1
Births...........................	9.6	8.0	9.4	11.5	11.2
Outpatient					
Emergency Outpatient Visits........	313.7	301.4	309.1	310.6	298.4
Other Outpatient Visits.............	741.4	683.0	696.6	752.4	816.5
Total Outpatient Visits	1,055.1	984.4	1,005.7	1,063.0	1,114.9
Outpatient Surgeries	32.1	36.0	39.0	39.5	38.4
Expense per Capita (per person).....	$1,522.3	$1,494.7	$1,484.2	$1,497.3	$1,495.8

TABLE **6**

NEW HAMPSHIRE

U.S. Registered Community Hospitals
(Nonfederal, short-term general and other special hospitals)

Overview 2008–2012

	2012	2011	2010	2009	2008
Total Community Hospitals in					
New Hampshire............................	28	28	28	28	28
Bed Size Category					
6-24	1	1	1	1	1
25-49	10	10	9	9	8
50-99	7	6	7	7	9
100-199	6	7	7	7	6
200-299	3	3	3	3	3
300-399	1	1	1	1	1
400-499	0	0	0	0	0
500 + ...	0	0	0	0	0
Location					
Hospitals Urban..........................	11	11	11	11	10
Hospitals Rural	17	17	17	17	18
Control					
State and Local Government................	0	0	0	0	0
Not for Profit	24	24	24	24	24
Investor owned	4	4	4	4	4
Physician Models					
Independent Practice Association	2	2	2	2	2
Group Practice without Walls...............	2	2	2	2	2
Open Physician-Hospital Organization	4	5	9	10	10
Closed Physician-Hospital Organization	0	0	0	0	1
Management Service Organization	0	0	0	1	0
Integrated Salary Model....................	19	20	17	16	16
Equity Model	0	0	0	0	0
Foundation...............................	0	0	0	0	1
Insurance Products					
Health Maintenance Organization	0	0	0	0	0
Preferred Provider Organization..............	0	0	0	0	1
Indemnity Fee for Service	0	0	0	0	0
Managed Care Contracts					
Health Maintenance Organization	19	20	23	26	25
Preferred Provider Organization..............	18	19	21	25	24
Affiliations					
Hospitals in a System......................	6	6	6	6	6
Hospitals in a Network	12	11	10	11	11
Hospitals in a Group Purchasing Organization..	25	25	26	27	26

TABLE 6

NEW HAMPSHIRE

U.S. Registered Community Hospitals
(Nonfederal, short-term general and other special hospitals)

Utilization, Personnel, Revenue and Expenses, Community Health Indicators 2008–2012

	2012	2011	2010	2009	2008
TOTAL FACILITY (Includes Hospital and Nursing Home Units)					
Utilization - Inpatient					
Beds	2,831	2,840	2,851	2,863	2,858
Admissions	119,814	122,341	119,971	122,959	124,184
Inpatient Days	627,784	634,954	624,399	655,015	664,659
Average Length of Stay.	5.2	5.2	5.2	5.3	5.4
Inpatient Surgeries	33,606	34,281	33,622	33,041	35,022
Births.	12,035	12,649	12,630	13,261	13,636
Utilization - Outpatient					
Emergency Outpatient Visits	652,190	677,358	667,605	627,769	623,814
Other Outpatient Visits.	4,330,937	4,318,549	4,109,910	4,097,077	3,844,709
Total Outpatient Visits	4,983,127	4,995,907	4,777,515	4,724,846	4,468,523
Outpatient Surgeries	90,715	91,348	92,450	91,495	91,320
Personnel					
Full Time RNs	4,460	4,282	4,298	4,191	4,181
Full Time LPNs	278	276	278	250	223
Part Time RNs	3,068	3,128	3,008	3,017	3,102
Part Time LPNs	128	126	139	176	156
Total Full Time	21,736	21,846	22,066	21,046	20,853
Total Part Time	10,229	10,000	10,151	10,294	10,452
Revenue - Inpatient					
Gross Inpatient Revenue.	$4,263,267,285	$4,150,081,268	$3,890,334,236	$3,730,906,874	$3,458,246,012
Revenue - Outpatient					
Gross Outpatient Revenue	$6,315,255,279	$5,916,747,273	$5,494,839,267	$4,960,506,458	$4,446,890,786
Revenue and Expenses - Totals					
(Includes Inpatient and Outpatient)					
Total Gross Revenue.	$10,578,522,564	$10,066,828,541	$9,385,173,503	$8,691,413,332	$7,905,136,798
Deductions from Revenue	6,389,949,615	5,928,255,856	5,410,431,600	4,934,553,834	4,413,714,285
Net Patient Revenue	4,188,572,949	4,138,572,685	3,974,741,903	3,756,859,498	3,491,422,513
Other Operating Revenue	172,037,917	129,629,985	106,982,372	93,662,673	87,274,249
Other Nonoperating Revenue	65,319,726	296,520	52,157,491	-52,943,319	-67,525,945
Total Net Revenue.	4,425,930,592	4,268,499,190	4,133,881,766	3,797,578,852	3,511,170,817
Total Expenses.	4,024,997,567	3,948,270,249	3,781,620,257	3,539,365,267	3,330,628,143
HOSPITAL UNIT (Excludes Separate Nursing Home Units)					
Utilization - Inpatient					
Beds	2,728	2,710	2,721	2,683	2,678
Admissions	119,684	121,996	119,391	122,334	123,622
Inpatient Days	592,483	593,304	577,175	602,460	605,089
Average Length of Stay.	5.0	4.9	4.8	4.9	4.9
Personnel					
Total Full Time	21,685	21,766	22,003	20,963	20,767
Total Part Time	10,202	9,960	10,110	10,246	10,380
Revenue and Expenses - Totals					
(Includes Inpatient and Outpatient)					
Total Net Revenue.	$4,417,200,764	$4,256,119,678	$4,120,469,030	$3,781,637,703	$3,496,911,705
Total Expenses.	4,017,253,998	3,938,257,684	3,770,403,066	3,528,118,615	3,319,098,045
COMMUNITY HEALTH INDICATORS PER 1000 POPULATION					
Total Population (in thousands)	1,321	1,318	1,324	1,325	1,322
Inpatient					
Beds	2.1	2.2	2.2	2.2	2.2
Admissions	90.7	92.8	90.6	92.8	93.9
Inpatient Days	475.3	481.7	471.8	494.5	502.8
Inpatient Surgeries	25.4	26.0	25.4	24.9	26.5
Births.	9.1	9.6	9.5	10.0	10.3
Outpatient					
Emergency Outpatient Visits	493.8	513.9	504.4	473.9	471.9
Other Outpatient Visits.	3,279.2	3,276.1	3,105.3	3,093.1	2,908.5
Total Outpatient Visits	3,773.0	3,790.0	3,609.7	3,567.1	3,380.5
Outpatient Surgeries	68.7	69.3	69.9	69.1	69.1
Expense per Capita (per person).	$3,047.6	$2,995.2	$2,857.2	$2,672.1	$2,519.6

States

TABLE 6

NEW JERSEY

U.S. Registered Community Hospitals
(Nonfederal, short-term general and other special hospitals)

Overview 2008–2012

	2012	2011	2010	2009	2008
Total Community Hospitals in New Jersey.....	77	73	73	74	73
Bed Size Category					
6-24	0	0	0	0	0
25-49	2	1	2	3	3
50-99	9	7	6	5	4
100-199	20	18	16	19	19
200-299	17	21	20	16	16
300-399	12	10	11	12	13
400-499	9	9	9	11	11
500 + ...	8	7	9	8	7
Location					
Hospitals Urban........................	77	73	73	74	73
Hospitals Rural	0	0	0	0	0
Control					
State and Local Government................	3	2	3	3	4
Not for Profit	60	61	62	64	61
Investor owned	14	10	8	7	8
Physician Models					
Independent Practice Association	11	10	12	14	16
Group Practice without Walls...............	5	1	3	3	2
Open Physician-Hospital Organization	5	3	4	7	10
Closed Physician-Hospital Organization	3	2	2	4	2
Management Service Organization	13	13	12	13	12
Integrated Salary Model....................	27	25	23	22	17
Equity Model	3	0	0	2	0
Foundation..............................	8	7	4	3	3
Insurance Products					
Health Maintenance Organization	12	7	6	3	4
Preferred Provider Organization..............	14	7	7	5	6
Indemnity Fee for Service	5	2	3	4	3
Managed Care Contracts					
Health Maintenance Organization	49	48	53	53	52
Preferred Provider Organization..............	49	47	53	54	53
Affiliations					
Hospitals in a System.....................	47	42	42	43	42
Hospitals in a Network	30	29	26	28	33
Hospitals in a Group Purchasing Organization..	54	53	54	55	61

States

TABLE 6

NEW JERSEY

U.S. Registered Community Hospitals
(Nonfederal, short-term general and other special hospitals)

Utilization, Personnel, Revenue and Expenses, Community Health Indicators 2008–2012

	2012	2011	2010	2009	2008
TOTAL FACILITY (Includes Hospital and Nursing Home Units)					
Utilization - Inpatient					
Beds	21,162	20,396	21,096	21,054	20,867
Admissions	1,047,545	1,050,828	1,067,267	1,094,810	1,086,445
Inpatient Days	5,370,619	5,344,077	5,433,359	5,565,763	5,595,966
Average Length of Stay	5.1	5.1	5.1	5.1	5.2
Inpatient Surgeries	243,512	243,218	254,003	250,689	255,641
Births	101,599	101,362	100,677	105,841	107,580
Utilization - Outpatient					
Emergency Outpatient Visits	3,703,899	3,474,457	3,360,970	3,484,463	3,350,786
Other Outpatient Visits	11,883,599	12,350,842	12,619,644	14,948,039	14,789,129
Total Outpatient Visits	15,587,498	15,825,299	15,980,614	18,432,502	18,139,915
Outpatient Surgeries	381,289	381,281	378,695	385,028	378,011
Personnel					
Full Time RNs	27,979	27,286	26,849	27,096	26,330
Full Time LPNs	763	881	976	948	988
Part Time RNs	13,111	14,084	12,933	11,792	11,559
Part Time LPNs	294	321	342	313	341
Total Full Time	101,341	100,956	101,574	102,243	100,758
Total Part Time	42,586	43,164	39,829	37,722	37,240
Revenue - Inpatient					
Gross Inpatient Revenue	$58,452,281,514	$56,915,377,319	$53,676,558,488	$53,769,546,685	$55,005,071,849
Revenue - Outpatient					
Gross Outpatient Revenue	$31,284,903,340	$27,132,937,292	$25,954,408,517	$23,718,074,694	$21,188,946,872
Revenue and Expenses - Totals					
(Includes Inpatient and Outpatient)					
Total Gross Revenue	$89,737,184,854	$84,048,314,611	$79,630,967,005	$77,487,621,379	$76,194,018,721
Deductions from Revenue	70,204,451,132	66,316,458,143	62,268,213,291	60,433,181,540	60,144,230,629
Net Patient Revenue	19,532,733,722	17,731,856,468	17,362,753,714	17,054,439,839	16,049,788,092
Other Operating Revenue	1,217,574,869	1,039,183,060	991,173,520	937,712,136	843,164,744
Other Nonoperating Revenue	398,816,960	157,790,540	355,140,452	506,772,443	-674,159,972
Total Net Revenue	21,149,125,551	18,928,830,068	18,709,067,686	18,498,924,418	16,218,792,864
Total Expenses	19,790,864,680	18,237,577,704	17,953,893,599	17,724,384,287	17,087,597,199
HOSPITAL UNIT (Excludes Separate Nursing Home Units)					
Utilization - Inpatient					
Beds	20,632	19,853	20,533	20,583	20,358
Admissions	1,043,187	1,046,456	1,061,552	1,091,384	1,082,467
Inpatient Days	5,189,878	5,168,493	5,258,495	5,408,363	5,429,164
Average Length of Stay	5.0	4.9	5.0	5.0	5.0
Personnel					
Total Full Time	100,839	100,398	100,902	101,537	99,958
Total Part Time	42,335	42,916	39,482	37,475	36,951
Revenue and Expenses - Totals					
(Includes Inpatient and Outpatient)					
Total Net Revenue	$21,088,046,402	$18,869,785,791	$18,584,183,240	$18,453,887,888	$16,159,968,959
Total Expenses	19,740,490,336	18,187,967,013	17,859,249,404	17,680,544,335	17,039,861,968
COMMUNITY HEALTH INDICATORS PER 1000 POPULATION					
Total Population (in thousands)	8,865	8,821	8,733	8,708	8,663
Inpatient					
Beds	2.4	2.3	2.4	2.4	2.4
Admissions	118.2	119.1	122.2	125.7	125.4
Inpatient Days	605.9	605.8	622.2	639.2	645.9
Inpatient Surgeries	27.5	27.6	29.1	28.8	29.5
Births	11.5	11.5	11.5	12.2	12.4
Outpatient					
Emergency Outpatient Visits	417.8	393.9	384.9	400.2	386.8
Other Outpatient Visits	1,340.6	1,400.1	1,445.1	1,716.6	1,707.1
Total Outpatient Visits	1,758.4	1,794.0	1,830.0	2,116.8	2,093.9
Outpatient Surgeries	43.0	43.2	43.4	44.2	43.6
Expense per Capita (per person)	$2,232.6	$2,067.5	$2,055.9	$2,035.5	$1,972.4

States

TABLE 6

NEW MEXICO

U.S. Registered Community Hospitals
(Nonfederal, short-term general and other special hospitals)

Overview 2008–2012

	2012	2011	2010	2009	2008
Total Community Hospitals in New Mexico	37	36	36	37	36
Bed Size Category					
6-24	5	4	4	4	4
25-49	9	8	8	8	9
50-99	10	12	12	14	10
100-199	6	7	8	8	10
200-299	5	3	2	1	1
300-399	0	0	0	0	0
400-499	1	0	0	0	0
500 + ...	1	2	2	2	2
Location					
Hospitals Urban..........................	14	14	14	15	14
Hospitals Rural	23	22	22	22	22
Control					
State and Local Government................	6	6	6	7	7
Not for Profit	15	15	16	14	14
Investor owned	16	15	14	16	15
Physician Models					
Independent Practice Association	3	3	4	4	3
Group Practice without Walls...............	0	0	0	1	0
Open Physician-Hospital Organization	4	4	3	4	4
Closed Physician-Hospital Organization	0	0	0	0	1
Management Service Organization	0	0	0	0	1
Integrated Salary Model....................	11	9	11	13	10
Equity Model	0	0	0	1	1
Foundation...............................	0	0	1	2	2
Insurance Products					
Health Maintenance Organization	8	7	6	7	7
Preferred Provider Organization..............	6	7	6	7	6
Indemnity Fee for Service	4	4	5	5	4
Managed Care Contracts					
Health Maintenance Organization	16	13	14	19	17
Preferred Provider Organization..............	16	13	15	19	19
Affiliations					
Hospitals in a System......................	29	28	28	30	28
Hospitals in a Network	11	11	11	10	7
Hospitals in a Group Purchasing Organization..	22	22	20	26	22

TABLE **6**

NEW MEXICO

U.S. Registered Community Hospitals
(Nonfederal, short-term general and other special hospitals)

Utilization, Personnel, Revenue and Expenses, Community Health Indicators 2008–2012

	2012	2011	2010	2009	2008
TOTAL FACILITY (Includes Hospital and Nursing Home Units)					
Utilization - Inpatient					
Beds	4,076	4,068	3,975	3,913	3,935
Admissions	177,744	175,112	186,092	183,116	174,169
Inpatient Days	850,391	861,109	831,384	844,787	809,916
Average Length of Stay.	4.8	4.9	4.5	4.6	4.7
Inpatient Surgeries.	47,292	53,331	49,435	51,319	48,698
Births.	23,924	21,537	23,767	26,224	24,127
Utilization - Outpatient					
Emergency Outpatient Visits	793,582	854,871	844,650	829,138	770,475
Other Outpatient Visits.	3,361,978	3,740,262	3,795,337	3,814,530	3,481,084
Total Outpatient Visits	4,155,560	4,595,133	4,639,987	4,643,668	4,251,559
Outpatient Surgeries	92,264	93,352	92,079	92,936	84,596
Personnel					
Full Time RNs	6,326	5,549	6,022	5,579	5,151
Full Time LPNs	353	292	391	455	401
Part Time RNs	2,254	2,092	2,065	2,213	1,997
Part Time LPNs	100	72	124	145	143
Total Full Time	21,672	19,318	20,493	21,568	19,610
Total Part Time	6,526	5,387	5,559	6,609	5,789
Revenue - Inpatient					
Gross Inpatient Revenue.	$6,068,430,416	$5,955,197,886	$5,597,578,195	$5,011,641,495	$4,955,498,423
Revenue - Outpatient					
Gross Outpatient Revenue	$6,116,116,964	$5,493,320,827	$5,288,644,232	$4,601,410,841	$4,098,164,016
Revenue and Expenses - Totals					
(Includes Inpatient and Outpatient)					
Total Gross Revenue.	$12,184,547,380	$11,448,518,713	$10,886,222,427	$9,613,052,336	$9,053,662,439
Deductions from Revenue	8,059,915,659	7,609,704,329	6,965,889,535	5,938,985,924	5,863,897,074
Net Patient Revenue	4,124,631,721	3,838,814,384	3,920,332,892	3,674,066,412	3,189,765,365
Other Operating Revenue	229,495,765	211,597,602	193,738,359	179,587,865	201,317,481
Other Nonoperating Revenue	21,327,949	53,311,105	32,566,260	22,192,097	25,179,087
Total Net Revenue.	4,375,455,435	4,103,723,091	4,146,637,511	3,875,846,374	3,416,261,933
Total Expenses.	4,003,331,871	3,713,540,269	3,540,766,412	3,378,281,656	3,078,569,624
HOSPITAL UNIT (Excludes Separate Nursing Home Units)					
Utilization - Inpatient					
Beds	4,076	4,068	3,928	3,863	3,838
Admissions	177,744	175,112	186,058	182,956	173,883
Inpatient Days	850,391	861,109	818,802	841,637	788,033
Average Length of Stay.	4.8	4.9	4.4	4.6	4.5
Personnel					
Total Full Time	21,499	19,318	20,450	21,545	19,566
Total Part Time	6,433	5,387	5,554	6,606	5,778
Revenue and Expenses - Totals					
(Includes Inpatient and Outpatient)					
Total Net Revenue.	$4,375,455,435	$4,103,723,091	$4,145,724,111	$3,872,546,211	$3,409,480,468
Total Expenses.	4,003,331,871	3,713,540,269	3,537,873,415	3,375,982,169	3,074,660,998
COMMUNITY HEALTH INDICATORS PER 1000 POPULATION					
Total Population (in thousands)	2,086	2,082	2,034	2,010	1,987
Inpatient					
Beds	2.0	2.0	2.0	1.9	2.0
Admissions	85.2	84.1	91.5	91.1	87.7
Inpatient Days	407.8	413.6	408.8	420.4	407.7
Inpatient Surgeries.	22.7	25.6	24.3	25.5	24.5
Births.	11.5	10.3	11.7	13.0	12.1
Outpatient					
Emergency Outpatient Visits	380.5	410.6	415.3	412.6	387.8
Other Outpatient Visits.	1,612.0	1,796.3	1,866.1	1,898.1	1,752.1
Total Outpatient Visits	1,992.6	2,206.8	2,281.4	2,310.7	2,139.9
Outpatient Surgeries	44.2	44.8	45.3	46.2	42.6
Expense per Capita (per person).	$1,919.6	$1,783.4	$1,740.9	$1,681.0	$1,549.5

TABLE 6

NEW YORK

U.S. Registered Community Hospitals
(Nonfederal, short-term general and other special hospitals)

Overview 2008–2012

	2012	2011	2010	2009	2008
Total Community Hospitals in New York	**178**	**182**	**185**	**189**	**194**
Bed Size Category					
6-24	7	6	5	4	5
25-49	7	7	7	7	9
50-99	16	19	18	19	19
100-199	40	41	40	45	47
200-299	39	36	44	40	38
300-399	22	26	25	28	29
400-499	12	14	13	15	14
500 + ...	35	33	33	31	33
Location					
Hospitals Urban..........................	140	145	147	150	158
Hospitals Rural	38	37	38	39	36
Control					
State and Local Government................	26	26	25	25	26
Not for Profit	152	156	160	164	167
Investor owned	0	0	0	0	1
Physician Models					
Independent Practice Association	38	35	35	32	38
Group Practice without Walls...............	7	5	6	4	5
Open Physician-Hospital Organization	15	14	12	9	13
Closed Physician-Hospital Organization	13	10	10	10	9
Management Service Organization	16	15	18	15	13
Integrated Salary Model...................	77	77	74	63	56
Equity Model	1	2	0	0	4
Foundation..............................	3	3	2	3	2
Insurance Products					
Health Maintenance Organization	42	48	45	39	50
Preferred Provider Organization.............	13	21	30	22	30
Indemnity Fee for Service	9	10	22	12	15
Managed Care Contracts					
Health Maintenance Organization	114	116	116	111	115
Preferred Provider Organization.............	108	111	109	101	105
Affiliations					
Hospitals in a System.....................	87	84	82	80	73
Hospitals in a Network....................	75	83	82	76	73
Hospitals in a Group Purchasing Organization..	128	134	128	116	116

TABLE 6

NEW YORK

U.S. Registered Community Hospitals
(Nonfederal, short-term general and other special hospitals)

Utilization, Personnel, Revenue and Expenses, Community Health Indicators 2008–2012

	2012	2011	2010	2009	2008
TOTAL FACILITY (Includes Hospital and Nursing Home Units)					
Utilization - Inpatient					
Beds	57,148	58,080	59,510	60,400	61,237
Admissions	2,444,350	2,491,403	2,509,980	2,533,577	2,528,191
Inpatient Days	16,783,079	16,924,697	17,226,868	17,474,823	17,973,047
Average Length of Stay	6.9	6.8	6.9	6.9	7.1
Inpatient Surgeries	615,646	615,656	683,336	653,545	660,660
Births	232,967	239,622	238,062	238,647	242,326
Utilization - Outpatient					
Emergency Outpatient Visits	8,379,030	8,432,260	8,063,821	8,542,392	8,114,078
Other Outpatient Visits	48,264,808	45,578,620	45,586,391	45,702,429	44,455,562
Total Outpatient Visits	56,643,838	54,010,880	53,650,212	54,244,821	52,569,640
Outpatient Surgeries	1,309,661	1,335,088	1,369,360	1,369,632	1,340,449
Personnel					
Full Time RNs	80,336	81,500	79,270	79,073	76,900
Full Time LPNs	5,110	5,403	5,095	5,781	5,964
Part Time RNs	23,613	23,368	24,090	21,651	22,118
Part Time LPNs	1,389	1,427	1,492	1,442	1,561
Total Full Time	354,362	350,923	333,121	344,168	340,045
Total Part Time	84,860	85,040	80,711	76,142	74,972
Revenue - Inpatient					
Gross Inpatient Revenue	$91,398,462,566	$86,312,444,902	$83,446,219,992	$79,742,230,648	$76,153,885,959
Revenue - Outpatient					
Gross Outpatient Revenue	$62,547,461,326	$56,035,192,523	$52,554,490,709	$48,142,548,531	$43,198,790,671
Revenue and Expenses - Totals					
(Includes Inpatient and Outpatient)					
Total Gross Revenue	$153,945,923,892	$142,347,637,425	$136,000,710,701	$127,884,779,179	$119,352,676,630
Deductions from Revenue	95,942,060,347	87,498,353,474	83,151,232,467	77,411,417,932	71,744,138,399
Net Patient Revenue	58,003,863,545	54,849,283,951	52,849,478,234	50,473,361,247	47,608,538,231
Other Operating Revenue	4,732,632,403	4,212,820,400	4,222,330,075	3,824,228,913	3,624,584,884
Other Nonoperating Revenue	758,391,592	541,024,602	925,916,282	1,020,046,507	-31,698,081
Total Net Revenue	63,494,887,540	59,603,128,953	57,997,724,591	55,317,636,667	51,201,425,034
Total Expenses	62,122,860,564	58,543,388,525	56,081,000,844	54,164,979,905	52,930,511,542
HOSPITAL UNIT (Excludes Separate Nursing Home Units)					
Utilization - Inpatient					
Beds	50,458	51,072	53,436	54,708	55,922
Admissions	2,426,083	2,471,603	2,494,952	2,518,427	2,514,606
Inpatient Days	14,420,693	14,460,605	15,107,729	15,475,231	16,133,356
Average Length of Stay	5.9	5.9	6.1	6.1	6.4
Personnel					
Total Full Time	348,723	346,182	329,655	339,060	334,474
Total Part Time	82,206	82,889	78,770	73,758	72,541
Revenue and Expenses - Totals					
(Includes Inpatient and Outpatient)					
Total Net Revenue	$62,830,487,679	$58,992,643,837	$57,401,240,974	$54,761,298,914	$50,719,366,889
Total Expenses	61,440,662,596	57,946,106,911	55,490,108,946	53,587,952,457	52,469,154,258
COMMUNITY HEALTH INDICATORS PER 1000 POPULATION					
Total Population (in thousands)	19,570	19,465	19,578	19,541	19,468
Inpatient					
Beds	2.9	3.0	3.0	3.1	3.1
Admissions	124.9	128.0	128.2	129.7	129.9
Inpatient Days	857.6	869.5	879.9	894.2	923.2
Inpatient Surgeries	31.5	31.6	34.9	33.4	33.9
Births	11.9	12.3	12.2	12.2	12.4
Outpatient					
Emergency Outpatient Visits	428.2	433.2	411.9	437.1	416.8
Other Outpatient Visits	2,466.2	2,341.5	2,328.5	2,338.7	2,283.5
Total Outpatient Visits	2,894.4	2,774.7	2,740.4	2,775.9	2,700.3
Outpatient Surgeries	66.9	68.6	69.9	70.1	68.9
Expense per Capita (per person)	$3,174.4	$3,007.6	$2,864.5	$2,771.8	$2,718.9

TABLE 6

NORTH CAROLINA

U.S. Registered Community Hospitals
(Nonfederal, short-term general and other special hospitals)

Overview 2008–2012

	2012	2011	2010	2009	2008
Total Community Hospitals in North Carolina..	118	117	117	115	116
Bed Size Category					
6-24	5	3	4	4	4
25-49	26	20	19	18	16
50-99	22	28	25	20	22
100-199	31	31	35	39	40
200-299	12	13	13	13	12
300-399	8	8	6	6	7
400-499	1	1	2	2	2
500 + ...	13	13	13	13	13
Location					
Hospitals Urban.	61	59	59	58	55
Hospitals Rural	57	58	58	57	61
Control					
State and Local Government.	30	30	32	32	32
Not for Profit	72	75	73	74	74
Investor owned	16	12	12	9	10
Physician Models					
Independent Practice Association	8	10	10	11	11
Group Practice without Walls.	2	1	2	3	2
Open Physician-Hospital Organization	9	9	10	11	10
Closed Physician-Hospital Organization	5	6	6	7	6
Management Service Organization	14	12	12	14	16
Integrated Salary Model	60	57	54	50	57
Equity Model	2	2	4	5	3
Foundation.	2	2	3	2	5
Insurance Products					
Health Maintenance Organization	5	6	7	4	7
Preferred Provider Organization.	14	16	14	10	10
Indemnity Fee for Service	2	6	5	2	2
Managed Care Contracts					
Health Maintenance Organization	75	71	70	71	80
Preferred Provider Organization.	83	77	75	80	89
Affiliations					
Hospitals in a System.	95	90	78	70	69
Hospitals in a Network	46	43	41	39	41
Hospitals in a Group Purchasing Organization..	99	94	90	90	102

TABLE **6**

NORTH CAROLINA

U.S. Registered Community Hospitals
(Nonfederal, short-term general and other special hospitals)

Utilization, Personnel, Revenue and Expenses, Community Health Indicators 2008–2012

	2012	2011	2010	2009	2008
TOTAL FACILITY (Includes Hospital and Nursing Home Units)					
Utilization - Inpatient					
Beds	22,708	23,136	23,012	22,830	23,140
Admissions	1,027,640	1,035,400	1,038,337	1,034,112	1,041,918
Inpatient Days	5,726,216	5,830,425	5,852,967	5,788,671	6,019,401
Average Length of Stay............	5.6	5.6	5.6	5.6	5.8
Inpatient Surgeries...............	281,357	287,065	293,323	296,668	292,208
Births..........................	114,140	115,013	117,422	122,588	126,934
Utilization - Outpatient					
Emergency Outpatient Visits........	4,636,192	4,448,191	4,259,853	4,249,375	4,166,718
Other Outpatient Visits.............	15,094,661	14,180,481	14,026,042	14,071,173	13,566,350
Total Outpatient Visits	19,730,853	18,628,672	18,285,895	18,320,548	17,733,068
Outpatient Surgeries	549,918	551,009	558,068	561,072	561,677
Personnel					
Full Time RNs	39,539	37,691	37,461	36,051	33,527
Full Time LPNs	1,454	1,457	1,585	1,567	1,847
Part Time RNs...................	13,727	13,740	13,790	13,892	15,014
Part Time LPNs	395	433	509	560	717
Total Full Time..................	138,663	134,652	130,456	128,117	127,114
Total Part Time	36,991	36,793	35,766	37,093	39,645
Revenue - Inpatient					
Gross Inpatient Revenue...........	$32,277,023,087	$30,029,780,874	$28,197,730,702	$25,877,825,356	$23,694,080,318
Revenue - Outpatient					
Gross Outpatient Revenue	$31,543,420,298	$27,738,748,951	$24,683,456,547	$22,124,796,442	$19,809,416,116
Revenue and Expenses - Totals					
(Includes Inpatient and Outpatient)					
Total Gross Revenue..............	$63,820,443,385	$57,768,529,825	$52,881,187,249	$48,002,621,798	$43,503,496,434
Deductions from Revenue..........	40,976,435,538	37,629,541,786	33,708,237,290	29,458,448,362	26,008,781,838
Net Patient Revenue	22,844,007,847	20,138,988,039	19,172,949,959	18,544,173,436	17,494,714,596
Other Operating Revenue	1,376,765,805	1,235,529,371	1,122,729,376	1,094,994,175	988,309,628
Other Nonoperating Revenue	664,882,512	273,053,042	492,730,856	213,265,535	-560,668,606
Total Net Revenue................	24,885,656,164	21,647,570,452	20,788,410,191	19,852,433,146	17,922,355,618
Total Expenses..................	22,659,692,061	20,062,914,117	18,847,920,294	18,590,518,185	17,662,604,664
HOSPITAL UNIT (Excludes Separate Nursing Home Units)					
Utilization - Inpatient					
Beds	20,823	21,041	20,841	20,811	20,496
Admissions	1,020,541	1,027,691	1,030,472	1,026,457	1,031,609
Inpatient Days	5,135,293	5,171,227	5,150,233	5,133,526	5,128,782
Average Length of Stay............	5.0	5.0	5.0	5.0	5.0
Personnel					
Total Full Time..................	137,311	133,321	128,958	126,542	125,088
Total Part Time	36,455	36,217	35,100	36,425	38,721
Revenue and Expenses - Totals					
(Includes Inpatient and Outpatient)					
Total Net Revenue................	$24,752,345,760	$21,508,952,533	$20,648,909,546	$19,725,156,052	$17,753,404,722
Total Expenses..................	22,524,391,595	19,925,373,321	18,715,167,064	18,471,921,787	17,488,022,607
COMMUNITY HEALTH INDICATORS PER 1000 POPULATION					
Total Population (in thousands)	9,752	9,656	9,459	9,381	9,247
Inpatient					
Beds	2.3	2.4	2.4	2.4	2.5
Admissions	105.4	107.2	109.8	110.2	112.7
Inpatient Days	587.2	603.8	618.8	617.1	650.9
Inpatient Surgeries...............	28.9	29.7	31.0	31.6	31.6
Births..........................	11.7	11.9	12.4	13.1	13.7
Outpatient					
Emergency Outpatient Visits........	475.4	460.6	450.4	453.0	450.6
Other Outpatient Visits.............	1,547.8	1,468.5	1,482.8	1,500.0	1,467.1
Total Outpatient Visits	2,023.2	1,929.2	1,933.2	1,953.0	1,917.7
Outpatient Surgeries	56.4	57.1	59.0	59.8	60.7
Expense per Capita (per person).....	$2,323.6	$2,077.7	$1,992.6	$1,981.7	$1,910.1

States

TABLE 6

NORTH DAKOTA

U.S. Registered Community Hospitals
(Nonfederal, short-term general and other special hospitals)

Overview 2008–2012

	2012	2011	2010	2009	2008
Total Community Hospitals in North Dakota ...	44	41	41	41	41
Bed Size Category					
6-24	14	13	10	10	11
25-49	15	14	15	15	12
50-99	8	7	8	9	11
100-199	2	2	3	2	2
200-299	3	3	3	3	3
300-399	0	0	0	0	0
400-499	1	1	1	1	1
500 + ...	1	1	1	1	1
Location					
Hospitals Urban...........................	8	8	8	8	7
Hospitals Rural	36	33	33	33	34
Control					
State and Local Government................	0	0	0	0	0
Not for Profit	41	39	39	39	39
Investor owned	3	2	2	2	2
Physician Models					
Independent Practice Association	3	3	4	4	4
Group Practice without Walls...............	1	0	0	0	0
Open Physician-Hospital Organization	2	1	1	2	3
Closed Physician-Hospital Organization	0	0	0	0	0
Management Service Organization	0	0	0	0	0
Integrated Salary Model....................	10	8	10	16	15
Equity Model	0	0	0	1	1
Foundation...............................	1	1	1	2	4
Insurance Products					
Health Maintenance Organization	2	0	1	0	0
Preferred Provider Organization..............	2	5	5	5	7
Indemnity Fee for Service	0	1	2	2	4
Managed Care Contracts					
Health Maintenance Organization	1	2	1	3	1
Preferred Provider Organization..............	10	11	13	17	16
Affiliations					
Hospitals in a System.....................	20	19	17	17	15
Hospitals in a Network	9	7	8	12	8
Hospitals in a Group Purchasing Organization..	22	17	19	28	25

TABLE 6

NORTH DAKOTA

U.S. Registered Community Hospitals
(Nonfederal, short-term general and other special hospitals)

Utilization, Personnel, Revenue and Expenses, Community Health Indicators 2008–2012

	2012	2011	2010	2009	2008
TOTAL FACILITY (Includes Hospital and Nursing Home Units)					
Utilization - Inpatient					
Beds	3,254	3,145	3,345	3,362	3,442
Admissions	92,940	94,125	94,436	92,593	89,225
Inpatient Days	727,855	701,723	718,950	751,653	744,876
Average Length of Stay	7.8	7.5	7.6	8.1	8.3
Inpatient Surgeries	26,617	28,285	29,558	27,732	26,451
Births	14,625	12,731	12,851	10,552	9,966
Utilization - Outpatient					
Emergency Outpatient Visits	419,652	408,870	353,557	303,190	289,070
Other Outpatient Visits	2,566,926	2,540,152	2,722,180	2,059,310	1,406,490
Total Outpatient Visits	2,986,578	2,949,022	3,075,737	2,362,500	1,695,560
Outpatient Surgeries	68,599	59,702	54,165	56,128	46,734
Personnel					
Full Time RNs	3,651	3,103	2,889	2,497	2,424
Full Time LPNs	514	501	514	599	512
Part Time RNs	2,791	2,485	2,452	2,163	2,002
Part Time LPNs	441	404	392	361	460
Total Full Time	16,049	14,606	13,962	13,326	12,312
Total Part Time	9,429	8,536	8,187	7,909	7,148
Revenue - Inpatient					
Gross Inpatient Revenue	$2,688,456,061	$2,320,300,120	$2,092,135,268	$2,019,340,609	$1,483,180,662
Revenue - Outpatient					
Gross Outpatient Revenue	$3,413,782,975	$2,783,603,262	$2,551,094,052	$2,583,127,227	$1,953,610,192
Revenue and Expenses - Totals					
(Includes Inpatient and Outpatient)					
Total Gross Revenue	$6,102,239,036	$5,103,903,382	$4,643,229,320	$4,602,467,836	$3,436,790,854
Deductions from Revenue	3,415,592,851	2,807,521,605	2,493,872,027	2,518,310,749	1,680,883,923
Net Patient Revenue	2,686,646,185	2,296,381,777	2,149,357,293	2,084,157,087	1,755,906,931
Other Operating Revenue	125,508,307	107,145,231	96,921,743	91,082,749	87,201,376
Other Nonoperating Revenue	24,882,062	22,983,677	33,585,013	13,376,054	-13,097,663
Total Net Revenue	2,837,036,554	2,426,510,685	2,279,864,049	2,188,615,890	1,830,010,644
Total Expenses	2,666,135,816	2,229,494,218	2,142,846,297	2,133,367,717	1,853,693,024
HOSPITAL UNIT (Excludes Separate Nursing Home Units)					
Utilization - Inpatient					
Beds	2,906	2,944	3,063	2,569	2,649
Admissions	91,966	92,902	92,796	90,862	86,795
Inpatient Days	613,301	633,852	634,164	485,393	479,593
Average Length of Stay	6.7	6.8	6.8	5.3	5.5
Personnel					
Total Full Time	15,785	14,472	13,822	12,820	11,728
Total Part Time	9,268	8,439	8,048	7,540	6,808
Revenue and Expenses - Totals					
(Includes Inpatient and Outpatient)					
Total Net Revenue	$2,813,596,727	$2,414,246,674	$2,258,523,169	$2,145,215,671	$1,780,423,431
Total Expenses	2,647,960,716	2,223,176,123	2,126,714,369	2,094,921,706	1,809,203,400
COMMUNITY HEALTH INDICATORS PER 1000 POPULATION					
Total Population (in thousands)	700	684	654	647	641
Inpatient					
Beds	4.7	4.6	5.1	5.2	5.4
Admissions	132.8	137.6	144.4	143.1	139.1
Inpatient Days	1,040.3	1,026.0	1,099.7	1,162.0	1,161.3
Inpatient Surgeries	38.0	41.4	45.2	42.9	41.2
Births	20.9	18.6	19.7	16.3	15.5
Outpatient					
Emergency Outpatient Visits	599.8	597.8	540.8	468.7	450.7
Other Outpatient Visits	3,669.0	3,714.0	4,163.8	3,183.6	2,192.8
Total Outpatient Visits	4,268.8	4,311.9	4,704.6	3,652.3	2,643.4
Outpatient Surgeries	98.1	87.3	82.8	86.8	72.9
Expense per Capita (per person)	$3,810.8	$3,259.8	$3,277.6	$3,298.1	$2,890.0

TABLE 6

OHIO

U.S. Registered Community Hospitals
(Nonfederal, short-term general and other special hospitals)

Overview 2008–2012

	2012	2011	2010	2009	2008
Total Community Hospitals in Ohio..........	185	183	183	183	181
Bed Size Category					
6-24	6	2	3	4	4
25-49	47	47	44	45	44
50-99	29	33	33	32	29
100-199	44	40	41	43	45
200-299	25	27	28	25	25
300-399	12	12	12	11	11
400-499	9	9	9	11	10
500 + ...	13	13	13	12	13
Location					
Hospitals Urban.........................	130	128	128	128	130
Hospitals Rural	55	55	55	55	51
Control					
State and Local Government................	19	19	21	22	21
Not for Profit	140	138	138	138	139
Investor owned	26	26	24	23	21
Physician Models					
Independent Practice Association	13	15	15	19	25
Group Practice without Walls...............	6	6	7	8	9
Open Physician-Hospital Organization	44	50	52	46	41
Closed Physician-Hospital Organization	15	15	9	10	13
Management Service Organization	19	33	35	39	49
Integrated Salary Model	78	70	71	64	68
Equity Model	8	8	9	7	8
Foundation.............................	20	29	31	28	27
Insurance Products					
Health Maintenance Organization	24	33	36	32	31
Preferred Provider Organization..............	31	39	43	44	34
Indemnity Fee for Service	10	14	16	15	11
Managed Care Contracts					
Health Maintenance Organization	121	114	113	120	112
Preferred Provider Organization..............	117	119	120	129	120
Affiliations					
Hospitals in a System.....................	122	118	114	111	107
Hospitals in a Network	77	76	77	77	74
Hospitals in a Group Purchasing Organization..	136	135	133	143	141

TABLE 6

OHIO

U.S. Registered Community Hospitals
(Nonfederal, short-term general and other special hospitals)

Utilization, Personnel, Revenue and Expenses, Community Health Indicators 2008–2012

	2012	2011	2010	2009	2008
TOTAL FACILITY (Includes Hospital and Nursing Home Units)					
Utilization - Inpatient					
Beds	33,659	33,828	34,316	33,994	33,860
Admissions	1,501,183	1,504,603	1,516,501	1,531,076	1,547,720
Inpatient Days	7,367,870	7,434,042	7,598,267	7,744,235	7,814,849
Average Length of Stay	4.9	4.9	5.0	5.1	5.0
Inpatient Surgeries	383,187	393,731	405,507	407,777	413,959
Births	128,393	128,695	133,946	141,295	143,941
Utilization - Outpatient					
Emergency Outpatient Visits	6,578,749	6,506,331	6,383,429	6,207,290	6,023,705
Other Outpatient Visits	30,377,613	29,390,397	29,375,819	28,033,655	26,868,157
Total Outpatient Visits	36,956,362	35,896,728	35,759,248	34,240,945	32,891,862
Outpatient Surgeries	810,268	803,825	817,556	800,882	787,850
Personnel					
Full Time RNs	54,347	52,672	51,255	48,681	45,914
Full Time LPNs	2,960	3,790	3,309	3,580	3,769
Part Time RNs	25,890	26,034	25,325	24,409	24,600
Part Time LPNs	1,785	1,788	1,808	1,859	2,080
Total Full Time	205,576	203,689	198,795	198,906	194,709
Total Part Time	76,463	78,003	76,929	75,934	76,454
Revenue - Inpatient					
Gross Inpatient Revenue	$55,828,522,139	$51,716,805,929	$49,069,396,749	$45,306,391,429	$41,893,875,454
Revenue - Outpatient					
Gross Outpatient Revenue	$52,981,694,494	$47,899,777,396	$44,283,440,488	$40,277,248,420	$35,108,967,663
Revenue and Expenses - Totals					
(Includes Inpatient and Outpatient)					
Total Gross Revenue	$108,810,216,633	$99,616,583,325	$93,352,837,237	$85,583,639,849	$77,002,843,117
Deductions from Revenue	73,204,925,076	67,235,879,337	61,559,545,620	55,069,727,140	48,579,748,500
Net Patient Revenue	35,605,291,557	32,380,703,988	31,793,291,617	30,513,912,709	28,423,094,617
Other Operating Revenue	2,642,307,155	2,439,029,875	2,302,711,954	2,204,346,362	1,902,066,455
Other Nonoperating Revenue	770,720,233	66,768,231	824,057,575	899,809,957	-1,531,882,065
Total Net Revenue	39,018,318,945	34,886,502,094	34,920,061,146	33,618,069,028	28,793,279,007
Total Expenses	35,772,141,755	32,605,625,518	32,374,139,783	30,929,648,514	29,074,986,966
HOSPITAL UNIT (Excludes Separate Nursing Home Units)					
Utilization - Inpatient					
Beds	32,901	32,734	33,157	32,613	32,422
Admissions	1,491,784	1,492,180	1,503,171	1,517,223	1,532,848
Inpatient Days	7,117,086	7,086,115	7,219,041	7,292,581	7,365,607
Average Length of Stay	4.8	4.7	4.8	4.8	4.8
Personnel					
Total Full Time	205,033	202,974	197,828	197,669	193,511
Total Part Time	76,040	77,530	76,311	75,222	75,671
Revenue and Expenses - Totals					
(Includes Inpatient and Outpatient)					
Total Net Revenue	$38,920,461,713	$34,777,592,693	$34,807,563,235	$33,478,190,434	$28,664,373,342
Total Expenses	35,672,905,913	32,496,965,573	32,265,651,508	30,795,620,302	28,951,022,330
COMMUNITY HEALTH INDICATORS PER 1000 POPULATION					
Total Population (in thousands)	11,544	11,545	11,532	11,543	11,528
Inpatient					
Beds	2.9	2.9	3.0	2.9	2.9
Admissions	130.0	130.3	131.5	132.6	134.3
Inpatient Days	638.2	643.9	658.9	670.9	677.9
Inpatient Surgeries	33.2	34.1	35.2	35.3	35.9
Births	11.1	11.1	11.6	12.2	12.5
Outpatient					
Emergency Outpatient Visits	569.9	563.6	553.5	537.8	522.5
Other Outpatient Visits	2,631.4	2,545.7	2,547.3	2,428.7	2,330.7
Total Outpatient Visits	3,201.3	3,109.3	3,100.8	2,966.5	2,853.2
Outpatient Surgeries	70.2	69.6	70.9	69.4	68.3
Expense per Capita (per person)	$3,098.7	$2,824.2	$2,807.3	$2,679.6	$2,522.1

States

TABLE **6**

OKLAHOMA

U.S. Registered Community Hospitals
(Nonfederal, short-term general and other special hospitals)

Overview 2008–2012

	2012	2011	2010	2009	2008
Total Community Hospitals in Oklahoma	117	115	113	116	115
Bed Size Category					
6-24	21	21	22	20	23
25-49	47	44	41	42	41
50-99	23	24	22	26	24
100-199	13	14	15	15	14
200-299	3	2	2	3	2
300-399	4	4	5	4	5
400-499	0	1	1	1	2
500 + ...	6	5	5	5	4
Location					
Hospitals Urban.	51	49	48	49	46
Hospitals Rural	66	66	65	67	69
Control					
State and Local Government.	40	41	44	45	45
Not for Profit	37	38	36	36	37
Investor owned	40	36	33	35	33
Physician Models					
Independent Practice Association	13	16	14	15	11
Group Practice without Walls.	5	4	6	6	4
Open Physician-Hospital Organization	12	11	9	11	11
Closed Physician-Hospital Organization	3	1	0	0	3
Management Service Organization	9	7	7	11	11
Integrated Salary Model	52	49	34	26	22
Equity Model	1	1	0	0	1
Foundation.	2	1	0	1	1
Insurance Products					
Health Maintenance Organization	13	13	8	7	5
Preferred Provider Organization.	12	16	10	8	8
Indemnity Fee for Service	5	8	4	4	3
Managed Care Contracts					
Health Maintenance Organization	52	48	38	38	41
Preferred Provider Organization.	76	76	63	62	64
Affiliations					
Hospitals in a System.	65	60	53	60	57
Hospitals in a Network	33	30	22	19	20
Hospitals in a Group Purchasing Organization. .	95	91	87	89	85

TABLE 6

OKLAHOMA

U.S. Registered Community Hospitals
(Nonfederal, short-term general and other special hospitals)

Utilization, Personnel, Revenue and Expenses, Community Health Indicators 2008–2012

	2012	2011	2010	2009	2008
TOTAL FACILITY (Includes Hospital and Nursing Home Units)					
Utilization - Inpatient					
Beds	11,349	11,303	11,170	11,316	10,988
Admissions	424,024	424,190	429,096	442,394	462,954
Inpatient Days	2,242,204	2,257,353	2,340,946	2,401,771	2,436,253
Average Length of Stay.	5.3	5.3	5.5	5.4	5.3
Inpatient Surgeries.	107,089	107,010	109,345	117,362	117,982
Births.	50,107	46,583	48,569	53,456	49,851
Utilization - Outpatient					
Emergency Outpatient Visits	1,908,047	1,847,389	1,762,821	1,743,802	1,645,625
Other Outpatient Visits.	4,866,096	4,175,877	3,895,891	3,827,100	3,785,996
Total Outpatient Visits	6,774,143	6,023,266	5,658,712	5,570,902	5,431,621
Outpatient Surgeries	223,225	211,753	206,440	200,043	198,007
Personnel					
Full Time RNs	12,313	11,500	11,105	10,929	10,585
Full Time LPNs	1,688	1,612	1,686	1,903	1,986
Part Time RNs.	4,277	4,046	3,984	3,654	3,684
Part Time LPNs	495	464	567	500	508
Total Full Time.	46,426	44,647	43,629	43,977	43,201
Total Part Time	13,623	13,085	13,056	12,159	12,279
Revenue - Inpatient					
Gross Inpatient Revenue.	$14,248,526,243	$13,445,502,051	$12,758,064,725	$12,064,230,137	$11,758,611,895
Revenue - Outpatient					
Gross Outpatient Revenue	$11,878,040,440	$10,390,808,413	$9,221,121,763	$8,258,194,596	$7,423,183,911
Revenue and Expenses - Totals					
(Includes Inpatient and Outpatient)					
Total Gross Revenue.	$26,126,566,683	$23,836,310,464	$21,979,186,488	$20,322,424,733	$19,181,795,806
Deductions from Revenue.	18,251,141,886	16,779,981,602	15,258,319,649	13,635,382,267	12,656,733,800
Net Patient Revenue	7,875,424,797	7,056,328,862	6,720,866,839	6,687,042,466	6,525,062,006
Other Operating Revenue	264,973,762	269,741,536	235,730,490	201,195,524	211,578,156
Other Nonoperating Revenue	27,381,522	185,667,771	102,371,200	-36,278,624	37,213,785
Total Net Revenue.	8,167,780,081	7,511,738,169	7,058,968,529	6,851,959,366	6,773,853,947
Total Expenses.	7,462,798,181	6,782,884,227	6,484,581,837	6,376,319,309	6,361,690,040
HOSPITAL UNIT (Excludes Separate Nursing Home Units)					
Utilization - Inpatient					
Beds	11,086	11,033	10,981	11,013	10,699
Admissions	422,856	423,362	427,982	440,886	461,577
Inpatient Days	2,164,883	2,183,306	2,280,666	2,277,293	2,339,600
Average Length of Stay.	5.1	5.2	5.3	5.2	5.1
Personnel					
Total Full Time.	46,159	44,486	43,532	43,684	42,916
Total Part Time	13,555	13,026	12,983	12,110	12,202
Revenue and Expenses - Totals					
(Includes Inpatient and Outpatient)					
Total Net Revenue.	$8,133,239,746	$7,501,813,546	$7,049,646,928	$6,836,200,847	$6,759,273,857
Total Expenses.	7,451,915,559	6,772,484,570	6,475,775,258	6,361,745,192	6,348,305,959
COMMUNITY HEALTH INDICATORS PER 1000 POPULATION					
Total Population (in thousands)	3,815	3,792	3,724	3,687	3,644
Inpatient					
Beds	3.0	3.0	3.0	3.1	3.0
Admissions	111.2	111.9	115.2	120.0	127.0
Inpatient Days	587.8	595.4	628.5	651.4	668.6
Inpatient Surgeries.	28.1	28.2	29.4	31.8	32.4
Births.	13.1	12.3	13.0	14.5	13.7
Outpatient					
Emergency Outpatient Visits	500.2	487.2	473.3	473.0	451.6
Other Outpatient Visits.	1,275.6	1,101.4	1,046.0	1,038.0	1,039.0
Total Outpatient Visits	1,775.7	1,588.6	1,519.3	1,510.9	1,490.6
Outpatient Surgeries	58.5	55.8	55.4	54.3	54.3
Expense per Capita (per person).	$1,956.3	$1,789.0	$1,741.1	$1,729.4	$1,745.8

States

TABLE 6

OREGON

U.S. Registered Community Hospitals
(Nonfederal, short-term general and other special hospitals)

Overview 2008–2012

	2012	2011	2010	2009	2008
Total Community Hospitals in Oregon	58	59	58	58	58
Bed Size Category					
6-24	8	9	9	8	8
25-49	20	20	20	19	19
50-99	9	10	10	12	11
100-199	10	9	9	9	9
200-299	4	4	4	4	5
300-399	2	2	1	1	0
400-499	3	3	3	3	4
500 + ...	2	2	2	2	2
Location					
Hospitals Urban..........................	30	30	29	29	26
Hospitals Rural	28	29	29	29	32
Control					
State and Local Government...............	11	12	12	12	13
Not for Profit	45	45	44	44	43
Investor owned	2	2	2	2	2
Physician Models					
Independent Practice Association	10	11	12	13	13
Group Practice without Walls................	8	9	9	8	8
Open Physician-Hospital Organization	5	6	6	6	6
Closed Physician-Hospital Organization	2	2	2	2	2
Management Service Organization	14	13	14	14	14
Integrated Salary Model	41	40	39	35	35
Equity Model	1	0	0	1	1
Foundation..............................	4	4	5	6	5
Insurance Products					
Health Maintenance Organization	14	16	15	15	14
Preferred Provider Organization..............	10	17	19	15	14
Indemnity Fee for Service	0	3	3	3	3
Managed Care Contracts					
Health Maintenance Organization	38	35	34	29	30
Preferred Provider Organization..............	49	52	51	51	51
Affiliations					
Hospitals in a System.....................	41	40	39	39	37
Hospitals in a Network....................	28	28	27	25	25
Hospitals in a Group Purchasing Organization..	56	58	57	56	56

TABLE 6

OREGON

U.S. Registered Community Hospitals
(Nonfederal, short-term general and other special hospitals)

Utilization, Personnel, Revenue and Expenses, Community Health Indicators 2008–2012

	2012	2011	2010	2009	2008
TOTAL FACILITY (Includes Hospital and Nursing Home Units)					
Utilization - Inpatient					
Beds	6,706	6,805	6,420	6,481	6,814
Admissions	336,677	342,649	321,334	323,733	348,600
Inpatient Days	1,429,092	1,468,277	1,387,082	1,437,561	1,551,894
Average Length of Stay	4.2	4.3	4.3	4.4	4.5
Inpatient Surgeries	119,276	123,292	114,683	114,337	120,048
Births	43,472	43,262	41,914	43,940	47,273
Utilization - Outpatient					
Emergency Outpatient Visits	1,402,280	1,404,165	1,229,539	1,312,068	1,330,142
Other Outpatient Visits	8,402,499	7,969,367	7,982,714	7,587,931	7,228,022
Total Outpatient Visits	9,804,779	9,373,532	9,212,253	8,899,999	8,558,164
Outpatient Surgeries	203,622	211,379	205,542	207,341	210,333
Personnel					
Full Time RNs	10,528	10,359	9,293	9,230	9,498
Full Time LPNs	162	185	189	212	214
Part Time RNs	7,366	7,692	7,003	7,068	7,753
Part Time LPNs	113	154	131	165	171
Total Full Time	38,512	39,278	35,968	35,768	37,581
Total Part Time	19,732	20,655	18,954	19,325	20,437
Revenue - Inpatient					
Gross Inpatient Revenue	$9,763,893,851	$9,510,397,093	$8,342,718,826	$7,965,180,365	$7,942,127,860
Revenue - Outpatient					
Gross Outpatient Revenue	$9,057,121,305	$8,564,788,044	$7,669,159,468	$7,028,661,629	$6,403,379,909
Revenue and Expenses - Totals					
(Includes Inpatient and Outpatient)					
Total Gross Revenue	$18,821,015,156	$18,075,185,137	$16,011,878,294	$14,993,841,994	$14,345,507,769
Deductions from Revenue	9,946,369,291	9,586,390,414	8,389,072,711	7,773,324,462	7,249,042,014
Net Patient Revenue	8,874,645,865	8,488,794,723	7,622,805,583	7,220,517,532	7,096,465,755
Other Operating Revenue	431,506,659	357,481,939	356,073,198	354,503,423	351,902,221
Other Nonoperating Revenue	120,073,921	115,998,119	164,944,836	-58,115,473	-55,685,102
Total Net Revenue	9,426,226,445	8,962,274,781	8,143,823,617	7,516,905,482	7,392,682,874
Total Expenses	9,102,609,637	8,726,772,182	7,875,937,042	7,402,240,332	7,376,298,400
HOSPITAL UNIT (Excludes Separate Nursing Home Units)					
Utilization - Inpatient					
Beds	6,538	6,618	6,233	6,228	6,551
Admissions	336,526	342,499	321,153	323,516	348,313
Inpatient Days	1,387,370	1,426,510	1,338,597	1,373,086	1,485,018
Average Length of Stay	4.1	4.2	4.2	4.2	4.3
Personnel					
Total Full Time	38,416	39,186	35,872	35,629	37,436
Total Part Time	19,687	20,579	18,863	19,243	20,381
Revenue and Expenses - Totals					
(Includes Inpatient and Outpatient)					
Total Net Revenue	$9,416,990,860	$8,952,622,279	$8,133,821,379	$7,504,259,729	$7,380,524,478
Total Expenses	9,094,089,019	8,718,381,099	7,866,577,239	7,391,642,279	7,366,061,834
COMMUNITY HEALTH INDICATORS PER 1000 POPULATION					
Total Population (in thousands)	3,899	3,872	3,856	3,826	3,783
Inpatient					
Beds	1.7	1.8	1.7	1.7	1.8
Admissions	86.3	88.5	83.3	84.6	92.1
Inpatient Days	366.5	379.2	359.8	375.8	410.2
Inpatient Surgeries	30.6	31.8	29.7	29.9	31.7
Births	11.1	11.2	10.9	11.5	12.5
Outpatient					
Emergency Outpatient Visits	359.6	362.7	318.9	343.0	351.6
Other Outpatient Visits	2,154.8	2,058.3	2,070.5	1,983.4	1,910.7
Total Outpatient Visits	2,514.5	2,420.9	2,389.4	2,326.4	2,262.3
Outpatient Surgeries	52.2	54.6	53.3	54.2	55.6
Expense per Capita (per person)	$2,334.4	$2,253.9	$2,042.8	$1,934.9	$1,949.9

States

TABLE 6

PENNSYLVANIA

U.S. Registered Community Hospitals
(Nonfederal, short-term general and other special hospitals)

Overview 2008–2012

	2012	2011	2010	2009	2008
Total Community Hospitals in Pennsylvania ...	192	194	196	194	201
Bed Size Category					
6-24	4	3	3	3	2
25-49	27	28	29	29	29
50-99	38	40	42	40	42
100-199	47	47	46	47	49
200-299	35	34	34	37	41
300-399	18	18	17	13	14
400-499	9	10	11	10	9
500 + ...	14	14	14	15	15
Location					
Hospitals Urban.........................	145	146	147	145	156
Hospitals Rural	47	48	49	49	45
Control					
State and Local Government...............	2	2	2	2	3
Not for Profit	142	145	151	153	160
Investor owned	48	47	43	39	38
Physician Models					
Independent Practice Association	12	8	7	8	9
Group Practice without Walls...............	5	6	8	13	13
Open Physician-Hospital Organization	22	22	24	25	32
Closed Physician-Hospital Organization	3	3	3	4	4
Management Service Organization	23	19	21	26	27
Integrated Salary Model....................	78	73	75	73	69
Equity Model	3	1	2	3	2
Foundation..............................	4	8	8	6	6
Insurance Products					
Health Maintenance Organization	37	35	29	24	29
Preferred Provider Organization..............	38	41	42	39	44
Indemnity Fee for Service	23	19	17	12	15
Managed Care Contracts					
Health Maintenance Organization	132	120	117	115	116
Preferred Provider Organization..............	128	116	115	109	112
Affiliations					
Hospitals in a System.....................	127	128	118	112	116
Hospitals in a Network....................	52	51	49	47	48
Hospitals in a Group Purchasing Organization..	141	134	139	134	131

TABLE 6

PENNSYLVANIA

U.S. Registered Community Hospitals
(Nonfederal, short-term general and other special hospitals)

Utilization, Personnel, Revenue and Expenses, Community Health Indicators 2008–2012

	2012	2011	2010	2009	2008
TOTAL FACILITY (Includes Hospital and Nursing Home Units)					
Utilization - Inpatient					
Beds	39,314	39,676	39,889	39,212	40,407
Admissions	1,692,087	1,766,191	1,809,935	1,841,550	1,901,417
Inpatient Days	9,287,033	9,659,186	9,769,701	9,865,210	10,353,793
Average Length of Stay	5.5	5.5	5.4	5.4	5.4
Inpatient Surgeries	545,302	526,338	534,919	540,046	558,918
Births	134,221	132,967	134,404	137,478	143,674
Utilization - Outpatient					
Emergency Outpatient Visits	6,239,042	6,221,333	6,120,131	6,009,572	6,006,841
Other Outpatient Visits	32,791,595	31,681,366	32,432,398	31,882,222	32,449,554
Total Outpatient Visits	39,030,637	37,902,699	38,552,529	37,891,794	38,456,395
Outpatient Surgeries	913,296	895,861	914,558	917,586	948,852
Personnel					
Full Time RNs	55,710	54,899	53,217	51,430	51,379
Full Time LPNs	3,035	3,115	3,406	3,769	4,183
Part Time RNs	25,187	25,473	24,947	25,315	25,909
Part Time LPNs	1,227	1,311	1,558	1,737	2,013
Total Full Time	212,082	211,563	207,153	203,289	211,389
Total Part Time	73,405	73,672	72,508	74,386	75,418
Revenue - Inpatient					
Gross Inpatient Revenue	$83,077,919,932	$81,435,847,151	$77,752,923,156	$73,916,497,474	$72,947,964,529
Revenue - Outpatient					
Gross Outpatient Revenue	$65,297,151,073	$58,909,827,289	$52,558,766,166	$47,748,195,221	$43,951,207,740
Revenue and Expenses - Totals					
(Includes Inpatient and Outpatient)					
Total Gross Revenue	$148,375,071,005	$140,345,674,440	$130,311,689,322	$121,664,692,695	$116,899,172,269
Deductions from Revenue	110,484,264,654	104,430,760,108	96,372,359,561	89,109,854,967	85,447,182,883
Net Patient Revenue	37,890,806,351	35,914,914,332	33,939,329,761	32,554,837,728	31,451,989,386
Other Operating Revenue	1,891,935,772	1,762,852,582	1,560,413,652	1,478,517,269	1,437,920,156
Other Nonoperating Revenue	244,155,533	671,813,569	355,838,893	-446,883,805	183,327,965
Total Net Revenue	40,026,897,656	38,349,580,483	35,855,582,306	33,586,471,192	33,073,237,507
Total Expenses	37,279,476,131	35,246,467,258	33,929,583,373	32,711,950,307	31,323,216,832
HOSPITAL UNIT (Excludes Separate Nursing Home Units)					
Utilization - Inpatient					
Beds	37,482	37,995	38,271	37,446	38,441
Admissions	1,674,103	1,748,683	1,793,060	1,822,836	1,880,413
Inpatient Days	8,740,926	9,116,795	9,324,956	9,383,976	9,836,158
Average Length of Stay	5.2	5.2	5.2	5.1	5.2
Personnel					
Total Full Time	211,038	210,543	205,956	201,932	209,962
Total Part Time	72,757	73,114	71,746	73,493	74,556
Revenue and Expenses - Totals					
(Includes Inpatient and Outpatient)					
Total Net Revenue	$39,806,434,073	$38,167,896,294	$35,657,261,435	$33,390,355,912	$32,864,948,434
Total Expenses	37,097,937,820	35,082,553,586	33,767,820,668	32,546,735,654	31,124,814,383
COMMUNITY HEALTH INDICATORS PER 1000 POPULATION					
Total Population (in thousands)	12,764	12,743	12,633	12,605	12,566
Inpatient					
Beds	3.1	3.1	3.2	3.1	3.2
Admissions	132.6	138.6	143.3	146.1	151.3
Inpatient Days	727.6	758.0	773.4	782.7	823.9
Inpatient Surgeries	42.7	41.3	42.3	42.8	44.5
Births	10.5	10.4	10.6	10.9	11.4
Outpatient					
Emergency Outpatient Visits	488.8	488.2	484.5	476.8	478.0
Other Outpatient Visits	2,569.2	2,486.2	2,567.3	2,529.4	2,582.3
Total Outpatient Visits	3,058.0	2,974.4	3,051.8	3,006.1	3,060.3
Outpatient Surgeries	71.6	70.3	72.4	72.8	75.5
Expense per Capita (per person)	$2,920.8	$2,766.0	$2,685.8	$2,595.2	$2,492.6

States

TABLE 6

RHODE ISLAND

U.S. Registered Community Hospitals
(Nonfederal, short-term general and other special hospitals)

Overview 2008–2012

	2012	2011	2010	2009	2008
Total Community Hospitals in Rhode Island ...	11	11	11	11	11
Bed Size Category					
6-24	0	0	0	0	0
25-49	0	0	0	0	0
50-99	1	1	1	1	1
100-199	5	5	5	5	6
200-299	3	3	3	3	2
300-399	1	1	1	1	1
400-499	0	0	0	0	0
500 +	1	1	1	1	1
Location					
Hospitals Urban	11	11	11	11	10
Hospitals Rural	0	0	0	0	1
Control					
State and Local Government	0	0	0	0	0
Not for Profit	11	11	11	11	11
Investor owned	0	0	0	0	0
Physician Models					
Independent Practice Association	4	5	5	4	6
Group Practice without Walls	1	1	0	0	0
Open Physician-Hospital Organization	4	5	6	6	7
Closed Physician-Hospital Organization	0	0	0	1	1
Management Service Organization	2	2	2	2	2
Integrated Salary Model	6	5	6	5	5
Equity Model	0	0	0	0	0
Foundation	2	2	2	2	3
Insurance Products					
Health Maintenance Organization	1	1	1	1	2
Preferred Provider Organization	0	1	0	0	1
Indemnity Fee for Service	0	0	0	0	0
Managed Care Contracts					
Health Maintenance Organization	6	6	7	7	9
Preferred Provider Organization	6	7	7	7	10
Affiliations					
Hospitals in a System	6	5	5	5	5
Hospitals in a Network	4	6	6	3	1
Hospitals in a Group Purchasing Organization	6	7	7	7	9

TABLE 6

RHODE ISLAND

U.S. Registered Community Hospitals
(Nonfederal, short-term general and other special hospitals)

Utilization, Personnel, Revenue and Expenses, Community Health Indicators 2008–2012

	2012	2011	2010	2009	2008
TOTAL FACILITY (Includes Hospital and Nursing Home Units)					
Utilization - Inpatient					
Beds	2,461	2,468	2,479	2,512	2,463
Admissions	117,051	120,407	123,188	126,761	127,413
Inpatient Days	580,207	611,837	621,614	654,695	666,745
Average Length of Stay	5.0	5.1	5.0	5.2	5.2
Inpatient Surgeries	32,119	32,737	32,612	39,752	38,970
Births	11,045	11,249	11,492	11,815	12,785
Utilization - Outpatient					
Emergency Outpatient Visits	578,431	542,625	495,149	502,224	494,817
Other Outpatient Visits	1,605,322	1,699,025	2,127,266	2,131,290	2,139,409
Total Outpatient Visits	2,183,753	2,241,650	2,622,415	2,633,514	2,634,226
Outpatient Surgeries	67,537	67,432	66,930	79,583	82,597
Personnel					
Full Time RNs	2,656	2,426	2,251	2,255	2,301
Full Time LPNs	71	70	58	87	92
Part Time RNs	2,780	2,737	2,771	2,705	3,147
Part Time LPNs	60	60	54	95	118
Total Full Time	12,871	12,810	12,686	12,928	12,908
Total Part Time	7,847	7,800	8,001	7,707	8,873
Revenue - Inpatient					
Gross Inpatient Revenue	$3,911,358,415	$3,763,721,393	$3,623,363,473	$3,585,072,822	$3,383,235,261
Revenue - Outpatient					
Gross Outpatient Revenue	$4,210,401,437	$3,841,600,497	$3,560,931,543	$3,292,773,520	$3,067,731,603
Revenue and Expenses - Totals					
(Includes Inpatient and Outpatient)					
Total Gross Revenue	$8,121,759,852	$7,605,321,890	$7,184,295,016	$6,877,846,342	$6,450,966,864
Deductions from Revenue	5,309,722,108	4,867,608,639	4,555,181,118	4,297,920,625	4,018,043,505
Net Patient Revenue	2,812,037,744	2,737,713,251	2,629,113,898	2,579,925,717	2,432,923,359
Other Operating Revenue	259,567,063	257,774,487	265,788,290	241,675,005	247,620,663
Other Nonoperating Revenue	26,181,940	10,927,762	6,408,073	6,908,048	6,024,220
Total Net Revenue	3,097,786,747	3,006,415,500	2,901,310,261	2,828,508,770	2,686,568,242
Total Expenses	3,067,815,218	3,021,867,827	2,883,693,916	2,812,067,020	2,649,565,524
HOSPITAL UNIT (Excludes Separate Nursing Home Units)					
Utilization - Inpatient					
Beds	2,461	2,468	2,479	2,512	2,439
Admissions	117,051	120,407	123,188	126,761	127,095
Inpatient Days	580,207	611,837	621,614	654,695	662,377
Average Length of Stay	5.0	5.1	5.0	5.2	5.2
Personnel					
Total Full Time	12,871	12,810	12,686	12,928	12,846
Total Part Time	7,847	7,800	8,001	7,707	8,790
Revenue and Expenses - Totals					
(Includes Inpatient and Outpatient)					
Total Net Revenue	$3,097,786,747	$3,006,415,500	$2,901,310,261	$2,828,508,770	$2,679,872,351
Total Expenses	3,067,815,218	3,021,867,827	2,883,693,916	2,812,067,020	2,643,600,577
COMMUNITY HEALTH INDICATORS PER 1000 POPULATION					
Total Population (in thousands)	1,050	1,051	1,057	1,053	1,054
Inpatient					
Beds	2.3	2.3	2.3	2.4	2.3
Admissions	111.4	114.5	116.6	120.4	120.9
Inpatient Days	552.4	582.0	588.2	621.6	632.9
Inpatient Surgeries	30.6	31.1	30.9	37.7	37.0
Births	10.5	10.7	10.9	11.2	12.1
Outpatient					
Emergency Outpatient Visits	550.7	516.1	468.5	476.9	469.7
Other Outpatient Visits	1,528.5	1,616.1	2,012.8	2,023.6	2,030.8
Total Outpatient Visits	2,079.2	2,132.3	2,481.3	2,500.5	2,500.4
Outpatient Surgeries	64.3	64.1	63.3	75.6	78.4
Expense per Capita (per person)	$2,920.9	$2,874.4	$2,728.5	$2,670.0	$2,515.0

States

TABLE 6

SOUTH CAROLINA

U.S. Registered Community Hospitals
(Nonfederal, short-term general and other special hospitals)

Overview 2008–2012

	2012	2011	2010	2009	2008
Total Community Hospitals in South Carolina..	67	66	67	70	69
Bed Size Category					
6-24	1	2	1	2	0
25-49	16	17	19	18	18
50-99	13	11	10	13	12
100-199	14	14	13	13	14
200-299	9	8	9	10	12
300-399	6	6	7	7	7
400-499	4	3	3	2	1
500 + ...	4	5	5	5	5
Location					
Hospitals Urban.	43	41	42	45	41
Hospitals Rural	24	25	25	25	28
Control					
State and Local Government.	18	19	17	20	20
Not for Profit	26	23	24	25	25
Investor owned	23	24	26	25	24
Physician Models					
Independent Practice Association	6	6	5	5	6
Group Practice without Walls.	1	1	1	1	3
Open Physician-Hospital Organization	5	4	4	7	8
Closed Physician-Hospital Organization	2	2	1	0	1
Management Service Organization	1	0	2	1	0
Integrated Salary Model.	20	20	19	15	14
Equity Model	2	1	0	0	0
Foundation.	0	0	0	0	0
Insurance Products					
Health Maintenance Organization	1	6	7	7	2
Preferred Provider Organization.	6	9	10	10	5
Indemnity Fee for Service	0	1	6	6	1
Managed Care Contracts					
Health Maintenance Organization	40	43	39	45	37
Preferred Provider Organization.	40	43	38	46	36
Affiliations					
Hospitals in a System.	50	44	44	47	45
Hospitals in a Network	12	12	12	12	15
Hospitals in a Group Purchasing Organization..	55	60	59	58	52

TABLE 6

SOUTH CAROLINA

U.S. Registered Community Hospitals
(Nonfederal, short-term general and other special hospitals)

Utilization, Personnel, Revenue and Expenses, Community Health Indicators 2008–2012

	2012	2011	2010	2009	2008
TOTAL FACILITY (Includes Hospital and Nursing Home Units)					
Utilization - Inpatient					
Beds	12,539	12,253	12,495	12,483	12,498
Admissions	506,072	508,652	522,793	528,204	528,872
Inpatient Days	2,861,439	2,878,860	3,002,541	2,960,134	2,962,830
Average Length of Stay	5.7	5.7	5.7	5.6	5.6
Inpatient Surgeries	197,921	194,171	194,895	205,119	196,304
Births	53,353	53,530	54,894	57,559	56,068
Utilization - Outpatient					
Emergency Outpatient Visits	1,435,010	1,687,578	1,453,696	2,171,925	1,954,264
Other Outpatient Visits	5,114,768	4,732,533	4,922,633	4,147,745	3,969,951
Total Outpatient Visits	6,549,778	6,420,111	6,376,329	6,319,670	5,924,215
Outpatient Surgeries	309,250	298,549	289,794	300,093	294,280
Personnel					
Full Time RNs	17,934	17,357	17,476	17,451	16,203
Full Time LPNs	775	947	1,062	1,170	1,292
Part Time RNs	4,652	4,897	5,184	5,246	5,834
Part Time LPNs	227	280	347	395	510
Total Full Time	60,411	58,183	58,567	58,933	58,372
Total Part Time	13,579	13,721	14,343	14,332	16,302
Revenue - Inpatient					
Gross Inpatient Revenue	$20,007,919,363	$19,216,509,155	$18,371,422,174	$17,448,319,308	$16,743,319,395
Revenue - Outpatient					
Gross Outpatient Revenue	$15,551,458,526	$14,306,685,453	$12,660,946,189	$11,900,471,047	$10,266,244,867
Revenue and Expenses - Totals					
(Includes Inpatient and Outpatient)					
Total Gross Revenue	$35,559,377,889	$33,523,194,608	$31,032,368,363	$29,348,790,355	$27,009,564,262
Deductions from Revenue	25,246,098,981	23,252,635,242	21,049,743,519	19,883,727,173	18,082,987,646
Net Patient Revenue	10,313,278,908	10,270,559,366	9,982,624,844	9,465,063,182	8,926,576,616
Other Operating Revenue	308,030,013	243,603,622	249,339,525	236,614,730	262,341,118
Other Nonoperating Revenue	277,725,354	141,294,623	210,607,769	190,176,135	85,822,937
Total Net Revenue	10,899,034,275	10,655,457,611	10,442,572,138	9,891,854,047	9,274,740,671
Total Expenses	9,729,644,756	9,707,103,556	9,349,824,264	9,264,970,348	8,890,465,525
HOSPITAL UNIT (Excludes Separate Nursing Home Units)					
Utilization - Inpatient					
Beds	11,656	11,479	11,611	11,739	11,728
Admissions	502,923	504,604	518,130	524,147	524,838
Inpatient Days	2,585,730	2,632,449	2,729,473	2,685,104	2,750,321
Average Length of Stay	5.1	5.2	5.3	5.1	5.2
Personnel					
Total Full Time	59,664	57,533	57,811	58,169	57,714
Total Part Time	13,328	13,382	14,118	13,998	16,043
Revenue and Expenses - Totals					
(Includes Inpatient and Outpatient)					
Total Net Revenue	$10,842,235,748	$10,577,543,806	$10,354,825,713	$9,821,499,987	$9,217,872,804
Total Expenses	9,666,217,448	9,635,628,294	9,272,925,368	9,204,773,809	8,842,007,632
COMMUNITY HEALTH INDICATORS PER 1000 POPULATION					
Total Population (in thousands)	4,724	4,679	4,597	4,561	4,503
Inpatient					
Beds	2.7	2.6	2.7	2.7	2.8
Admissions	107.1	108.7	113.7	115.8	117.4
Inpatient Days	605.8	615.2	653.2	649.0	657.9
Inpatient Surgeries	41.9	41.5	42.4	45.0	43.6
Births	11.3	11.4	11.9	12.6	12.5
Outpatient					
Emergency Outpatient Visits	303.8	360.7	316.2	476.2	434.0
Other Outpatient Visits	1,082.8	1,011.4	1,070.8	909.3	881.6
Total Outpatient Visits	1,386.6	1,372.0	1,387.1	1,385.5	1,315.5
Outpatient Surgeries	65.5	63.8	63.0	65.8	65.3
Expense per Capita (per person)	$2,059.7	$2,074.5	$2,033.9	$2,031.2	$1,974.2

States

TABLE 6

SOUTH DAKOTA

U.S. Registered Community Hospitals
(Nonfederal, short-term general and other special hospitals)

Overview 2008–2012

	2012	2011	2010	2009	2008
Total Community Hospitals in South Dakota...	54	53	53	53	53
Bed Size Category					
6-24	19	19	17	16	18
25-49	13	12	14	14	12
50-99	10	10	10	11	11
100-199	7	7	7	7	7
200-299	2	2	2	2	1
300-399	1	1	1	1	2
400-499	1	2	2	2	2
500 + ...	1	0	0	0	0
Location					
Hospitals Urban..........................	11	11	11	11	9
Hospitals Rural	43	42	42	42	44
Control					
State and Local Government...............	4	4	4	3	5
Not for Profit............................	46	45	45	46	44
Investor owned	4	4	4	4	4
Physician Models					
Independent Practice Association	9	10	8	12	11
Group Practice without Walls................	2	2	1	3	3
Open Physician-Hospital Organization	3	4	3	6	6
Closed Physician-Hospital Organization	3	3	2	3	3
Management Service Organization	2	3	1	2	2
Integrated Salary Model....................	25	27	23	28	25
Equity Model	3	2	1	2	2
Foundation...............................	3	3	2	1	1
Insurance Products					
Health Maintenance Organization	13	13	16	17	17
Preferred Provider Organization..............	12	13	11	10	13
Indemnity Fee for Service	5	8	6	9	8
Managed Care Contracts					
Health Maintenance Organization	27	25	23	24	24
Preferred Provider Organization..............	31	30	27	29	32
Affiliations					
Hospitals in a System.....................	39	37	37	38	38
Hospitals in a Network	23	24	21	22	22
Hospitals in a Group Purchasing Organization..	43	46	39	45	45

TABLE **6**

SOUTH DAKOTA

U.S. Registered Community Hospitals
(Nonfederal, short-term general and other special hospitals)

Utilization, Personnel, Revenue and Expenses, Community Health Indicators 2008–2012

	2012	2011	2010	2009	2008
TOTAL FACILITY (Includes Hospital and Nursing Home Units)					
Utilization - Inpatient					
Beds	4,188	4,084	4,108	4,142	4,113
Admissions	108,263	101,867	101,128	102,335	102,116
Inpatient Days	960,652	956,044	935,410	1,005,265	1,005,766
Average Length of Stay.	8.9	9.4	9.2	9.8	9.8
Inpatient Surgeries.	29,636	31,220	30,363	32,416	31,715
Births.	12,242	11,976	11,437	11,848	12,258
Utilization - Outpatient					
Emergency Outpatient Visits	282,899	251,769	259,364	240,618	239,192
Other Outpatient Visits.	1,979,362	1,862,618	1,782,993	1,698,830	1,618,764
Total Outpatient Visits	2,262,261	2,114,387	2,042,357	1,939,448	1,857,956
Outpatient Surgeries	76,606	69,535	67,743	71,571	71,162
Personnel					
Full Time RNs	4,457	4,068	3,633	3,596	3,160
Full Time LPNs	267	270	216	191	185
Part Time RNs	1,948	1,951	1,736	2,003	2,253
Part Time LPNs	124	144	129	132	131
Total Full Time.	16,543	15,443	14,483	15,119	14,488
Total Part Time	6,807	6,954	6,316	7,357	8,067
Revenue - Inpatient					
Gross Inpatient Revenue.	$3,259,110,943	$2,969,819,139	$2,779,376,912	$2,534,795,960	$2,293,166,775
Revenue - Outpatient					
Gross Outpatient Revenue	$3,103,567,011	$2,643,342,592	$2,405,199,211	$2,107,192,538	$1,875,244,749
Revenue and Expenses - Totals					
(Includes Inpatient and Outpatient)					
Total Gross Revenue.	$6,362,677,954	$5,613,161,731	$5,184,576,123	$4,641,988,498	$4,168,411,524
Deductions from Revenue.	3,649,680,422	3,130,649,704	2,884,612,400	2,468,508,414	2,187,095,692
Net Patient Revenue	2,712,997,532	2,482,512,027	2,299,963,723	2,173,480,084	1,981,315,832
Other Operating Revenue	146,318,931	129,361,349	122,786,678	113,185,811	103,615,596
Other Nonoperating Revenue	34,097,686	101,197,230	34,907,740	-20,449,611	30,994,497
Total Net Revenue.	2,893,414,149	2,713,070,606	2,457,658,141	2,266,216,284	2,115,925,925
Total Expenses.	2,494,970,877	2,353,418,704	2,194,315,958	2,075,750,158	1,919,761,533
HOSPITAL UNIT (Excludes Separate Nursing Home Units)					
Utilization - Inpatient					
Beds	2,847	2,602	2,869	2,728	2,671
Admissions	106,941	100,451	99,824	100,901	100,555
Inpatient Days	503,324	443,426	505,190	507,150	509,176
Average Length of Stay.	4.7	4.4	5.1	5.0	5.1
Personnel					
Total Full Time.	15,690	14,561	13,753	14,238	13,650
Total Part Time	6,221	6,292	5,684	6,607	7,369
Revenue and Expenses - Totals					
(Includes Inpatient and Outpatient)					
Total Net Revenue.	$2,806,088,891	$2,626,079,779	$2,382,414,150	$2,185,615,059	$2,035,881,683
Total Expenses.	2,410,336,333	2,278,140,332	2,128,257,681	2,002,334,795	1,848,451,464
COMMUNITY HEALTH INDICATORS PER 1000 POPULATION					
Total Population (in thousands)	833	824	820	812	805
Inpatient					
Beds	5.0	5.0	5.0	5.1	5.1
Admissions	129.9	123.6	123.3	126.0	126.9
Inpatient Days	1,152.8	1,160.1	1,140.6	1,237.4	1,250.1
Inpatient Surgeries.	35.6	37.9	37.0	39.9	39.4
Births.	14.7	14.5	13.9	14.6	15.2
Outpatient					
Emergency Outpatient Visits	339.5	305.5	316.3	296.2	297.3
Other Outpatient Visits.	2,375.2	2,260.2	2,174.2	2,091.2	2,012.1
Total Outpatient Visits	2,714.6	2,565.7	2,490.4	2,387.4	2,309.4
Outpatient Surgeries	91.9	84.4	82.6	88.1	88.5
Expense per Capita (per person).	$2,993.9	$2,855.8	$2,675.7	$2,555.1	$2,386.2

States

TABLE 6

TENNESSEE

U.S. Registered Community Hospitals
(Nonfederal, short-term general and other special hospitals)

Overview 2008–2012

	2012	2011	2010	2009	2008
Total Community Hospitals in Tennessee	132	133	134	137	137
Bed Size Category					
6-24	9	7	6	6	7
25-49	34	36	35	36	36
50-99	31	32	32	32	32
100-199	26	26	29	30	29
200-299	13	13	12	13	12
300-399	7	7	6	7	7
400-499	3	3	5	6	5
500 + ...	9	9	9	7	9
Location					
Hospitals Urban..........................	77	78	78	81	71
Hospitals Rural	55	55	56	56	66
Control					
State and Local Government................	21	21	20	22	22
Not for Profit	49	50	56	59	60
Investor owned	62	62	58	56	55
Physician Models					
Independent Practice Association	16	17	19	17	14
Group Practice without Walls...............	4	5	4	3	4
Open Physician-Hospital Organization	17	11	11	11	19
Closed Physician-Hospital Organization	4	3	3	3	5
Management Service Organization	14	17	16	18	15
Integrated Salary Model	30	29	31	26	19
Equity Model	0	0	0	0	0
Foundation..............................	2	3	4	7	8
Insurance Products					
Health Maintenance Organization	9	8	8	5	14
Preferred Provider Organization.............	13	17	17	16	26
Indemnity Fee for Service	7	3	3	2	10
Managed Care Contracts					
Health Maintenance Organization	56	68	66	67	86
Preferred Provider Organization.............	62	69	72	75	87
Affiliations					
Hospitals in a System.....................	107	105	101	103	104
Hospitals in a Network....................	31	38	41	41	45
Hospitals in a Group Purchasing Organization..	68	70	69	77	89

TABLE 6

TENNESSEE

U.S. Registered Community Hospitals
(Nonfederal, short-term general and other special hospitals)

Utilization, Personnel, Revenue and Expenses, Community Health Indicators 2008–2012

	2012	2011	2010	2009	2008
TOTAL FACILITY (Includes Hospital and Nursing Home Units)					
Utilization - Inpatient					
Beds	20,154	20,042	20,830	20,959	21,102
Admissions	823,781	805,805	832,554	859,191	859,344
Inpatient Days	4,500,597	4,465,285	4,579,402	4,799,858	4,911,215
Average Length of Stay	5.5	5.5	5.5	5.6	5.7
Inpatient Surgeries	241,056	234,368	249,367	255,557	243,820
Births	64,660	64,202	70,685	79,804	83,978
Utilization - Outpatient					
Emergency Outpatient Visits	3,260,802	3,113,164	3,130,660	3,301,872	3,251,592
Other Outpatient Visits	8,519,980	7,799,873	8,299,669	8,281,474	7,995,403
Total Outpatient Visits	11,780,782	10,913,037	11,430,329	11,583,346	11,246,995
Outpatient Surgeries	448,279	405,105	411,688	413,202	385,344
Personnel					
Full Time RNs	26,169	25,298	24,475	25,846	24,727
Full Time LPNs	2,252	2,503	2,706	2,938	3,286
Part Time RNs	9,110	9,124	9,222	8,514	8,891
Part Time LPNs	610	652	767	742	881
Total Full Time	91,851	89,424	88,145	93,028	90,902
Total Part Time	25,175	23,382	25,539	24,476	25,311
Revenue - Inpatient					
Gross Inpatient Revenue	$28,979,229,922	$27,704,113,354	$26,846,357,974	$25,367,667,093	$24,012,198,547
Revenue - Outpatient					
Gross Outpatient Revenue	$24,221,902,571	$20,574,396,531	$19,276,589,146	$17,453,642,146	$15,732,131,119
Revenue and Expenses - Totals					
(Includes Inpatient and Outpatient)					
Total Gross Revenue	$53,201,132,493	$48,278,509,885	$46,122,947,120	$42,821,309,239	$39,744,329,666
Deductions from Revenue	37,978,697,915	34,865,417,816	32,931,211,533	29,947,998,235	27,469,500,901
Net Patient Revenue	15,222,434,578	13,413,092,069	13,191,735,587	12,873,311,004	12,274,828,765
Other Operating Revenue	546,985,739	445,637,920	409,743,303	432,326,528	496,258,779
Other Nonoperating Revenue	108,447,768	158,051,242	268,674,837	-81,972,728	81,614,397
Total Net Revenue	15,877,868,085	14,016,781,231	13,870,153,727	13,223,664,804	12,852,701,941
Total Expenses	14,708,134,735	12,769,264,645	12,699,265,618	12,694,504,650	11,996,245,958
HOSPITAL UNIT (Excludes Separate Nursing Home Units)					
Utilization - Inpatient					
Beds	19,052	19,080	19,750	19,682	19,467
Admissions	816,107	797,947	825,283	850,278	849,060
Inpatient Days	4,178,131	4,182,726	4,244,905	4,400,598	4,396,275
Average Length of Stay	5.1	5.2	5.1	5.2	5.2
Personnel					
Total Full Time	90,895	88,534	87,258	91,886	89,529
Total Part Time	24,986	23,260	25,367	24,274	25,004
Revenue and Expenses - Totals					
(Includes Inpatient and Outpatient)					
Total Net Revenue	$15,793,027,961	$13,930,291,003	$13,791,578,759	$13,131,489,651	$12,735,644,514
Total Expenses	14,632,776,271	12,708,497,514	12,630,190,370	12,619,381,549	11,896,072,460
COMMUNITY HEALTH INDICATORS PER 1000 POPULATION					
Total Population (in thousands)	6,456	6,403	6,338	6,296	6,240
Inpatient					
Beds	3.1	3.1	3.3	3.3	3.4
Admissions	127.6	125.8	131.4	136.5	137.7
Inpatient Days	697.1	697.3	722.5	762.3	787.0
Inpatient Surgeries	37.3	36.6	39.3	40.6	39.1
Births	10.0	10.0	11.2	12.7	13.5
Outpatient					
Emergency Outpatient Visits	505.1	486.2	493.9	524.4	521.1
Other Outpatient Visits	1,319.6	1,218.1	1,309.5	1,315.3	1,281.2
Total Outpatient Visits	1,824.7	1,704.3	1,803.4	1,839.7	1,802.3
Outpatient Surgeries	69.4	63.3	65.0	65.6	61.7
Expense per Capita (per person)	$2,278.1	$1,994.2	$2,003.6	$2,016.2	$1,922.3

States

TABLE **6**

TEXAS

U.S. Registered Community Hospitals
(Nonfederal, short-term general and other special hospitals)

Overview 2008–2012

	2012	2011	2010	2009	2008
Total Community Hospitals in Texas..........	**425**	**420**	**426**	**428**	**426**
Bed Size Category					
6-24	74	70	73	69	63
25-49	107	109	107	111	111
50-99	87	82	86	79	87
100-199	55	58	61	66	64
200-299	42	43	41	43	44
300-399	23	19	20	21	20
400-499	13	15	14	16	14
500 + ...	24	24	24	23	23
Location					
Hospitals Urban..........................	276	269	275	277	265
Hospitals Rural	149	151	151	151	161
Control					
State and Local Government...............	106	110	113	116	117
Not for Profit	151	149	148	147	152
Investor owned	168	161	165	165	157
Physician Models					
Independent Practice Association	58	62	72	69	67
Group Practice without Walls...............	15	15	15	24	14
Open Physician-Hospital Organization	83	79	82	84	90
Closed Physician-Hospital Organization	26	20	19	18	17
Management Service Organization	62	71	73	74	63
Integrated Salary Model....................	115	114	97	95	91
Equity Model	8	9	13	13	12
Foundation...............................	37	37	35	33	34
Insurance Products					
Health Maintenance Organization	60	65	66	62	49
Preferred Provider Organization..............	50	79	84	75	66
Indemnity Fee for Service	13	22	26	22	23
Managed Care Contracts					
Health Maintenance Organization	331	318	318	323	314
Preferred Provider Organization..............	362	357	358	361	361
Affiliations					
Hospitals in a System......................	283	272	278	286	281
Hospitals in a Network.....................	116	115	114	106	104
Hospitals in a Group Purchasing Organization..	407	399	398	386	385

States

TABLE 6

TEXAS

U.S. Registered Community Hospitals
(Nonfederal, short-term general and other special hospitals)

Utilization, Personnel, Revenue and Expenses, Community Health Indicators 2008–2012

	2012	2011	2010	2009	2008
TOTAL FACILITY (Includes Hospital and Nursing Home Units)					
Utilization - Inpatient					
Beds	61,290	60,755	61,357	62,069	61,039
Admissions	2,548,864	2,534,688	2,580,401	2,621,436	2,585,680
Inpatient Days	13,170,816	13,062,644	13,331,491	13,590,044	13,430,355
Average Length of Stay	5.2	5.2	5.2	5.2	5.2
Inpatient Surgeries	729,749	736,841	761,437	781,093	763,867
Births	369,860	364,901	381,038	397,979	390,274
Utilization - Outpatient					
Emergency Outpatient Visits	10,439,383	9,889,631	9,739,066	9,438,151	8,819,272
Other Outpatient Visits	30,271,030	29,375,051	28,541,761	26,584,907	25,999,796
Total Outpatient Visits	40,710,413	39,264,682	38,280,827	36,023,058	34,819,068
Outpatient Surgeries	1,024,211	1,034,126	1,061,053	1,049,368	1,030,039
Personnel					
Full Time RNs	83,746	79,968	82,490	80,537	73,086
Full Time LPNs	7,679	8,278	9,113	9,798	10,227
Part Time RNs	22,853	22,557	20,107	20,901	21,580
Part Time LPNs	1,674	1,683	2,103	2,416	2,487
Total Full Time	278,323	274,534	280,656	280,533	266,604
Total Part Time	64,880	63,938	59,204	61,186	63,288
Revenue - Inpatient					
Gross Inpatient Revenue	$114,321,510,363	$105,598,575,282	$100,476,401,353	$95,184,048,332	$87,141,175,562
Revenue - Outpatient					
Gross Outpatient Revenue	$82,221,757,827	$72,395,257,221	$66,131,968,217	$58,578,510,903	$49,826,890,592
Revenue and Expenses - Totals					
(Includes Inpatient and Outpatient)					
Total Gross Revenue	$196,543,268,190	$177,993,832,503	$166,608,369,570	$153,762,559,235	$136,968,066,154
Deductions from Revenue	144,431,424,185	132,820,105,328	122,345,151,455	111,061,711,464	97,866,719,468
Net Patient Revenue	52,111,844,005	45,173,727,175	44,263,218,115	42,700,847,771	39,101,346,686
Other Operating Revenue	5,301,391,230	4,676,074,781	4,492,462,311	4,384,346,385	4,040,612,362
Other Nonoperating Revenue	842,027,514	1,373,986,299	1,120,744,597	304,258,670	310,546,108
Total Net Revenue	58,255,262,749	51,223,788,255	49,876,425,023	47,389,452,826	43,452,505,156
Total Expenses	51,154,019,956	45,556,147,376	44,225,750,333	43,410,205,109	40,396,037,477
HOSPITAL UNIT (Excludes Separate Nursing Home Units)					
Utilization - Inpatient					
Beds	60,350	59,835	60,497	61,160	59,947
Admissions	2,539,148	2,525,028	2,570,756	2,610,941	2,574,309
Inpatient Days	12,898,573	12,794,132	13,090,722	13,329,807	13,117,477
Average Length of Stay	5.1	5.1	5.1	5.1	5.1
Personnel					
Total Full Time	277,484	273,785	279,998	279,502	265,647
Total Part Time	64,773	63,837	59,051	61,033	62,914
Revenue and Expenses - Totals					
(Includes Inpatient and Outpatient)					
Total Net Revenue	$58,163,406,060	$51,125,792,174	$49,780,310,157	$47,305,885,374	$43,361,995,590
Total Expenses	51,073,523,904	45,465,619,488	44,132,923,562	43,327,541,508	40,292,698,073
COMMUNITY HEALTH INDICATORS PER 1000 POPULATION					
Total Population (in thousands)	26,059	25,675	25,213	24,782	24,304
Inpatient					
Beds	2.4	2.4	2.4	2.5	2.5
Admissions	97.8	98.7	102.3	105.8	106.4
Inpatient Days	505.4	508.8	528.7	548.4	552.6
Inpatient Surgeries	28.0	28.7	30.2	31.5	31.4
Births	14.2	14.2	15.1	16.1	16.1
Outpatient					
Emergency Outpatient Visits	400.6	385.2	386.3	380.8	362.9
Other Outpatient Visits	1,161.6	1,144.1	1,132.0	1,072.7	1,069.8
Total Outpatient Visits	1,562.2	1,529.3	1,518.3	1,453.6	1,432.6
Outpatient Surgeries	39.3	40.3	42.1	42.3	42.4
Expense per Capita (per person)	$1,963.0	$1,774.4	$1,754.1	$1,751.7	$1,662.1

States

TABLE **6**

UTAH

U.S. Registered Community Hospitals
(Nonfederal, short-term general and other special hospitals)

Overview 2008–2012

	2012	2011	2010	2009	2008
Total Community Hospitals in Utah...........	47	46	44	44	43
Bed Size Category					
6-24	9	8	8	6	6
25-49	16	16	15	15	14
50-99	3	4	3	6	6
100-199	10	9	8	8	9
200-299	4	4	5	4	4
300-399	3	3	3	3	2
400-499	1	2	2	1	1
500 + ...	1	0	0	1	1
Location					
Hospitals Urban..........................	28	28	26	26	21
Hospitals Rural	19	18	18	18	22
Control					
State and Local Government................	6	6	6	6	5
Not for Profit	26	25	23	23	23
Investor owned	15	15	15	15	15
Physician Models					
Independent Practice Association	4	4	4	6	2
Group Practice without Walls...............	2	2	1	1	0
Open Physician-Hospital Organization	1	1	1	3	2
Closed Physician-Hospital Organization	2	3	2	2	1
Management Service Organization	2	2	2	2	1
Integrated Salary Model	19	18	13	13	13
Equity Model	1	1	1	1	0
Foundation..............................	1	1	1	2	1
Insurance Products					
Health Maintenance Organization	16	17	15	15	16
Preferred Provider Organization..............	9	15	13	13	12
Indemnity Fee for Service	4	7	5	7	7
Managed Care Contracts					
Health Maintenance Organization	13	12	14	13	14
Preferred Provider Organization..............	18	18	17	17	19
Affiliations					
Hospitals in a System......................	38	38	36	36	37
Hospitals in a Network	8	11	11	16	15
Hospitals in a Group Purchasing Organization..	21	25	22	21	19

TABLE 6

UTAH

U.S. Registered Community Hospitals
(Nonfederal, short-term general and other special hospitals)

Utilization, Personnel, Revenue and Expenses, Community Health Indicators 2008–2012

	2012	2011	2010	2009	2008
TOTAL FACILITY (Includes Hospital and Nursing Home Units)					
Utilization - Inpatient					
Beds	5,212	5,135	5,086	4,973	4,874
Admissions	241,436	236,131	224,264	226,239	226,376
Inpatient Days	992,015	993,098	979,963	1,003,710	1,015,945
Average Length of Stay	4.1	4.2	4.4	4.4	4.5
Inpatient Surgeries	71,909	71,272	70,503	71,568	67,840
Births	51,575	52,695	49,392	52,189	55,088
Utilization - Outpatient					
Emergency Outpatient Visits	894,661	855,152	834,897	865,286	856,277
Other Outpatient Visits	5,459,212	4,999,514	4,642,827	4,609,086	4,449,171
Total Outpatient Visits	6,353,873	5,854,666	5,477,724	5,474,372	5,305,448
Outpatient Surgeries	166,063	174,376	166,870	155,162	152,105
Personnel					
Full Time RNs	7,273	7,462	7,303	6,961	6,780
Full Time LPNs	299	337	358	367	378
Part Time RNs	4,801	4,362	4,353	4,454	4,620
Part Time LPNs	171	181	187	222	277
Total Full Time	26,395	26,733	26,111	26,390	26,648
Total Part Time	14,612	13,696	13,418	14,135	14,535
Revenue - Inpatient					
Gross Inpatient Revenue	$8,253,048,052	$7,051,376,726	$6,581,097,114	$5,718,543,491	$5,428,255,474
Revenue - Outpatient					
Gross Outpatient Revenue	$6,983,551,734	$6,027,847,868	$5,300,499,527	$4,667,222,276	$4,060,507,024
Revenue and Expenses - Totals					
(Includes Inpatient and Outpatient)					
Total Gross Revenue	$15,236,599,786	$13,079,224,594	$11,881,596,641	$10,385,765,767	$9,488,762,498
Deductions from Revenue	9,233,540,993	7,638,050,195	6,906,546,426	5,568,409,487	5,093,986,033
Net Patient Revenue	6,003,058,793	5,441,174,399	4,975,050,215	4,817,356,280	4,394,776,465
Other Operating Revenue	221,419,572	265,484,132	243,975,154	228,925,055	207,762,710
Other Nonoperating Revenue	9,983,495	10,166,250	31,741,257	12,752,174	20,119,824
Total Net Revenue	6,234,461,860	5,716,824,781	5,250,766,626	5,059,033,509	4,622,658,999
Total Expenses	5,117,473,502	4,679,558,728	4,470,510,613	4,263,844,434	4,041,481,901
HOSPITAL UNIT (Excludes Separate Nursing Home Units)					
Utilization - Inpatient					
Beds	5,080	5,008	4,931	4,808	4,720
Admissions	240,784	235,615	223,117	224,928	225,065
Inpatient Days	951,874	954,737	935,962	961,475	976,402
Average Length of Stay	4.0	4.1	4.2	4.3	4.3
Personnel					
Total Full Time	26,322	26,670	26,037	26,296	26,562
Total Part Time	14,549	13,647	13,364	14,068	14,449
Revenue and Expenses - Totals					
(Includes Inpatient and Outpatient)					
Total Net Revenue	$6,225,430,738	$5,708,620,280	$5,239,992,029	$5,050,316,084	$4,612,854,633
Total Expenses	5,110,023,379	4,672,187,702	4,461,414,330	4,255,351,046	4,034,303,806
COMMUNITY HEALTH INDICATORS PER 1000 POPULATION					
Total Population (in thousands)	2,855	2,817	2,831	2,785	2,727
Inpatient					
Beds	1.8	1.8	1.8	1.8	1.8
Admissions	84.6	83.8	79.2	81.2	83.0
Inpatient Days	347.4	352.5	346.2	360.5	372.5
Inpatient Surgeries	25.2	25.3	24.9	25.7	24.9
Births	18.1	18.7	17.4	18.7	20.2
Outpatient					
Emergency Outpatient Visits	313.3	303.5	294.9	310.7	314.0
Other Outpatient Visits	1,912.0	1,774.6	1,640.1	1,655.2	1,631.3
Total Outpatient Visits	2,225.3	2,078.2	1,935.1	1,966.0	1,945.3
Outpatient Surgeries	58.2	61.9	58.9	55.7	55.8
Expense per Capita (per person)	$1,792.3	$1,661.1	$1,579.3	$1,531.2	$1,481.8

TABLE **6**

VERMONT

U.S. Registered Community Hospitals
(Nonfederal, short-term general and other special hospitals)

Overview 2008–2012

	2012	2011	2010	2009	2008
Total Community Hospitals in Vermont	14	14	14	14	14
Bed Size Category					
6-24	2	2	1	1	1
25-49	6	6	6	6	6
50-99	3	3	4	4	4
100-199	1	1	1	1	1
200-299	1	1	1	1	1
300-399	0	0	0	0	0
400-499	1	1	1	1	1
500 + ...	0	0	0	0	0
Location					
Hospitals Urban..........................	2	2	2	2	2
Hospitals Rural	12	12	12	12	12
Control					
State and Local Government................	0	0	0	0	0
Not for Profit	14	14	14	14	14
Investor owned	0	0	0	0	0
Physician Models					
Independent Practice Association	0	0	0	0	0
Group Practice without Walls................	0	0	0	0	0
Open Physician-Hospital Organization	3	3	3	2	3
Closed Physician-Hospital Organization	0	1	1	1	1
Management Service Organization	0	0	0	0	0
Integrated Salary Model	6	7	8	7	9
Equity Model	0	0	0	0	0
Foundation..............................	0	0	0	0	0
Insurance Products					
Health Maintenance Organization	2	2	2	3	3
Preferred Provider Organization..............	1	1	0	0	0
Indemnity Fee for Service	2	1	0	0	0
Managed Care Contracts					
Health Maintenance Organization	2	5	6	6	7
Preferred Provider Organization..............	3	5	5	4	6
Affiliations					
Hospitals in a System.....................	1	1	1	1	1
Hospitals in a Network	5	5	5	5	5
Hospitals in a Group Purchasing Organization..	10	10	10	10	12

States

TABLE 6

VERMONT

U.S. Registered Community Hospitals
(Nonfederal, short-term general and other special hospitals)

Utilization, Personnel, Revenue and Expenses, Community Health Indicators 2008–2012

	2012	2011	2010	2009	2008
TOTAL FACILITY (Includes Hospital and Nursing Home Units)					
Utilization - Inpatient					
Beds	1,231	1,218	1,288	1,296	1,302
Admissions	48,887	48,941	49,449	50,922	51,301
Inpatient Days	307,154	310,510	305,289	321,741	328,506
Average Length of Stay	6.3	6.3	6.2	6.3	6.4
Inpatient Surgeries	13,036	13,258	13,950	15,557	14,160
Births	5,250	12,755	5,604	5,829	5,982
Utilization - Outpatient					
Emergency Outpatient Visits	302,030	296,666	352,808	357,793	304,717
Other Outpatient Visits	2,740,382	2,788,192	2,999,812	2,997,816	3,001,378
Total Outpatient Visits	3,042,412	3,084,858	3,352,620	3,355,609	3,306,095
Outpatient Surgeries	46,671	48,381	48,158	48,673	47,401
Personnel					
Full Time RNs	1,852	1,720	1,748	1,671	1,690
Full Time LPNs	148	159	166	163	218
Part Time RNs	1,553	1,595	1,311	1,262	1,239
Part Time LPNs	104	128	149	110	160
Total Full Time	9,967	9,724	9,629	9,738	9,611
Total Part Time	4,590	4,930	4,078	3,920	3,763
Revenue - Inpatient					
Gross Inpatient Revenue	$1,089,276,425	$1,055,321,773	$1,154,115,173	$1,055,165,310	$903,264,654
Revenue - Outpatient					
Gross Outpatient Revenue	$3,001,872,051	$2,665,042,545	$2,538,622,333	$2,313,816,425	$2,017,330,510
Revenue and Expenses - Totals					
(Includes Inpatient and Outpatient)					
Total Gross Revenue	$4,091,148,476	$3,720,364,318	$3,692,737,506	$3,368,981,735	$2,920,595,164
Deductions from Revenue	2,173,153,296	1,901,314,973	1,982,861,871	1,719,852,956	1,383,550,785
Net Patient Revenue	1,917,995,180	1,819,049,345	1,709,875,635	1,649,128,779	1,537,044,379
Other Operating Revenue	71,915,614	57,250,217	56,110,764	51,534,989	46,804,137
Other Nonoperating Revenue	39,281,120	18,547,865	35,893,255	-10,009,965	-27,559,443
Total Net Revenue	2,029,191,914	1,894,847,427	1,801,879,654	1,690,653,803	1,556,289,073
Total Expenses	1,931,290,820	1,776,728,126	1,714,899,646	1,660,403,783	1,558,572,905
HOSPITAL UNIT (Excludes Separate Nursing Home Units)					
Utilization - Inpatient					
Beds	1,053	1,010	1,080	1,118	1,061
Admissions	48,477	48,523	49,078	50,549	51,001
Inpatient Days	248,986	241,161	233,003	259,463	245,411
Average Length of Stay	5.1	5.0	4.7	5.1	4.8
Personnel					
Total Full Time	9,791	9,591	9,493	9,397	9,218
Total Part Time	4,502	4,811	3,963	3,708	3,538
Revenue and Expenses - Totals					
(Includes Inpatient and Outpatient)					
Total Net Revenue	$2,012,967,016	$1,876,507,339	$1,783,366,299	$1,669,557,556	$1,536,579,410
Total Expenses	1,915,144,417	1,759,323,094	1,697,709,912	1,635,099,616	1,540,919,362
COMMUNITY HEALTH INDICATORS PER 1000 POPULATION					
Total Population (in thousands)	626	626	622	622	621
Inpatient					
Beds	2.0	1.9	2.1	2.1	2.1
Admissions	78.1	78.1	79.4	81.9	82.6
Inpatient Days	490.7	495.7	490.5	517.5	529.0
Inpatient Surgeries	20.8	21.2	22.4	25.0	22.8
Births	8.4	20.4	9.0	9.4	9.6
Outpatient					
Emergency Outpatient Visits	482.5	473.6	566.8	575.5	490.6
Other Outpatient Visits	4,377.5	4,450.9	4,819.5	4,821.5	4,832.8
Total Outpatient Visits	4,860.0	4,924.5	5,386.3	5,397.0	5,323.4
Outpatient Surgeries	74.6	77.2	77.4	78.3	76.3
Expense per Capita (per person)	$3,085.1	$2,836.3	$2,755.2	$2,670.5	$2,509.6

States

TABLE 6

VIRGINIA

U.S. Registered Community Hospitals
(Nonfederal, short-term general and other special hospitals)

Overview 2008–2012

	2012	2011	2010	2009	2008
Total Community Hospitals in Virginia	94	89	89	90	90
Bed Size Category					
6-24	5	5	5	3	4
25-49	16	15	14	15	15
50-99	17	15	15	17	16
100-199	26	23	25	27	25
200-299	12	13	12	11	13
300-399	5	6	6	5	5
400-499	5	5	5	5	4
500 + ...	8	7	7	7	8
Location					
Hospitals Urban..........................	64	59	59	60	55
Hospitals Rural	30	30	30	30	35
Control					
State and Local Government................	5	4	4	4	4
Not for Profit	65	65	64	66	65
Investor owned	24	20	21	20	21
Physician Models					
Independent Practice Association	13	12	13	12	11
Group Practice without Walls...............	9	9	10	8	10
Open Physician-Hospital Organization	14	8	9	7	13
Closed Physician-Hospital Organization	2	2	2	1	1
Management Service Organization	16	17	18	15	10
Integrated Salary Model....................	45	47	51	40	39
Equity Model	9	8	8	7	7
Foundation..............................	2	2	1	1	2
Insurance Products					
Health Maintenance Organization	18	18	15	13	17
Preferred Provider Organization..............	15	20	18	12	18
Indemnity Fee for Service	9	9	2	1	5
Managed Care Contracts					
Health Maintenance Organization	55	59	55	48	50
Preferred Provider Organization..............	57	61	59	54	56
Affiliations					
Hospitals in a System.....................	78	73	70	69	60
Hospitals in a Network....................	41	44	44	37	38
Hospitals in a Group Purchasing Organization..	64	65	70	57	60

TABLE 6

VIRGINIA

U.S. Registered Community Hospitals
(Nonfederal, short-term general and other special hospitals)

Utilization, Personnel, Revenue and Expenses, Community Health Indicators 2008–2012

	2012	2011	2010	2009	2008
TOTAL FACILITY (Includes Hospital and Nursing Home Units)					
Utilization - Inpatient					
Beds	18,150	17,797	17,747	17,538	17,648
Admissions	796,004	788,441	776,678	793,145	795,578
Inpatient Days	4,516,303	4,391,769	4,310,430	4,375,451	4,452,740
Average Length of Stay	5.7	5.6	5.5	5.5	5.6
Inpatient Surgeries	209,255	210,890	223,354	234,981	235,678
Births	93,114	98,141	99,623	96,209	98,991
Utilization - Outpatient					
Emergency Outpatient Visits	3,600,733	3,407,824	3,256,956	3,199,466	3,091,131
Other Outpatient Visits	11,952,608	10,710,596	10,524,980	10,959,387	10,223,288
Total Outpatient Visits	15,553,341	14,118,420	13,781,936	14,158,853	13,314,419
Outpatient Surgeries	451,407	446,691	439,146	448,650	463,342
Personnel					
Full Time RNs	24,712	24,546	24,035	23,711	23,382
Full Time LPNs	2,104	2,062	2,226	2,231	2,460
Part Time RNs	10,964	11,202	11,030	10,025	10,075
Part Time LPNs	611	614	703	684	861
Total Full Time	83,946	83,312	82,310	82,332	83,178
Total Part Time	29,934	29,682	30,091	28,083	28,749
Revenue - Inpatient					
Gross Inpatient Revenue	$28,228,430,166	$25,657,236,400	$24,373,894,322	$22,941,847,825	$22,555,481,294
Revenue - Outpatient					
Gross Outpatient Revenue	$25,551,564,541	$22,821,731,869	$21,205,056,723	$18,818,269,487	$17,042,951,627
Revenue and Expenses - Totals					
(Includes Inpatient and Outpatient)					
Total Gross Revenue	$53,779,994,707	$48,478,968,269	$45,578,951,045	$41,760,117,312	$39,598,432,921
Deductions from Revenue	36,089,745,615	32,415,072,411	30,139,978,214	26,616,556,088	25,464,931,182
Net Patient Revenue	17,690,249,092	16,063,895,858	15,438,972,831	15,143,561,224	14,133,501,739
Other Operating Revenue	614,154,152	538,832,905	425,128,846	422,020,787	404,136,415
Other Nonoperating Revenue	354,593,302	170,711,732	253,492,718	10,537,285	-269,241,513
Total Net Revenue	18,658,996,546	16,773,440,495	16,117,594,395	15,576,119,296	14,268,396,641
Total Expenses	16,505,378,259	15,341,349,476	14,709,796,266	14,456,123,508	13,800,772,246
HOSPITAL UNIT (Excludes Separate Nursing Home Units)					
Utilization - Inpatient					
Beds	16,467	16,091	16,163	16,422	16,478
Admissions	789,746	781,788	770,195	788,427	790,203
Inpatient Days	3,951,225	3,823,198	3,775,706	3,995,348	4,052,958
Average Length of Stay	5.0	4.9	4.9	5.1	5.1
Personnel					
Total Full Time	82,960	82,422	81,441	81,316	82,241
Total Part Time	29,503	29,292	29,637	27,710	28,385
Revenue and Expenses - Totals					
(Includes Inpatient and Outpatient)					
Total Net Revenue	$18,515,704,755	$16,629,452,446	$15,986,427,239	$15,479,330,448	$14,180,093,186
Total Expenses	16,368,213,160	15,208,955,950	14,592,391,811	14,367,593,188	13,713,829,141
COMMUNITY HEALTH INDICATORS PER 1000 POPULATION					
Total Population (in thousands)	8,186	8,097	7,952	7,883	7,795
Inpatient					
Beds	2.2	2.2	2.2	2.2	2.3
Admissions	97.2	97.4	97.7	100.6	102.1
Inpatient Days	551.7	542.4	542.0	555.1	571.2
Inpatient Surgeries	25.6	26.0	28.1	29.8	30.2
Births	11.4	12.1	12.5	12.2	12.7
Outpatient					
Emergency Outpatient Visits	439.9	420.9	409.6	405.9	396.5
Other Outpatient Visits	1,460.2	1,322.9	1,323.5	1,390.3	1,311.4
Total Outpatient Visits	1,900.0	1,743.7	1,733.1	1,796.2	1,708.0
Outpatient Surgeries	55.1	55.2	55.2	56.9	59.4
Expense per Capita (per person)	$2,016.3	$1,894.8	$1,849.8	$1,833.9	$1,770.4

TABLE **6**

WASHINGTON

U.S. Registered Community Hospitals
(Nonfederal, short-term general and other special hospitals)

Overview 2008–2012

	2012	2011	2010	2009	2008
Total Community Hospitals in Washington	87	85	86	87	86
Bed Size Category					
6-24	8	8	7	7	4
25-49	27	27	29	30	31
50-99	14	11	10	11	12
100-199	15	16	16	16	14
200-299	12	12	13	13	15
300-399	4	5	6	5	8
400-499	5	4	3	3	0
500 + ...	2	2	2	2	2
Location					
Hospitals Urban........................	55	53	53	53	45
Hospitals Rural	32	32	33	34	41
Control					
State and Local Government................	38	38	39	41	42
Not for Profit	42	41	42	41	40
Investor owned	7	6	5	5	4
Physician Models					
Independent Practice Association	1	1	2	2	2
Group Practice without Walls...............	3	4	4	4	2
Open Physician-Hospital Organization	3	6	5	4	5
Closed Physician-Hospital Organization	1	1	0	0	0
Management Service Organization	3	4	6	6	3
Integrated Salary Model....................	39	40	39	42	34
Equity Model	3	3	4	4	0
Foundation..............................	4	4	5	7	7
Insurance Products					
Health Maintenance Organization	4	7	4	5	4
Preferred Provider Organization..............	9	14	11	12	12
Indemnity Fee for Service	2	1	0	1	1
Managed Care Contracts					
Health Maintenance Organization	38	35	34	36	33
Preferred Provider Organization..............	40	37	38	44	37
Affiliations					
Hospitals in a System......................	40	39	35	32	31
Hospitals in a Network	17	20	19	19	19
Hospitals in a Group Purchasing Organization..	44	51	48	60	47

TABLE 6

WASHINGTON

U.S. Registered Community Hospitals
(Nonfederal, short-term general and other special hospitals)

Utilization, Personnel, Revenue and Expenses, Community Health Indicators 2008–2012

	2012	2011	2010	2009	2008
TOTAL FACILITY (Includes Hospital and Nursing Home Units)					
Utilization - Inpatient					
Beds	12,132	11,670	11,537	11,322	11,348
Admissions	597,338	576,214	588,855	588,889	578,856
Inpatient Days	2,731,437	2,613,217	2,638,779	2,660,901	2,663,704
Average Length of Stay	4.6	4.5	4.5	4.5	4.6
Inpatient Surgeries	165,978	167,254	170,895	185,833	184,234
Births	76,089	77,238	78,216	80,667	82,557
Utilization - Outpatient					
Emergency Outpatient Visits	2,390,525	2,321,612	2,290,953	2,509,243	2,385,734
Other Outpatient Visits	10,576,020	10,136,318	9,515,677	8,996,667	8,992,320
Total Outpatient Visits	12,966,545	12,457,930	11,806,630	11,505,910	11,378,054
Outpatient Surgeries	265,920	261,623	261,997	266,107	263,762
Personnel					
Full Time RNs	18,981	16,121	16,109	15,789	13,202
Full Time LPNs	946	774	825	870	805
Part Time RNs	12,219	13,423	13,848	13,205	13,466
Part Time LPNs	509	560	616	665	696
Total Full Time	75,760	65,087	68,163	64,767	59,789
Total Part Time	37,294	39,667	39,185	36,879	40,524
Revenue - Inpatient					
Gross Inpatient Revenue	$25,728,322,501	$21,352,251,400	$21,516,174,379	$19,988,875,344	$17,882,046,988
Revenue - Outpatient					
Gross Outpatient Revenue	$22,312,583,270	$19,065,026,947	$18,594,056,137	$16,200,972,533	$13,659,739,047
Revenue and Expenses - Totals					
(Includes Inpatient and Outpatient)					
Total Gross Revenue	$48,040,905,771	$40,417,278,347	$40,110,230,516	$36,189,847,877	$31,541,786,035
Deductions from Revenue	31,116,500,841	25,612,881,399	25,534,351,330	22,273,010,097	19,034,411,541
Net Patient Revenue	16,924,404,930	14,804,396,948	14,575,879,186	13,916,837,780	12,507,374,494
Other Operating Revenue	972,579,978	842,178,249	804,026,112	755,280,721	664,009,322
Other Nonoperating Revenue	210,144,087	300,691,951	226,341,197	188,342,686	-98,368,171
Total Net Revenue	18,107,128,995	15,947,267,148	15,606,246,495	14,860,461,187	13,073,015,645
Total Expenses	16,739,742,990	14,869,963,274	14,641,932,019	13,773,406,044	12,327,733,007
HOSPITAL UNIT (Excludes Separate Nursing Home Units)					
Utilization - Inpatient					
Beds	11,914	11,453	11,382	10,974	10,959
Admissions	597,051	575,796	587,786	587,527	576,765
Inpatient Days	2,655,788	2,530,869	2,589,013	2,549,787	2,539,914
Average Length of Stay	4.4	4.4	4.4	4.3	4.4
Personnel					
Total Full Time	75,610	64,968	68,113	64,470	59,483
Total Part Time	37,137	39,509	39,097	36,649	40,227
Revenue and Expenses - Totals					
(Includes Inpatient and Outpatient)					
Total Net Revenue	$18,084,028,525	$15,927,548,095	$15,586,259,128	$14,821,016,445	$13,032,710,190
Total Expenses	16,718,398,352	14,852,332,389	14,623,738,440	13,737,554,929	12,289,499,219
COMMUNITY HEALTH INDICATORS PER 1000 POPULATION					
Total Population (in thousands)	6,897	6,830	6,746	6,664	6,566
Inpatient					
Beds	1.8	1.7	1.7	1.7	1.7
Admissions	86.6	84.4	87.3	88.4	88.2
Inpatient Days	396.0	382.6	391.2	399.3	405.7
Inpatient Surgeries	24.1	24.5	25.3	27.9	28.1
Births	11.0	11.3	11.6	12.1	12.6
Outpatient					
Emergency Outpatient Visits	346.6	339.9	339.6	376.5	363.3
Other Outpatient Visits	1,533.4	1,484.1	1,410.5	1,350.0	1,369.5
Total Outpatient Visits	1,880.0	1,824.0	1,750.1	1,726.5	1,732.9
Outpatient Surgeries	38.6	38.3	38.8	39.9	40.2
Expense per Capita (per person)	$2,427.1	$2,177.1	$2,170.4	$2,066.8	$1,877.5

States

TABLE 6

WEST VIRGINIA

U.S. Registered Community Hospitals
(Nonfederal, short-term general and other special hospitals)

Overview 2008–2012

	2012	2011	2010	2009	2008
Total Community Hospitals in West Virginia . . .	55	55	56	56	56
Bed Size Category					
6-24	3	3	3	3	3
25-49	16	15	14	14	13
50-99	12	13	13	13	14
100-199	12	11	14	14	14
200-299	7	8	9	8	8
300-399	2	2	1	2	2
400-499	1	1	0	0	0
500 + ...	2	2	2	2	2
Location					
Hospitals Urban.	26	26	27	27	20
Hospitals Rural	29	29	29	29	36
Control					
State and Local Government.	8	8	8	10	10
Not for Profit	33	33	34	32	32
Investor owned	14	14	14	14	14
Physician Models					
Independent Practice Association	2	2	3	4	4
Group Practice without Walls.	0	0	0	0	0
Open Physician-Hospital Organization	12	14	13	14	14
Closed Physician-Hospital Organization	1	1	3	3	3
Management Service Organization	2	2	2	3	5
Integrated Salary Model	27	25	25	25	25
Equity Model	0	0	0	0	0
Foundation.	0	0	0	0	0
Insurance Products					
Health Maintenance Organization	5	5	6	5	3
Preferred Provider Organization.	6	10	10	9	7
Indemnity Fee for Service	4	2	3	2	2
Managed Care Contracts					
Health Maintenance Organization	31	28	31	31	27
Preferred Provider Organization.	40	40	42	42	38
Affiliations					
Hospitals in a System.	30	30	29	25	23
Hospitals in a Network	20	21	21	22	20
Hospitals in a Group Purchasing Organization. .	53	52	53	53	52

States

TABLE 6

WEST VIRGINIA

U.S. Registered Community Hospitals
(Nonfederal, short-term general and other special hospitals)

Utilization, Personnel, Revenue and Expenses, Community Health Indicators 2008–2012

	2012	2011	2010	2009	2008
TOTAL FACILITY (Includes Hospital and Nursing Home Units)					
Utilization - Inpatient					
Beds	7,212	7,365	7,298	7,408	7,470
Admissions	276,114	282,194	278,221	280,252	283,673
Inpatient Days	1,587,250	1,632,308	1,612,811	1,648,197	1,665,076
Average Length of Stay	5.7	5.8	5.8	5.9	5.9
Inpatient Surgeries	82,602	82,491	83,992	80,776	79,916
Births	20,758	20,639	20,487	21,010	20,856
Utilization - Outpatient					
Emergency Outpatient Visits	1,224,551	1,216,780	1,207,918	1,221,485	1,183,158
Other Outpatient Visits	5,585,774	5,544,015	5,446,482	5,463,158	5,431,951
Total Outpatient Visits	6,810,325	6,760,795	6,654,400	6,684,643	6,615,109
Outpatient Surgeries	228,957	222,505	212,434	215,853	212,489
Personnel					
Full Time RNs	8,852	8,593	8,532	8,282	8,084
Full Time LPNs	1,130	1,099	1,217	1,298	1,387
Part Time RNs	3,251	3,252	3,395	3,447	3,392
Part Time LPNs	332	396	419	403	435
Total Full Time	34,272	33,119	33,349	32,751	32,463
Total Part Time	10,125	9,903	10,143	10,082	10,244
Revenue - Inpatient					
Gross Inpatient Revenue	$6,272,466,443	$6,028,967,872	$5,597,580,327	$5,174,519,813	$4,927,056,831
Revenue - Outpatient					
Gross Outpatient Revenue	$6,361,117,278	$5,824,592,215	$5,444,045,714	$5,161,162,251	$4,531,051,911
Revenue and Expenses - Totals					
(Includes Inpatient and Outpatient)					
Total Gross Revenue	$12,633,583,721	$11,853,560,087	$11,041,626,041	$10,335,682,064	$9,458,108,742
Deductions from Revenue	7,391,004,309	7,049,221,237	6,386,501,669	5,787,332,486	5,198,077,289
Net Patient Revenue	5,242,579,412	4,804,338,850	4,655,124,372	4,548,349,578	4,260,031,453
Other Operating Revenue	182,070,517	133,361,426	126,269,003	168,034,621	71,741,101
Other Nonoperating Revenue	86,836,379	-338,296	63,579,778	54,115,339	-125,408,354
Total Net Revenue	5,511,486,308	4,937,361,980	4,844,973,153	4,770,499,538	4,206,364,200
Total Expenses	5,151,427,691	4,724,080,410	4,689,352,987	4,584,221,488	4,289,258,433
HOSPITAL UNIT (Excludes Separate Nursing Home Units)					
Utilization - Inpatient					
Beds	6,423	6,554	6,454	6,575	6,587
Admissions	271,352	277,659	272,471	274,341	277,157
Inpatient Days	1,329,793	1,378,567	1,340,666	1,371,913	1,381,747
Average Length of Stay	4.9	5.0	4.9	5.0	5.0
Personnel					
Total Full Time	33,683	32,566	32,752	32,152	31,838
Total Part Time	9,785	9,508	9,781	9,787	9,825
Revenue and Expenses - Totals					
(Includes Inpatient and Outpatient)					
Total Net Revenue	$5,439,544,951	$4,873,165,838	$4,774,505,282	$4,700,079,381	$4,123,228,602
Total Expenses	5,097,076,501	4,670,781,412	4,637,567,799	4,529,683,828	4,229,627,238
COMMUNITY HEALTH INDICATORS PER 1000 POPULATION					
Total Population (in thousands)	1,855	1,855	1,826	1,820	1,815
Inpatient					
Beds	3.9	4.0	4.0	4.1	4.1
Admissions	148.8	152.1	152.4	154.0	156.3
Inpatient Days	855.5	879.8	883.5	905.7	917.5
Inpatient Surgeries	44.5	44.5	46.0	44.4	44.0
Births	11.2	11.1	11.2	11.5	11.5
Outpatient					
Emergency Outpatient Visits	660.0	655.8	661.7	671.2	651.9
Other Outpatient Visits	3,010.5	2,988.1	2,983.5	3,002.1	2,993.0
Total Outpatient Visits	3,670.5	3,643.9	3,645.2	3,673.3	3,644.9
Outpatient Surgeries	123.4	119.9	116.4	118.6	117.1
Expense per Capita (per person)	$2,776.4	$2,546.2	$2,568.8	$2,519.1	$2,363.4

States

TABLE 6

WISCONSIN

U.S. Registered Community Hospitals
(Nonfederal, short-term general and other special hospitals)

Overview 2008–2012

	2012	2011	2010	2009	2008
Total Community Hospitals in Wisconsin......	**128**	**125**	**124**	**126**	**126**
Bed Size Category					
6-24	21	15	13	12	12
25-49	33	36	37	37	36
50-99	33	31	31	32	32
100-199	20	22	21	25	24
200-299	11	11	13	11	13
300-399	7	7	5	6	6
400-499	0	1	2	2	2
500 + ...	3	2	2	1	1
Location					
Hospitals Urban..........................	72	69	68	69	62
Hospitals Rural	56	56	56	57	64
Control					
State and Local Government................	2	2	2	2	2
Not for Profit	121	119	117	118	119
Investor owned	5	4	5	6	5
Physician Models					
Independent Practice Association	11	11	9	13	13
Group Practice without Walls...............	0	3	3	3	2
Open Physician-Hospital Organization	6	4	4	3	3
Closed Physician-Hospital Organization	3	4	4	2	3
Management Service Organization	2	2	2	3	2
Integrated Salary Model....................	62	56	38	34	32
Equity Model	7	6	9	12	17
Foundation...............................	2	2	2	2	2
Insurance Products					
Health Maintenance Organization	41	36	20	23	23
Preferred Provider Organization..............	41	36	31	35	36
Indemnity Fee for Service	19	15	15	16	15
Managed Care Contracts					
Health Maintenance Organization	118	118	116	116	116
Preferred Provider Organization..............	121	120	118	118	120
Affiliations					
Hospitals in a System......................	75	72	72	74	72
Hospitals in a Network	44	43	37	36	39
Hospitals in a Group Purchasing Organization..	126	123	118	116	118

TABLE **6**

WISCONSIN

U.S. Registered Community Hospitals
(Nonfederal, short-term general and other special hospitals)

Utilization, Personnel, Revenue and Expenses, Community Health Indicators 2008–2012

	2012	2011	2010	2009	2008
TOTAL FACILITY (Includes Hospital and Nursing Home Units)					
Utilization - Inpatient					
Beds	13,020	13,134	13,520	13,637	13,707
Admissions	578,239	573,077	588,592	609,329	617,295
Inpatient Days	2,855,397	2,873,295	2,966,909	3,125,349	3,172,566
Average Length of Stay	4.9	5.0	5.0	5.1	5.1
Inpatient Surgeries	214,146	214,111	228,469	256,942	233,044
Births	65,632	66,783	67,843	70,129	69,465
Utilization - Outpatient					
Emergency Outpatient Visits	2,171,739	2,130,925	2,160,341	2,080,601	2,066,654
Other Outpatient Visits	13,957,038	13,379,041	12,444,617	12,847,067	12,136,773
Total Outpatient Visits	16,128,777	15,509,966	14,604,958	14,927,668	14,203,427
Outpatient Surgeries	526,585	531,355	522,864	535,955	491,040
Personnel					
Full Time RNs	15,095	15,048	14,476	14,345	14,522
Full Time LPNs	537	622	673	711	707
Part Time RNs	15,972	14,982	15,552	16,139	15,398
Part Time LPNs	645	706	794	908	927
Total Full Time	63,722	63,544	63,254	63,168	63,883
Total Part Time	48,388	46,533	48,472	51,235	47,517
Revenue - Inpatient					
Gross Inpatient Revenue	$17,011,582,655	$16,185,500,212	$15,357,857,584	$15,634,706,846	$13,612,135,956
Revenue - Outpatient					
Gross Outpatient Revenue	$20,638,540,030	$18,798,615,788	$16,468,660,136	$14,805,407,754	$13,162,259,140
Revenue and Expenses - Totals					
(Includes Inpatient and Outpatient)					
Total Gross Revenue	$37,650,122,685	$34,984,116,000	$31,826,517,720	$30,440,114,600	$26,774,395,096
Deductions from Revenue	21,459,464,213	19,455,297,266	16,996,231,064	16,618,465,592	13,709,265,312
Net Patient Revenue	16,190,658,472	15,528,818,734	14,830,286,656	13,821,649,008	13,065,129,784
Other Operating Revenue	751,235,572	644,957,778	630,341,533	716,584,248	643,332,317
Other Nonoperating Revenue	322,542,557	288,307,316	285,539,514	-26,443,242	-30,738,485
Total Net Revenue	17,264,436,601	16,462,083,828	15,746,167,703	14,511,790,014	13,677,723,616
Total Expenses	15,601,708,952	14,997,018,589	14,230,620,575	13,496,778,176	12,923,890,000
HOSPITAL UNIT (Excludes Separate Nursing Home Units)					
Utilization - Inpatient					
Beds	11,775	11,814	12,092	12,049	12,067
Admissions	575,966	570,650	586,022	606,542	614,395
Inpatient Days	2,439,508	2,453,855	2,511,474	2,597,929	2,629,527
Average Length of Stay	4.2	4.3	4.3	4.3	4.3
Personnel					
Total Full Time	63,255	62,919	62,460	62,376	63,068
Total Part Time	47,770	45,754	47,543	50,255	46,533
Revenue and Expenses - Totals					
(Includes Inpatient and Outpatient)					
Total Net Revenue	$17,182,065,794	$16,360,856,116	$15,640,069,501	$14,399,372,197	$13,576,550,948
Total Expenses	15,523,090,630	14,902,736,502	14,124,128,291	13,393,867,097	12,830,682,268
COMMUNITY HEALTH INDICATORS PER 1000 POPULATION					
Total Population (in thousands)	5,726	5,712	5,669	5,655	5,628
Inpatient					
Beds	2.3	2.3	2.4	2.4	2.4
Admissions	101.0	100.3	103.8	107.8	109.7
Inpatient Days	498.6	503.0	523.4	552.7	563.8
Inpatient Surgeries	37.4	37.5	40.3	45.4	41.4
Births	11.5	11.7	12.0	12.4	12.3
Outpatient					
Emergency Outpatient Visits	379.3	373.1	381.1	367.9	367.2
Other Outpatient Visits	2,437.3	2,342.4	2,195.4	2,271.9	2,156.6
Total Outpatient Visits	2,816.6	2,715.4	2,576.5	2,639.8	2,523.9
Outpatient Surgeries	92.0	93.0	92.2	94.8	87.3
Expense per Capita (per person)	$2,724.5	$2,625.6	$2,510.5	$2,386.8	$2,296.5

States

TABLE **6**

WYOMING

U.S. Registered Community Hospitals
(Nonfederal, short-term general and other special hospitals)

Overview 2008–2012

	2012	2011	2010	2009	2008
Total Community Hospitals in Wyoming.......	24	24	24	24	24
Bed Size Category					
6-24	0	0	0	0	0
25-49	11	11	11	11	10
50-99	6	6	6	6	7
100-199	5	4	4	4	4
200-299	2	3	3	3	3
300-399	0	0	0	0	0
400-499	0	0	0	0	0
500 + ...	0	0	0	0	0
Location					
Hospitals Urban.........................	2	2	2	2	2
Hospitals Rural	22	22	22	22	22
Control					
State and Local Government................	16	16	16	16	16
Not for Profit	5	5	5	5	5
Investor owned	3	3	3	3	3
Physician Models					
Independent Practice Association	2	2	2	3	3
Group Practice without Walls...............	0	0	0	0	0
Open Physician-Hospital Organization	1	1	1	1	1
Closed Physician-Hospital Organization	1	1	1	1	1
Management Service Organization	2	1	2	2	1
Integrated Salary Model	10	9	10	11	11
Equity Model	0	0	0	0	0
Foundation.............................	0	0	0	0	0
Insurance Products					
Health Maintenance Organization	2	2	1	1	1
Preferred Provider Organization.............	1	3	3	1	1
Indemnity Fee for Service	0	0	0	0	0
Managed Care Contracts					
Health Maintenance Organization	5	4	3	4	4
Preferred Provider Organization.............	17	14	14	14	14
Affiliations					
Hospitals in a System.....................	12	12	12	12	11
Hospitals in a Network....................	5	4	4	5	5
Hospitals in a Group Purchasing Organization..	22	21	21	21	23

TABLE 6

WYOMING

U.S. Registered Community Hospitals
(Nonfederal, short-term general and other special hospitals)

Utilization, Personnel, Revenue and Expenses, Community Health Indicators 2008–2012

	2012	2011	2010	2009	2008
TOTAL FACILITY (Includes Hospital and Nursing Home Units)					
Utilization - Inpatient					
Beds	1,923	1,958	1,958	2,002	2,073
Admissions	44,180	45,697	49,704	52,232	52,628
Inpatient Days	375,036	378,227	398,850	411,717	414,463
Average Length of Stay	8.5	8.3	8.0	7.9	7.9
Inpatient Surgeries	11,959	12,872	14,159	13,801	14,162
Births	6,364	6,363	6,920	7,305	7,303
Utilization - Outpatient					
Emergency Outpatient Visits	229,649	228,140	231,261	236,213	234,384
Other Outpatient Visits	976,926	890,706	866,984	823,944	774,610
Total Outpatient Visits	1,206,575	1,118,846	1,098,245	1,060,157	1,008,994
Outpatient Surgeries	28,021	29,019	29,260	26,180	25,183
Personnel					
Full Time RNs	1,798	1,721	1,680	1,561	1,664
Full Time LPNs	113	116	117	127	130
Part Time RNs	578	556	455	526	504
Part Time LPNs	50	52	54	76	57
Total Full Time	7,546	7,404	7,338	7,094	7,291
Total Part Time	2,166	2,067	2,005	2,310	1,892
Revenue - Inpatient					
Gross Inpatient Revenue	$1,129,646,064	$1,079,479,758	$1,072,618,270	$967,170,829	$951,929,394
Revenue - Outpatient					
Gross Outpatient Revenue	$1,327,536,898	$1,216,235,177	$1,103,760,780	$946,462,599	$801,309,584
Revenue and Expenses - Totals					
(Includes Inpatient and Outpatient)					
Total Gross Revenue	$2,457,182,962	$2,295,714,935	$2,176,379,050	$1,913,633,428	$1,753,238,978
Deductions from Revenue	1,211,190,965	1,180,144,790	1,096,026,956	955,291,698	802,095,376
Net Patient Revenue	1,245,991,997	1,115,570,145	1,080,352,094	958,341,730	951,143,602
Other Operating Revenue	74,346,388	69,049,844	74,157,196	66,460,224	55,280,832
Other Nonoperating Revenue	4,294,457	26,792,888	19,130,354	-798,016	21,606,525
Total Net Revenue	1,324,632,842	1,211,412,877	1,173,639,644	1,024,003,938	1,028,030,959
Total Expenses	1,182,216,845	1,046,675,080	1,031,425,657	980,632,479	949,368,614
HOSPITAL UNIT (Excludes Separate Nursing Home Units)					
Utilization - Inpatient					
Beds	1,245	1,281	1,303	1,303	1,335
Admissions	43,484	44,155	48,206	50,673	51,146
Inpatient Days	167,355	169,461	196,510	188,014	183,585
Average Length of Stay	3.8	3.8	4.1	3.7	3.6
Personnel					
Total Full Time	7,150	7,004	6,925	6,618	6,767
Total Part Time	1,957	1,888	1,841	2,117	1,696
Revenue and Expenses - Totals					
(Includes Inpatient and Outpatient)					
Total Net Revenue	$1,282,240,814	$1,170,074,150	$1,133,360,264	$984,238,688	$988,170,246
Total Expenses	1,141,742,073	1,006,052,821	991,627,019	938,219,346	907,237,150
COMMUNITY HEALTH INDICATORS PER 1000 POPULATION					
Total Population (in thousands)	576	568	548	544	533
Inpatient					
Beds	3.3	3.4	3.6	3.7	3.9
Admissions	76.6	80.4	90.8	96.0	98.7
Inpatient Days	650.6	665.7	728.3	756.5	777.6
Inpatient Surgeries	20.7	22.7	25.9	25.4	26.6
Births	11.0	11.2	12.6	13.4	13.7
Outpatient					
Emergency Outpatient Visits	398.4	401.5	422.3	434.0	439.8
Other Outpatient Visits	1,694.8	1,567.7	1,583.1	1,513.9	1,453.4
Total Outpatient Visits	2,093.3	1,969.3	2,005.4	1,947.9	1,893.1
Outpatient Surgeries	48.6	51.1	53.4	48.1	47.2
Expense per Capita (per person)	$2,051.0	$1,842.2	$1,883.4	$1,801.7	$1,781.2

Table 7

Table	Page
7	Facilities and Services in the U. S. Census Divisions and States for 2012 155

The facilities and services presented in Table 7 are listed below in alphabetical order by major heading (where applicable).

Table 7

2012 Facilities and Services in the U.S. Census Divisions and States

These data include only hospital-based facilities and services as reported by responding hospitals in Section C of the 2012 AHA Annual Survey, beginning on page 215. All hospitals are represented with Community Hospitals listed separately under United States. No estimates have been made for nonresponding hospitals. Definitions of facilities and services are listed in the Glossary, page 201.

CLASSIFICATION	HOSPITALS REPORTING	ADULT DAY CARE PROGRAM Number	Percent	AIRBORNE INFECTION ISOLATION ROOM Number	Percent	ALCOHOL/DRUG ABUSE OR DEPENDENCY INPATIENT CARE UNITS Number	Percent	ALCOHOL/DRUG ABUSE OR DEPENDENCY OUTPATIENT SERVICES Number	Percent	ALZHEIMER CENTER Number	Percent	AMBULANCE SERVICE Number	Percent	AMBULATORY SURGERY CENTER Number	Percent	ARTHRITIS TREATMENT CENTER Number	Percent	ASSISTED LIVING Number	Percent
UNITED STATES	4,774	212	4.4	3,609	75.6	478	10.0	695	14.6	208	4.4	723	15.1	1,203	25.2	285	6.0	184	3.9
COMMUNITY HOSPITALS	4,054	182	4.5	3,297	81.3	325	8.0	524	12.9	188	4.6	705	17.4	1,140	28.1	267	6.6	168	4.1
CENSUS DIVISION 1, NEW ENGLAND	187	10	5.3	136	72.7	20	10.7	58	31.0	15	8.0	27	14.4	71	38.0	18	9.6	6	3.2
Connecticut	32	3	9.4	24	75.0	6	18.8	16	50.0	4	12.5	5	15.6	19	59.4	5	15.6	1	3.1
Maine	39	1	2.6	29	74.4	6	15.4	14	35.9	4	10.3	8	20.5	13	33.3	0	0.0	3	7.7
Massachusetts	68	4	5.9	46	67.6	6	8.8	22	32.4	4	5.9	8	11.8	24	35.3	8	11.8	0	0.0
New Hampshire	26	2	7.7	23	88.5	0	0.0	2	7.7	1	3.8	4	15.4	6	23.1	3	11.5	1	3.8
Rhode Island	9	0	0.0	6	66.7	1	11.1	2	22.2	1	11.1	1	11.1	4	44.4	0	0.0	0	0.0
Vermont	13	0	0.0	8	61.5	1	7.7	2	15.4	1	7.7	1	7.7	5	38.5	2	15.4	1	7.7
CENSUS DIVISION 2, MIDDLE ATLANTIC	420	35	8.3	330	78.6	74	17.6	107	25.5	32	7.6	71	16.9	181	43.1	59	14.0	14	3.3
New Jersey	72	8	11.1	51	70.8	10	13.9	19	26.4	6	8.3	19	26.4	24	33.3	8	11.1	3	4.2
New York	159	21	13.2	131	82.4	49	30.8	61	38.4	15	9.4	26	16.4	102	64.2	32	20.1	1	0.6
Pennsylvania	189	6	3.2	148	78.3	15	7.9	27	14.3	11	5.8	26	13.8	55	29.1	19	10.1	10	5.3
CENSUS DIVISION 3, SOUTH ATLANTIC	671	24	3.6	544	81.1	76	11.3	103	15.4	33	4.9	92	13.7	163	24.3	45	6.7	19	2.8
Delaware	7	2	28.6	5	71.4	0	0.0	1	14.3	1	14.3	2	28.6	4	57.1	1	14.3	0	0.0
District of Columbia	11	0	0.0	10	90.9	1	9.1	3	27.3	1	9.1	1	9.1	4	36.4	3	27.3	1	9.1
Florida	152	3	2.0	128	84.2	16	10.5	14	9.2	10	6.6	14	9.2	47	30.9	9	5.9	1	0.7
Georgia	107	3	2.8	81	75.7	14	13.1	15	14.0	4	3.7	20	18.7	22	20.6	3	2.8	5	4.7
Maryland	51	4	7.8	40	78.4	6	11.8	16	31.4	4	7.8	2	3.9	14	27.5	8	15.7	3	5.9
North Carolina	120	4	3.3	102	85.0	15	12.5	19	15.8	5	4.2	23	19.2	34	28.3	8	6.7	5	4.2
South Carolina	82	2	2.4	62	75.6	14	17.1	11	13.4	3	3.7	12	14.6	10	12.2	3	3.7	0	0.0
Virginia	80	5	6.3	70	87.5	8	10.0	18	22.5	5	6.3	12	15.0	21	26.3	6	7.5	4	5.0
West Virginia	61	1	1.6	46	75.4	2	3.3	6	9.8	0	0.0	6	9.8	7	11.5	4	6.6	0	0.0
CENSUS DIVISION 4, EAST NORTH CENTRAL	726	36	5.0	595	82.0	95	13.1	156	21.5	57	7.9	107	14.7	199	27.4	66	9.1	28	3.9
Illinois	159	14	8.8	135	84.9	19	11.9	38	23.9	10	6.3	21	13.2	35	22.0	14	8.8	3	1.9
Indiana	124	2	1.6	92	74.2	14	11.3	23	18.5	2	1.6	28	22.6	34	27.4	4	3.2	5	4.0
Michigan	135	5	3.7	113	83.7	14	10.4	29	21.5	8	5.9	19	14.1	31	23.0	14	10.4	3	2.2
Ohio	161	7	4.3	138	85.7	15	9.3	31	19.3	11	6.8	25	15.5	53	32.9	16	9.9	3	1.9
Wisconsin	147	8	5.4	117	79.6	33	22.4	35	23.8	26	17.7	14	9.5	46	31.3	18	12.2	14	9.5
CENSUS DIVISION 5, EAST SOUTH CENTRAL	398	12	3.0	272	68.3	44	11.1	38	9.5	5	1.3	53	13.3	73	18.3	7	1.8	7	1.8
Alabama	106	2	1.9	71	67.0	12	11.3	9	8.5	2	1.9	10	9.4	20	18.9	2	1.9	2	1.9
Kentucky	90	4	4.4	75	83.3	8	8.9	9	10.0	1	1.1	10	11.1	16	17.8	2	2.2	1	1.1
Mississippi	112	1	0.9	59	52.7	15	13.4	8	7.1	1	0.9	17	15.2	14	12.5	0	0.0	2	1.8
Tennessee	90	5	5.6	67	74.4	9	10.0	12	13.3	1	1.1	16	17.8	23	25.6	3	3.3	2	2.2
CENSUS DIVISION 6, WEST NORTH CENTRAL	670	33	4.9	469	70.0	57	8.5	72	10.7	21	3.1	165	24.6	116	17.3	24	3.6	61	9.1
Iowa	126	4	3.2	85	67.5	11	8.7	18	14.3	4	3.2	56	44.4	25	19.8	3	2.4	12	9.5
Kansas	151	9	6.0	105	69.5	4	2.6	4	2.6	3	2.0	22	14.6	14	9.3	2	1.3	11	7.3
Minnesota	106	10	9.4	76	71.7	16	15.1	16	15.1	4	3.8	34	32.1	27	25.5	4	3.8	14	13.2
Missouri	151	1	0.7	118	78.1	23	15.2	21	13.9	4	2.6	26	17.2	24	15.9	9	6.0	2	1.3
Nebraska	60	1	1.7	36	60.0	3	5.0	5	8.3	2	3.3	9	15.0	11	18.3	2	3.3	5	8.3
North Dakota	29	2	6.9	18	62.1	4	13.8	3	10.3	0	0.0	7	24.1	5	17.2	3	10.3	3	10.3
South Dakota	47	6	12.8	31	66.0	1	2.1	5	10.6	4	8.5	11	23.4	10	21.3	1	2.1	14	29.8
CENSUS DIVISION 7, WEST SOUTH CENTRAL	900	13	1.4	678	75.3	45	5.0	55	6.1	8	0.9	103	11.4	144	16.0	19	2.1	18	2.0
Arkansas	80	3	3.8	65	81.3	4	5.0	6	7.5	1	1.3	11	13.8	13	16.3	2	2.5	1	1.3
Louisiana	118	4	3.4	67	56.8	5	4.2	7	5.9	1	0.8	8	6.8	27	22.9	6	5.1	2	1.7
Oklahoma	129	2	1.6	99	76.7	4	3.1	9	7.0	1	0.8	17	13.2	27	20.9	2	1.6	3	2.3
Texas	573	4	0.7	447	78.0	32	5.6	33	5.8	5	0.9	67	11.7	77	13.4	9	1.6	12	2.1
CENSUS DIVISION 8, MOUNTAIN	338	24	7.1	240	71.0	27	8.0	44	13.0	17	5.0	65	19.2	88	26.0	16	4.7	19	5.6
Arizona	54	0	0.0	38	70.4	3	5.6	10	18.5	2	3.7	1	1.9	14	25.9	2	3.7	0	0.0
Colorado	68	3	4.4	58	85.3	5	7.4	9	13.2	3	4.4	15	22.1	18	26.5	4	5.9	4	5.9
Idaho	35	4	11.4	22	62.9	4	11.4	5	14.3	0	0.0	11	31.4	14	40.0	3	8.6	2	5.7
Montana	55	14	25.5	36	65.5	2	3.6	3	5.5	4	7.3	13	23.6	10	18.2	1	1.8	10	18.2
Nevada	34	1	2.9	16	47.1	3	8.8	5	14.7	1	2.9	3	8.8	5	14.7	0	0.0	1	2.9
New Mexico	30	0	0.0	22	73.3	2	6.7	3	10.0	0	0.0	6	20.0	11	36.7	3	10.0	0	0.0
Utah	35	1	2.9	28	80.0	5	14.3	5	14.3	2	5.7	6	17.1	13	37.1	3	8.6	0	0.0
Wyoming	27	1	3.7	20	74.1	3	11.1	4	14.8	5	18.5	10	37.0	3	11.1	0	0.0	2	7.4
CENSUS DIVISION 9, PACIFIC	464	25	5.4	345	74.4	40	8.6	62	13.4	20	4.3	40	8.6	168	36.2	31	6.7	12	2.6
Alaska	14	0	0.0	7	50.0	1	7.1	5	35.7	0	0.0	1	7.1	2	14.3	0	0.0	0	0.0
California	296	16	5.4	220	74.3	29	9.8	41	13.9	18	6.1	20	6.8	109	36.8	21	7.1	4	1.4
Hawaii	21	1	4.8	14	66.7	2	9.5	2	4.8	0	0.0	0	0.0	5	23.8	0	0.0	0	0.0
Oregon	58	3	5.2	50	86.2	1	1.7	6	10.3	1	1.7	7	12.1	13	22.4	4	6.9	2	3.4
Washington	75	5	6.7	54	72.0	7	9.3	9	12.0	1	1.3	12	16.0	39	52.0	5	6.7	6	8.0

Table 7 (Continued)

These data include only hospital-based facilities and services as reported by responding hospitals in Section C of the 2012 AHA Annual Survey, beginning on page 215. All hospitals are represented with Community Hospitals listed separately under United States. No estimates have been made for nonresponding hospitals. Definitions of facilities and services are listed in the Glossary, page 201.

CLASSIFICATION	HOSPITALS REPORTING	AUXILIARY		BARIATRIC/ WEIGHT CONTROL SERVICES		BIRTHING/ LDR/ LDRP ROOM		BLOOD DONOR CENTER		BREAST CANCER SCREENING		BURN CARE UNITS		CASE MANAGEMENT		CHAPLAINCY/ PASTORAL CARE SERVICES		CHEMOTHERAPY	
		Number	Percent	Number	Percent	Number	Percent	Number	Percent	Number	Percent	Number	Percent	Number	Percent	Number	Percent	Number	Percent
UNITED STATES	4,774	2,712	56.8	1,178	24.7	2,540	53.2	311	6.5	3,272	68.5	197	4.1	4,083	85.5	3,111	65.2	2,423	50.8
COMMUNITY HOSPITALS	4,054	2,639	65.1	1,108	27.3	2,517	62.1	303	7.5	3,194	78.8	185	4.6	3,617	89.2	2,825	69.7	2,333	57.5
CENSUS DIVISION 1, NEW ENGLAND	187	109	58.3	63	33.7	123	65.8	30	16.0	146	78.1	12	6.4	175	93.6	151	80.7	131	70.1
Connecticut	32	19	59.4	16	50.0	23	71.9	4	12.5	24	75.0	1	3.1	29	90.6	30	93.8	24	75.0
Maine	39	25	64.1	7	17.9	29	74.4	0	0.0	34	87.2	2	5.1	39	100.0	29	74.4	27	69.2
Massachusetts	68	33	48.5	30	44.1	39	57.4	21	30.9	49	72.1	6	8.8	61	89.7	55	80.9	45	66.2
New Hampshire	26	17	65.4	6	23.1	18	69.2	4	15.4	22	84.6	1	3.8	25	96.2	20	76.9	19	73.1
Rhode Island	9	6	66.7	2	22.2	5	55.6	0	0.0	7	77.8	1	11.1	9	100.0	7	77.8	7	77.8
Vermont	13	9	69.2	2	15.4	9	69.2	1	7.7	10	76.9	1	7.7	12	92.3	10	76.9	9	69.2
CENSUS DIVISION 2, MIDDLE ATLANTIC	420	264	62.9	177	42.1	237	56.4	66	15.7	325	77.4	24	5.7	384	91.4	327	77.9	272	64.8
New Jersey	72	51	70.8	39	54.2	43	59.7	11	15.3	51	70.8	5	6.9	64	88.9	59	81.9	51	70.8
New York	159	104	65.4	70	44.0	105	66.0	35	22.0	137	86.2	12	7.5	154	96.9	134	84.3	115	72.3
Pennsylvania	189	109	57.7	68	36.0	89	47.1	20	10.6	137	72.5	7	3.7	166	87.8	134	70.9	106	56.1
CENSUS DIVISION 3, SOUTH ATLANTIC	671	421	62.7	176	26.2	367	54.7	47	7.0	502	74.8	28	4.2	608	90.6	526	78.4	372	55.4
Delaware	7	5	71.4	4	57.1	4	57.1	0	0.0	4	57.1	0	0.0	5	71.4	5	71.4	5	71.4
District of Columbia	11	3	27.3	6	54.5	7	63.6	3	27.3	7	63.6	1	9.1	10	90.9	11	100.0	7	63.6
Florida	152	91	59.9	45	29.6	73	48.0	7	4.6	108	71.1	9	5.9	143	94.1	123	80.9	99	65.1
Georgia	107	73	68.2	26	24.3	58	54.2	5	4.7	85	79.4	3	2.8	96	89.7	78	72.9	46	43.0
Maryland	51	39	76.5	16	31.4	30	58.8	12	23.5	37	72.5	3	5.9	46	90.2	46	90.2	41	80.4
North Carolina	120	72	60.0	33	27.5	79	65.8	6	5.0	89	74.2	5	4.2	107	89.2	97	80.8	74	61.7
South Carolina	82	44	53.7	14	17.1	44	53.7	5	6.1	58	70.7	2	2.4	72	87.8	53	64.6	30	36.6
Virginia	80	57	71.3	23	28.8	43	53.8	9	11.3	66	82.5	4	5.0	76	95.0	68	85.0	47	58.8
West Virginia	61	37	60.7	9	14.8	29	47.5	0	0.0	48	78.7	1	1.6	53	86.9	45	73.8	23	37.7
CENSUS DIVISION 4, EAST NORTH CENTRAL	726	456	62.8	194	26.7	439	60.5	38	5.2	576	79.3	33	4.5	646	89.0	532	73.3	451	62.1
Illinois	159	109	68.6	49	30.8	102	64.2	11	6.9	138	86.8	8	5.0	149	93.7	130	81.8	113	71.1
Indiana	124	57	46.0	24	19.4	74	59.7	3	2.4	90	72.6	3	2.4	109	87.9	91	73.4	70	56.5
Michigan	135	96	71.1	50	37.0	75	55.6	8	5.9	110	81.5	7	5.2	116	85.9	95	70.4	90	66.7
Ohio	161	110	68.3	38	23.6	92	57.1	12	7.5	130	80.7	9	5.6	145	90.1	129	80.1	108	67.1
Wisconsin	147	84	57.1	33	22.4	96	65.3	4	2.7	108	73.5	6	4.1	127	86.4	87	59.2	70	47.6
CENSUS DIVISION 5, EAST SOUTH CENTRAL	398	179	45.0	77	19.3	176	44.2	11	2.8	266	66.8	15	3.8	330	82.9	235	59.0	142	35.7
Alabama	106	54	50.9	27	25.5	51	48.1	4	3.8	70	66.0	6	5.7	90	84.9	63	59.4	35	33.0
Kentucky	90	56	62.2	23	25.6	43	47.8	4	4.4	74	82.2	7	7.8	85	94.4	73	81.1	44	48.9
Mississippi	112	29	25.9	11	9.8	42	37.5	1	0.9	56	50.0	1	0.9	72	64.3	32	28.6	23	20.5
Tennessee	90	40	44.4	16	17.8	40	44.4	2	2.2	66	73.3	1	1.1	83	92.2	67	74.4	40	44.4
CENSUS DIVISION 6, WEST NORTH CENTRAL	670	430	64.2	121	18.1	359	53.6	19	2.8	479	71.5	29	4.3	491	73.3	352	52.5	363	54.2
Iowa	126	110	87.3	17	13.5	78	61.9	3	2.4	113	89.7	6	4.8	105	83.3	68	42.9	87	69.0
Kansas	151	78	51.7	22	14.6	70	46.4	1	0.7	80	53.0	5	3.3	94	62.3	60	45.0	52	34.4
Minnesota	106	77	72.6	27	25.5	78	73.6	5	4.7	93	87.7	5	4.7	77	72.6	60	56.6	77	72.6
Missouri	151	100	66.2	29	19.2	70	46.4	6	4.0	103	68.2	8	5.3	132	87.4	106	70.2	73	48.3
Nebraska	60	30	50.0	15	25.0	34	56.7	1	1.7	44	73.3	3	5.0	39	65.0	30	50.0	38	63.3
North Dakota	29	15	51.7	5	17.2	10	34.5	1	3.4	17	58.6	2	6.9	18	62.1	15	51.7	11	37.9
South Dakota	47	20	42.6	6	12.8	19	40.4	2	4.3	29	61.7	0	0.0	26	55.3	19	40.4	25	53.2
CENSUS DIVISION 7, WEST SOUTH CENTRAL	900	406	45.1	170	18.9	350	38.9	32	3.6	426	47.3	23	2.6	759	84.3	461	51.2	241	26.8
Arkansas	80	51	63.8	11	13.8	33	41.3	5	6.3	46	57.5	2	2.5	70	87.5	39	48.8	27	33.8
Louisiana	118	43	36.4	22	18.6	43	36.4	7	5.9	65	55.1	6	5.1	95	80.5	58	49.2	40	33.9
Oklahoma	129	59	45.7	16	12.4	53	41.1	4	3.1	66	51.2	2	1.6	108	83.7	70	54.3	27	20.9
Texas	573	253	44.2	121	21.1	221	38.6	16	2.8	249	43.5	13	2.3	486	84.8	294	51.3	147	25.7
CENSUS DIVISION 8, MOUNTAIN	338	195	57.7	74	21.9	202	59.8	18	5.3	229	67.8	8	2.4	278	82.2	188	55.6	172	50.9
Arizona	54	33	61.1	13	24.1	28	51.9	3	5.6	34	63.0	2	3.7	52	96.3	37	68.5	29	53.7
Colorado	68	47	69.1	23	33.8	46	67.6	9	13.2	54	79.4	1	1.5	60	88.2	46	67.6	49	72.1
Idaho	35	24	68.6	10	28.6	21	60.0	2	5.7	22	62.9	1	2.9	28	80.0	22	62.9	15	42.9
Montana	55	32	58.2	4	7.3	27	49.1	0	0.0	35	63.6	0	0.0	34	61.8	23	41.8	20	36.4
Nevada	34	8	23.5	8	23.5	12	35.3	1	2.9	17	50.0	1	2.9	26	76.5	14	41.2	14	41.2
New Mexico	30	19	63.3	2	6.7	22	73.3	1	3.3	19	63.3	2	6.7	27	90.0	21	70.0	12	40.0
Utah	35	15	42.9	10	28.6	27	77.1	2	5.7	28	80.0	1	2.9	28	80.0	13	37.1	19	54.3
Wyoming	27	17	63.0	4	14.8	19	70.4	0	0.0	20	74.1	0	0.0	23	85.2	12	44.4	14	51.9
CENSUS DIVISION 9, PACIFIC	464	252	54.3	126	27.2	287	61.9	50	10.8	323	69.6	25	5.4	412	88.8	339	73.1	279	60.1
Alaska	14	6	42.9	2	14.3	9	64.3	0	0.0	8	57.1	1	7.1	10	71.4	9	64.3	10	71.4
California	296	157	53.0	88	29.7	175	59.1	47	15.9	200	67.6	17	5.7	269	90.9	215	72.6	182	61.5
Hawaii	21	6	28.6	5	23.8	6	28.6	0	0.0	11	52.4	3	14.3	15	71.4	9	42.9	11	52.4
Oregon	58	44	75.9	15	25.9	50	86.2	1	1.7	52	89.7	1	1.7	51	87.9	47	81.0	36	62.1
Washington	75	39	52.0	16	21.3	47	62.7	2	2.7	52	69.3	3	4.0	67	89.3	59	78.7	40	53.3

Table 7 (Continued)

These data include only hospital-based facilities and services as reported by responding hospitals in Section C of the 2012 AHA Annual Survey, beginning on page 215. All hospitals are represented with Community Hospitals listed separately under United States. No estimates have been made for nonresponding hospitals. Definitions of facilities and services are listed in the Glossary, page 201.

CLASSIFICATION	HOSPITALS REPORTING	CHILDREN'S WELLNESS PROGRAM		CHIROPRACTIC SERVICES		COMMUNITY OUTREACH		COMPLEMENTARY AND ALTERNATIVE MEDICINE SERVICES		COMPUTER ASSISTED ORTHOPEDIC SURGERY (CAOS)		CRISIS PREVENTION		DENTAL SERVICES		ENABLING SERVICES		ENROLLMENT ASSISTANCE SERVICES		EXTRACORPOREAL SHOCK WAVE LITHOTRIPTER (ESWL)	
		Number	Percent	Number	Percent	Number	Percent	Number	Percent	Number	Percent	Number	Percent	Number	Percent	Number	Percent	Number	Percent	Number	Percent
UNITED STATES	4,774	904	18.9	133	2.8	3,218	67.4	907	19.0	702	14.7	1,021	21.4	1,015	21.3	1,169	24.5	2,508	52.5	1,270	26.6
COMMUNITY HOSPITALS	4,054	879	21.7	98	2.4	2,990	73.8	845	20.8	685	16.9	886	21.9	856	21.1	1,097	27.1	2,334	57.6	1,215	30.0
CENSUS DIVISION 1, NEW ENGLAND	187	65	34.8	8	4.3	149	79.7	83	44.4	34	18.2	67	35.8	51	27.3	71	38.0	139	74.3	97	51.9
Connecticut	32	13	40.6	2	6.3	27	84.4	21	65.6	8	25.0	21	65.6	16	50.0	13	40.6	27	84.4	19	59.4
Maine	39	11	28.2	1	2.6	31	79.5	14	35.9	3	7.7	8	20.5	3	7.7	12	30.8	25	64.1	18	46.2
Massachusetts	68	25	36.8	3	4.4	52	76.5	26	38.2	15	22.1	23	33.8	16	23.5	26	38.2	53	77.9	37	54.4
New Hampshire	26	12	46.2	1	3.8	22	84.6	14	53.8	6	23.1	9	34.6	10	38.5	12	46.2	20	76.9	13	50.0
Rhode Island	9	2	22.2	1	11.1	9	100.0	3	33.3	1	11.1	4	44.4	2	22.2	3	33.3	6	66.7	5	55.6
Vermont	13	2	15.4	0	0.0	8	61.5	5	38.5	1	7.7	2	15.4	4	30.8	5	38.5	8	61.5	5	38.5
CENSUS DIVISION 2, MIDDLE ATLANTIC	420	140	33.3	22	5.2	321	76.4	117	27.9	87	20.7	169	40.2	164	39.0	153	36.4	272	64.8	150	35.7
New Jersey	72	29	40.3	3	4.2	51	70.8	20	27.8	17	23.6	39	54.2	27	37.5	32	44.4	44	61.1	23	31.9
New York	159	64	40.3	14	8.8	139	87.4	58	36.5	34	21.4	77	48.4	81	50.9	56	35.2	114	71.7	61	38.4
Pennsylvania	189	47	24.9	5	2.6	131	69.3	39	20.6	36	19.0	53	28.0	56	29.6	65	34.4	114	60.3	66	34.9
CENSUS DIVISION 3, SOUTH ATLANTIC	671	109	16.2	11	1.6	494	73.6	124	18.5	126	18.8	153	22.8	160	23.8	199	29.7	396	59.0	218	32.5
Delaware	7	5	71.4	0	0.0	5	71.4	3	42.9	1	14.3	4	57.1	2	28.6	2	28.6	5	71.4	3	42.9
District of Columbia	11	5	45.5	0	0.0	9	81.8	3	27.3	3	27.3	6	54.5	6	54.5	5	45.5	7	63.6	2	18.2
Florida	152	14	9.2	6	3.9	110	72.4	24	15.8	39	25.7	28	18.4	23	15.1	42	27.6	85	55.9	69	45.4
Georgia	107	9	8.4	1	0.9	71	66.4	15	14.0	22	20.6	24	22.4	18	16.8	29	27.1	66	61.7	31	29.0
Maryland	51	16	31.4	1	2.0	42	82.4	24	47.1	14	27.5	22	43.1	20	39.2	25	49.0	39	76.5	23	45.1
North Carolina	120	19	15.8	1	0.8	86	71.7	20	16.7	16	13.3	24	20.0	36	30.0	37	30.8	65	54.2	20	16.7
South Carolina	82	15	18.3	0	0.0	66	80.5	4	4.9	9	11.0	8	9.8	16	19.5	9	11.0	37	45.1	20	24.4
Virginia	80	13	16.3	1	1.3	64	80.0	25	31.3	19	23.8	29	36.3	25	31.3	37	46.3	63	78.8	33	41.3
West Virginia	61	13	21.3	1	1.6	41	67.2	6	9.8	3	4.9	11	18.0	14	23.0	13	21.3	29	47.5	17	27.9
CENSUS DIVISION 4, EAST NORTH CENTRAL	726	190	26.2	31	4.3	557	76.7	232	32.0	131	18.0	210	28.9	178	24.5	266	36.6	455	62.7	217	29.9
Illinois	159	48	30.2	7	4.4	128	80.5	47	29.6	39	24.5	59	37.1	45	28.3	61	38.4	103	64.8	41	25.8
Indiana	124	32	25.8	4	3.2	96	77.4	25	20.2	11	8.9	27	21.8	20	16.1	22	17.7	74	59.7	33	26.6
Michigan	135	48	35.6	6	4.4	107	79.3	50	37.0	24	17.8	45	33.3	35	25.9	66	48.9	97	71.9	47	34.8
Ohio	161	36	22.4	10	6.2	134	83.2	48	29.8	35	21.7	44	27.3	52	32.3	64	39.8	105	65.2	61	37.9
Wisconsin	147	26	17.7	4	2.7	92	62.6	62	42.2	22	15.0	35	23.8	26	17.7	53	36.1	76	51.7	35	23.8
CENSUS DIVISION 5, EAST SOUTH CENTRAL	398	45	11.3	5	1.3	254	63.8	22	5.5	41	10.3	50	12.6	74	18.6	57	14.3	163	41.0	98	24.6
Alabama	106	12	11.3	2	1.9	60	56.6	5	4.7	10	9.4	12	11.3	9	8.5	9	8.5	49	46.2	28	26.4
Kentucky	90	12	13.3	1	1.1	67	74.4	8	8.9	12	13.3	10	11.1	16	17.8	20	22.2	54	60.0	25	27.8
Mississippi	112	12	10.7	1	0.9	66	58.9	3	2.7	7	6.3	9	8.0	33	29.5	6	5.4	19	17.0	18	16.1
Tennessee	90	9	10.0	1	1.1	61	67.8	6	6.7	12	13.3	19	21.1	16	17.8	22	24.4	41	45.6	27	30.0
CENSUS DIVISION 6, WEST NORTH CENTRAL	670	109	16.3	22	3.3	413	61.6	106	15.8	54	8.1	120	17.9	116	17.3	126	18.8	284	42.4	108	16.1
Iowa	126	25	19.8	3	2.4	94	74.6	28	22.2	12	9.5	30	23.8	22	17.5	33	26.2	69	54.8	15	11.9
Kansas	151	13	8.6	1	0.7	59	39.1	8	5.3	5	3.3	7	4.6	13	8.6	12	7.9	45	29.8	21	13.9
Minnesota	106	23	21.7	9	8.5	73	68.9	29	27.4	9	8.5	24	22.6	17	16.0	17	16.0	43	40.6	20	18.9
Missouri	151	28	18.5	5	3.3	99	65.6	25	16.6	13	8.6	35	23.2	45	29.8	46	30.5	75	49.7	36	23.8
Nebraska	60	9	15.0	1	1.7	40	66.7	7	11.7	11	18.3	13	21.7	11	18.3	11	18.3	25	41.7	9	15.0
North Dakota	29	6	20.7	3	10.3	15	51.7	4	13.8	3	10.3	4	13.8	2	6.9	4	13.8	15	51.7	2	6.9
South Dakota	47	5	10.6	0	0.0	33	70.2	5	10.6	1	2.1	7	14.9	6	12.8	3	6.4	12	25.5	5	10.6
CENSUS DIVISION 7, WEST SOUTH CENTRAL	900	100	11.1	8	0.9	440	48.9	53	5.9	94	10.4	83	9.2	124	13.8	115	12.8	341	37.9	166	18.4
Arkansas	80	8	10.0	0	0.0	45	56.3	4	5.0	4	5.0	10	12.5	8	10.0	7	8.8	32	40.0	13	16.3
Louisiana	118	18	15.3	2	1.7	61	51.7	8	6.8	15	12.7	21	17.8	17	14.4	12	10.2	51	43.2	19	16.1
Oklahoma	129	12	9.3	2	1.6	61	47.3	5	3.9	10	7.8	8	6.2	20	15.5	9	7.0	44	34.1	22	17.1
Texas	573	62	10.8	4	0.7	273	47.6	36	6.3	65	11.3	44	7.7	79	13.8	87	15.2	214	37.3	112	19.5
CENSUS DIVISION 8, MOUNTAIN	538	63	18.6	10	3.0	239	70.7	68	20.1	52	15.4	74	21.9	63	18.6	62	18.3	187	55.3	65	19.2
Arizona	54	11	20.4	1	1.9	40	74.1	17	31.5	12	22.2	14	25.9	10	18.5	10	18.5	37	68.5	17	31.5
Colorado	68	8	11.8	4	5.9	55	80.9	22	32.4	15	22.1	13	19.1	14	20.6	17	25.0	45	66.2	14	20.6
Idaho	35	7	20.0	2	5.7	27	77.1	6	17.1	9	25.7	6	17.1	7	20.0	6	17.1	18	51.4	3	8.6
Montana	55	13	23.6	1	1.8	34	61.8	9	16.4	5	9.1	9	16.4	3	5.5	6	10.9	31	56.4	6	10.9
Nevada	34	6	17.6	2	5.9	17	50.0	1	2.9	2	5.9	6	17.6	5	14.7	7	20.6	11	32.4	1	2.9
New Mexico	30	6	20.0	0	0.0	23	76.7	4	13.3	2	6.7	5	16.7	8	26.7	4	13.3	18	60.0	8	26.7
Utah	35	9	25.7	0	0.0	26	74.3	6	17.1	6	17.1	16	45.7	12	34.3	12	34.3	21	60.0	11	31.4
Wyoming	27	3	11.1	0	0.0	17	63.0	3	11.1	1	3.7	5	18.5	4	14.8	1	3.7	6	22.2	5	18.5
CENSUS DIVISION 9, PACIFIC	464	83	17.9	16	3.4	351	75.6	102	22.0	83	17.9	95	20.5	85	18.3	120	25.9	271	58.4	151	32.5
Alaska	14	3	21.4	0	0.0	9	64.3	1	7.1	1	7.1	5	35.7	1	7.1	2	14.3	8	57.1	4	28.6
California	296	51	17.2	9	3.0	225	76.0	64	21.6	48	16.2	56	18.9	64	21.6	77	26.0	164	55.4	105	35.5
Hawaii	21	1	4.8	0	0.0	11	52.4	2	9.5	1	4.8	4	19.0	2	9.5	3	14.3	10	47.6	5	23.8
Oregon	58	12	20.7	2	3.4	52	89.7	16	27.6	19	32.8	10	17.2	4	6.9	18	31.0	44	75.9	17	29.3
Washington	75	16	21.3	5	6.7	54	72.0	19	25.3	14	18.7	22	29.3	13	17.3	20	26.7	45	60.0	20	26.7

Table 7 (Continued)

These data include only hospital-based facilities and services as reported by responding hospitals in Section C of the 2012 AHA Annual Survey, beginning on page 215. All hospitals are represented with Community Hospitals listed separately under United States. No estimates have been made for nonresponding hospitals. Definitions of facilities and services are listed in the Glossary, page 201.

CLASSIFICATION	HOSPITALS REPORTING	FERTILITY CLINIC		FITNESS CENTER		FREESTANDING OUTPATIENT CARE CENTER		GENETIC TESTING/ COUNSELING		GERIATRIC SERVICES		HEALTH FAIR		COMMUNITY HEALTH EDUCATION		HEALTH RESEARCH		HEALTH SCREENINGS		HEMODIALYSIS		HIV/AIDS SERVICES	
		Number	Percent	Number	Percent	Number	Percent	Number	Percent	Number	Percent	Number	Percent	Number	Percent	Number	Percent	Number	Percent	Number	Percent	Number	Percent
UNITED STATES	4,774	234	4.9	1,361	28.5	1,475	30.9	694	14.5	1,818	38.1	3,438	72.0	3,469	72.7	1,112	23.3	3,547	74.3	1,459	30.6	1,069	22.4
COMMUNITY HOSPITALS	4,054	230	5.7	1,261	31.1	1,358	33.5	673	16.6	1,638	40.4	3,242	80.0	3,245	80.0	1,017	25.1	3,339	82.4	1,361	33.6	978	24.1
CENSUS DIVISION 1, NEW ENGLAND	187	23	12.3	55	29.4	87	46.5	53	28.3	88	47.1	149	79.7	159	85.0	77	41.2	159	85.0	63	33.7	81	43.3
Connecticut	32	6	18.8	13	40.6	21	65.6	13	40.6	18	56.3	27	84.4	28	87.5	22	68.8	29	90.6	13	40.6	21	65.6
Maine	39	3	7.7	14	35.9	16	41.0	7	17.9	13	33.3	30	76.9	33	84.6	10	25.6	35	89.7	7	17.9	14	35.9
Massachusetts	68	9	13.2	11	16.2	31	45.6	23	33.8	32	47.1	54	79.4	53	77.9	29	42.6	54	79.4	32	47.1	29	42.6
New Hampshire	26	2	7.7	8	30.8	11	42.3	5	19.2	15	57.7	23	88.5	23	88.5	7	26.9	23	88.5	3	11.5	11	42.3
Rhode Island	9	1	11.1	4	44.4	5	55.6	2	22.2	6	66.7	8	88.9	8	88.9	5	55.6	8	88.9	5	55.6	3	33.3
Vermont	13	2	15.4	5	38.5	3	23.1	3	23.1	4	30.8	7	53.8	12	92.3	4	30.8	10	76.9	3	23.1	3	23.1
CENSUS DIVISION 2, MIDDLE ATLANTIC	420	44	10.5	119	28.3	222	52.9	132	31.4	238	56.7	335	79.8	334	79.5	160	38.1	341	81.2	209	49.8	175	41.7
New Jersey	72	10	13.9	20	27.8	32	44.4	31	43.1	45	62.5	50	69.4	53	73.6	34	47.2	57	79.2	46	63.9	35	48.6
New York	159	23	14.5	44	27.7	103	64.8	59	37.1	99	62.3	144	90.6	141	88.7	67	42.1	140	88.1	103	64.8	84	52.8
Pennsylvania	189	11	5.8	55	29.1	87	46.0	42	22.2	94	49.7	141	74.6	140	74.1	59	31.2	144	76.2	60	31.7	56	29.6
CENSUS DIVISION 3, SOUTH ATLANTIC	671	31	4.6	201	30.0	267	39.8	114	17.0	247	36.8	533	79.4	520	77.5	183	27.3	539	80.3	274	40.8	199	29.7
Delaware	7	0	0.0	2	28.6	4	57.1	4	57.1	2	28.6	4	57.1	5	71.4	4	57.1	5	71.4	4	57.1	4	57.1
District of Columbia	11	1	9.1	2	18.2	5	45.5	5	45.5	5	45.5	7	63.6	9	81.8	7	63.6	8	72.7	6	54.5	7	63.6
Florida	152	7	4.6	50	32.9	62	40.8	34	22.4	52	34.2	118	77.6	125	82.2	57	37.5	123	80.9	79	52.0	44	28.9
Georgia	107	3	2.8	31	29.0	43	40.2	10	9.3	34	31.8	78	72.9	77	72.0	25	23.4	85	79.4	42	39.3	25	23.4
Maryland	51	5	9.8	15	29.4	21	41.2	23	45.1	32	62.7	45	88.2	41	80.4	26	51.0	45	88.2	34	66.7	23	45.1
North Carolina	120	6	5.0	40	33.3	48	40.0	14	11.7	42	35.0	94	78.3	96	80.0	26	21.7	97	80.8	37	30.8	29	24.2
South Carolina	82	2	2.4	19	23.2	24	29.3	5	6.1	33	40.2	63	76.8	58	70.7	11	13.4	66	72.0	29	35.4	26	31.7
Virginia	80	5	6.3	21	26.3	40	50.0	14	17.5	29	36.3	70	87.5	63	78.8	21	26.3	66	82.5	28	35.0	30	37.5
West Virginia	61	2	3.3	21	34.4	20	32.8	5	8.2	18	29.5	54	88.5	46	75.4	6	9.8	51	83.6	15	24.6	11	18.0
CENSUS DIVISION 4, EAST NORTH CENTRAL	726	43	5.9	255	35.1	276	38.0	119	16.4	351	48.3	561	77.3	601	82.8	227	31.3	592	81.5	226	31.1	173	23.8
Illinois	159	11	6.9	47	29.6	64	40.3	26	16.4	83	52.2	138	86.8	140	88.1	55	34.6	143	89.9	45	28.3	48	30.2
Indiana	124	5	4.0	35	28.2	39	31.5	15	12.1	40	32.3	91	73.4	93	75.0	31	25.0	95	76.6	32	25.8	20	16.1
Michigan	135	10	7.4	49	36.3	62	45.9	27	20.0	70	51.9	108	80.0	112	83.0	57	42.2	116	85.9	50	37.0	49	36.3
Ohio	161	11	6.8	68	42.2	66	41.0	30	18.6	63	39.1	134	83.2	140	87.0	61	37.9	140	87.0	70	43.5	49	30.4
Wisconsin	147	6	4.1	56	38.1	45	30.6	21	14.3	95	64.6	90	61.2	116	78.9	23	15.6	98	66.7	29	19.7	7	4.8
CENSUS DIVISION 5, EAST SOUTH CENTRAL	398	12	3.0	104	26.1	81	20.4	26	6.5	124	31.2	262	65.8	248	62.3	59	14.8	258	64.8	97	24.4	65	16.3
Alabama	106	4	3.8	33	31.1	21	19.8	5	4.7	36	34.0	74	69.8	63	59.4	16	15.1	73	68.9	35	33.0	13	12.3
Kentucky	90	2	2.2	19	21.1	24	26.7	8	8.9	29	32.2	75	83.3	77	85.6	18	20.0	76	84.4	21	23.3	11	12.2
Mississippi	112	2	1.8	32	28.6	11	9.8	2	1.8	21	18.8	46	41.1	49	43.8	6	5.4	43	38.4	13	11.6	22	19.6
Tennessee	90	4	4.4	20	22.2	25	27.8	11	12.2	38	42.2	67	74.4	59	65.6	19	21.1	66	73.3	28	31.1	19	21.1
CENSUS DIVISION 6, WEST NORTH CENTRAL	670	30	4.5	240	35.8	103	15.4	61	9.1	242	36.1	464	69.3	486	72.5	91	13.6	523	78.1	137	20.4	112	16.7
Iowa	126	3	2.4	49	38.9	16	12.7	7	5.6	54	42.9	107	84.9	105	83.3	14	11.1	119	94.4	25	19.8	26	20.6
Kansas	151	3	2.0	42	27.8	9	6.0	10	6.6	42	27.8	78	51.7	78	51.7	9	6.0	87	57.6	16	10.6	16	10.6
Minnesota	106	6	5.7	38	35.8	23	21.7	14	13.2	46	43.4	73	68.9	91	85.8	18	17.0	84	79.2	19	17.9	19	17.9
Missouri	151	10	6.6	59	39.1	40	26.5	19	12.6	54	35.8	107	70.9	107	70.9	30	19.9	116	76.8	48	31.8	36	23.8
Nebraska	60	4	6.7	25	41.7	10	16.7	6	10.0	19	31.7	45	75.0	46	76.7	11	18.3	50	83.3	12	20.0	8	13.3
North Dakota	29	3	10.3	10	34.5	3	10.3	3	10.3	12	41.4	19	65.5	22	75.9	4	13.8	21	72.4	6	20.7	3	10.3
South Dakota	47	1	2.1	17	36.2	2	4.3	2	4.3	15	31.9	35	74.5	37	78.7	5	10.6	46	97.9	11	23.4	4	8.5
CENSUS DIVISION 7, WEST SOUTH CENTRAL	900	17	1.9	190	21.1	183	20.3	58	6.4	251	27.9	543	60.3	513	57.0	103	11.4	529	58.8	188	20.9	97	10.8
Arkansas	80	0	0.0	20	25.0	14	17.5	4	5.0	29	36.3	61	76.3	46	57.5	8	10.0	59	73.8	14	17.5	12	15.0
Louisiana	118	1	0.8	20	16.9	30	25.4	9	7.6	39	33.1	70	59.3	72	61.0	19	16.1	61	51.7	25	21.2	19	16.1
Oklahoma	129	3	2.3	21	16.3	20	15.5	5	3.9	30	23.3	74	57.4	81	62.8	14	10.9	81	62.8	22	17.1	9	7.0
Texas	573	13	2.3	129	22.5	119	20.8	40	7.0	153	26.7	338	59.0	314	54.8	62	10.8	328	57.2	127	22.2	57	9.9
CENSUS DIVISION 8, MOUNTAIN	338	11	3.3	93	27.5	93	27.5	46	13.6	113	33.4	261	77.2	255	75.4	67	19.8	264	78.1	91	26.9	59	17.5
Arizona	54	3	5.6	18	33.3	16	29.6	9	16.7	17	31.5	32	59.3	44	81.5	20	37.0	42	77.8	26	48.1	14	25.9
Colorado	68	2	2.9	27	39.7	24	35.3	21	30.9	18	26.5	55	80.9	59	86.8	20	29.4	56	82.4	20	29.4	16	23.5
Idaho	35	1	2.9	10	28.6	11	31.4	5	14.3	10	28.6	31	88.6	31	88.6	6	17.1	28	80.0	6	17.1	4	11.4
Montana	55	1	1.8	7	12.7	8	14.5	3	5.5	27	49.1	48	87.3	37	67.3	6	10.9	48	87.3	5	9.1	8	14.5
Nevada	34	0	0.0	9	26.5	7	20.6	2	5.9	8	23.5	20	58.8	16	47.1	5	14.7	17	50.0	8	23.5	5	14.7
New Mexico	30	0	0.0	9	30.0	9	30.0	0	0.0	7	23.3	24	80.0	18	60.0	1	3.3	22	73.3	6	20.0	3	10.0
Utah	35	4	11.4	15	42.9	15	42.9	6	17.1	16	45.7	29	82.9	29	82.9	9	25.7	28	80.0	13	37.1	7	20.0
Wyoming	27	0	0.0	5	18.5	3	11.1	0	0.0	10	37.0	22	81.5	21	77.8	0	0.0	23	85.2	7	25.9	2	7.4
CENSUS DIVISION 9, PACIFIC	464	23	5.0	104	22.4	163	35.1	85	18.3	164	35.3	330	71.1	353	76.1	145	31.3	342	73.7	174	37.5	108	23.3
Alaska	14	0	0.0	4	22.4	2	14.3	1	7.1	2	14.3	8	57.1	11	78.6	1	7.1	11	78.6	1	7.1	0	0.0
California	296	18	6.1	65	22.0	110	37.2	61	20.6	110	37.2	203	68.6	212	71.6	100	33.8	207	69.9	129	43.6	81	27.4
Hawaii	21	0	0.0	7	4.8	4	19.0	2	9.5	6	28.6	12	57.1	15	71.4	7	33.3	14	66.7	6	28.6	3	14.3
Oregon	58	1	1.7	19	32.8	20	34.5	4	6.9	20	34.5	48	82.8	53	91.4	11	19.0	49	84.5	16	27.6	12	20.7
Washington	75	4	5.3	15	20.0	27	36.0	17	22.7	26	34.7	59	78.7	62	82.7	28	37.3	61	81.3	22	29.3	12	16.0

Table 7 (Continued)

These data include only hospital-based facilities and services as reported by responding hospitals in Section C of the 2012 AHA Annual Survey, beginning on page 215. All hospitals are represented with Community Hospitals listed separately under United States. No estimates have been made for nonresponding hospitals. Definitions of facilities and services are listed in the Glossary, page 201.

CLASSIFICATION	HOSPITALS REPORTING	HOME HEALTH SERVICES Number	Percent	HOSPICE Number	Percent	HOSPITAL-BASED OUTPATIENT CARE CENTER SERVICES Number	Percent	IMMUNIZATION PROGRAM Number	Percent	INDIGENT CARE CLINIC Number	Percent	LINGUISTIC/TRANSLATION SERVICES Number	Percent	MEALS ON WHEELS Number	Percent	MOBILE HEALTH SERVICES Number	Percent	NEONATAL INTERMEDIATE CARE UNITS Number	Percent	NEUROLOGICAL SERVICES Number	Percent	NUTRITION PROGRAMS CENTER Number	Percent
UNITED STATES	4,774	1,253	26.2	961	20.1	3,448	72.2	1,871	39.2	759	15.9	2,599	54.4	404	8.5	517	10.8	705	14.8	2,298	48.1	3,492	73.1
COMMUNITY HOSPITALS	4,054	1,186	29.3	893	22.0	3,198	78.9	1,718	42.4	721	17.8	2,385	58.8	392	9.7	481	11.9	693	17.1	2,148	53.0	3,158	77.9
CENSUS DIVISION 1, NEW ENGLAND	187	37	19.8	50	26.7	160	85.6	112	59.9	48	25.7	128	68.4	5	2.7	24	12.8	28	15.0	129	69.0	172	92.0
Connecticut	32	8	25.0	16	50.0	27	84.4	21	65.6	16	50.0	23	71.9	0	0.0	6	18.8	4	12.5	27	84.4	29	90.6
Maine	39	6	15.4	6	15.4	32	82.1	29	74.4	8	20.5	20	51.3	2	5.1	3	7.7	4	10.3	18	46.2	38	97.4
Massachusetts	68	15	22.1	14	20.6	58	85.3	36	52.9	12	17.6	54	79.4	1	1.5	8	11.8	14	20.6	50	73.5	61	89.7
New Hampshire	26	6	23.1	8	30.8	25	96.2	15	57.7	7	26.9	16	61.5	1	3.8	4	15.4	3	11.5	20	76.9	26	100.0
Rhode Island	9	0	0.0	2	22.2	8	88.9	5	55.6	3	33.3	7	77.8	0	0.0	2	22.2	2	22.2	7	77.8	8	88.9
Vermont	13	2	15.4	4	30.8	10	76.9	6	46.2	2	15.4	8	61.5	1	7.7	1	7.7	1	7.7	7	53.8	10	76.9
CENSUS DIVISION 2, MIDDLE ATLANTIC	420	117	27.9	109	26.0	342	81.4	225	53.6	153	36.4	269	64.0	38	9.0	67	16.0	111	26.4	300	71.4	342	81.4
New Jersey	72	15	20.8	14	19.4	59	81.9	36	50.0	40	55.6	55	76.4	11	15.3	18	25.0	40	55.6	58	80.6	57	79.2
New York	159	40	25.2	47	29.6	138	86.8	99	62.3	71	44.7	116	73.0	15	9.4	36	22.6	47	29.6	124	78.0	137	86.2
Pennsylvania	189	62	32.8	48	25.4	145	76.7	90	47.6	42	22.2	98	51.9	12	6.3	13	6.9	24	12.7	118	62.4	148	78.3
CENSUS DIVISION 3, SOUTH ATLANTIC	671	163	24.3	126	18.8	509	75.9	240	35.8	117	17.4	388	57.8	28	4.2	103	15.4	147	21.9	388	57.8	521	77.6
Delaware	11	3	42.9	1	14.3	4	57.1	9	57.1	1	14.3	5	71.4	0	0.0	0	0.0	4	14.3	5	71.4	5	71.4
District of Columbia	11	1	9.1	1	9.1	10	90.9	9	81.8	5	45.5	9	81.8	1	9.1	4	36.4	4	36.4	11	100.0	11	100.0
Florida	152	38	25.0	20	13.2	108	71.1	43	28.3	29	19.1	90	59.2	1	0.7	21	13.8	30	19.7	108	71.1	114	75.0
Georgia	107	15	14.0	15	14.0	70	65.4	26	24.3	14	13.1	65	60.7	1	0.9	13	12.1	28	26.2	53	49.5	81	75.7
Maryland	51	10	19.6	14	27.5	46	90.2	32	62.7	22	43.1	35	68.6	5	9.8	13	25.5	6	11.8	40	78.4	45	88.2
North Carolina	120	32	26.7	24	20.0	95	79.2	40	33.3	18	15.0	67	55.8	5	4.2	20	16.7	36	30.0	60	50.0	91	75.8
South Carolina	82	16	19.5	10	12.2	60	73.2	22	26.8	6	7.3	37	45.1	4	4.9	9	11.0	27	32.9	35	42.7	61	74.4
Virginia	80	32	40.0	34	42.5	66	82.5	32	40.0	16	20.0	57	71.3	7	8.8	19	23.8	13	16.3	47	58.8	67	83.8
West Virginia	61	16	26.2	7	11.5	50	82.0	32	52.5	6	9.8	23	37.7	4	6.6	4	6.6	2	3.3	29	47.5	46	75.4
CENSUS DIVISION 4, EAST NORTH CENTRAL	726	214	29.5	187	25.8	555	76.4	331	45.6	147	20.2	442	60.9	122	16.8	88	12.1	80	11.0	411	56.6	614	84.6
Illinois	159	52	32.7	49	30.8	129	81.1	68	42.8	32	20.1	100	62.9	28	17.6	17	10.7	30	18.9	101	63.5	133	83.6
Indiana	124	38	30.6	31	25.0	80	64.5	47	37.9	21	16.9	71	57.3	24	19.4	15	12.1	17	13.7	60	48.4	93	75.0
Michigan	135	44	32.6	44	32.6	109	80.7	82	60.7	34	25.2	87	64.4	12	8.9	15	11.1	9	6.7	80	59.3	117	86.7
Ohio	161	53	32.9	45	28.0	121	75.2	74	46.0	45	28.0	101	62.7	24	14.9	24	14.9	24	14.9	106	65.8	142	88.2
Wisconsin	147	27	18.4	18	12.2	116	78.9	60	40.8	15	10.2	83	56.5	34	23.1	17	11.6	0	0.0	64	43.5	129	87.8
CENSUS DIVISION 5, EAST SOUTH CENTRAL	398	90	22.6	48	12.1	234	58.8	86	21.6	30	7.5	167	42.0	9	2.3	29	7.3	70	17.6	157	39.4	226	56.8
Alabama	106	27	25.5	12	11.3	71	67.0	21	19.8	7	6.6	46	43.4	4	3.8	5	4.7	11	10.4	44	41.5	57	53.8
Kentucky	90	29	32.2	13	14.4	69	76.7	17	18.9	10	11.1	49	54.4	4	4.4	11	12.2	19	21.1	44	48.9	63	70.0
Mississippi	112	10	8.9	7	6.3	39	34.8	28	25.0	6	5.4	27	24.1	0	0.0	5	4.5	29	25.9	28	25.0	41	36.6
Tennessee	90	24	26.7	16	17.8	55	61.1	20	22.2	7	7.8	45	50.0	1	1.1	8	8.9	11	12.2	41	45.6	65	72.2
CENSUS DIVISION 6, WEST NORTH CENTRAL	670	254	37.9	175	26.1	511	76.3	273	40.7	56	8.4	316	47.2	111	16.6	65	9.7	78	11.6	200	29.9	462	69.0
Iowa	126	58	46.0	53	42.1	110	87.3	61	48.4	11	8.7	68	54.0	32	25.4	11	8.7	10	7.9	34	27.0	111	88.1
Kansas	151	48	31.8	16	10.6	111	73.5	36	23.8	5	3.3	56	37.1	30	19.9	6	4.0	14	9.3	27	17.9	78	51.7
Minnesota	106	43	40.6	41	38.7	85	80.2	51	48.1	9	8.5	52	49.1	16	15.1	11	10.4	12	11.3	31	29.2	75	70.8
Missouri	151	52	34.4	30	19.9	108	71.5	64	42.4	20	13.2	84	55.6	16	10.6	21	13.9	30	19.9	73	48.3	120	79.5
Nebraska	60	27	45.0	18	30.0	46	76.7	24	40.0	4	6.7	32	53.3	6	10.0	4	6.7	5	8.3	22	36.7	40	66.7
North Dakota	29	6	20.7	6	20.7	19	65.5	13	44.8	4	13.8	11	37.9	3	10.3	5	17.2	4	13.8	4	13.8	13	44.8
South Dakota	47	20	42.6	11	23.4	32	68.1	24	51.1	3	6.4	13	27.7	7	14.9	7	14.9	3	6.4	9	19.1	25	53.2
CENSUS DIVISION 7, WEST SOUTH CENTRAL	900	167	18.6	83	9.2	550	61.1	257	28.6	68	7.6	391	43.4	40	4.4	54	6.0	91	10.1	319	35.4	558	62.0
Arkansas	80	30	37.5	8	10.0	51	63.8	16	20.0	0	0.0	35	43.8	4	5.0	6	7.5	10	12.5	25	31.3	51	63.8
Louisiana	118	12	10.2	6	5.1	65	55.1	37	31.4	13	11.0	37	31.4	2	1.7	8	6.8	9	7.6	40	33.9	71	60.2
Oklahoma	129	37	28.7	16	12.4	75	58.1	40	31.0	8	6.2	55	42.6	16	12.4	8	6.2	6	4.7	37	28.7	58	45.0
Texas	573	88	15.4	53	9.2	359	62.7	164	28.6	47	8.2	264	46.1	18	3.1	32	5.6	66	11.5	217	37.9	378	66.0
CENSUS DIVISION 8, MOUNTAIN	338	80	23.7	75	22.2	240	71.0	129	38.2	44	13.0	194	57.4	28	8.3	24	7.1	43	12.7	138	40.8	247	73.1
Arizona	54	8	14.8	11	20.4	37	68.5	17	31.5	6	11.1	36	66.7	3	5.6	4	7.4	9	16.7	33	61.1	43	79.6
Colorado	68	16	23.5	10	14.7	56	82.4	24	35.3	14	20.6	51	75.0	8	11.8	6	8.8	11	16.2	36	52.9	56	82.4
Idaho	35	6	17.1	8	22.9	26	74.3	14	40.0	3	8.6	20	57.1	4	11.4	5	14.3	1	2.9	11	31.4	23	65.7
Montana	55	17	30.9	19	34.5	41	74.5	30	54.5	7	12.7	20	36.4	10	18.2	1	1.8	2	3.6	12	21.8	39	70.9
Nevada	34	6	17.6	3	8.8	16	47.1	9	26.5	4	11.8	14	41.2	0	0.0	2	5.9	4	11.8	15	44.1	20	58.8
New Mexico	30	9	30.0	7	23.3	21	70.0	11	36.7	3	10.0	20	66.7	1	3.3	2	6.7	6	20.0	8	26.7	20	66.7
Utah	35	8	22.9	10	28.6	27	77.1	15	42.9	5	14.3	23	65.7	1	2.9	2	5.7	7	20.0	15	42.9	28	80.0
Wyoming	27	10	37.0	7	25.9	16	59.3	9	33.3	2	7.4	10	37.0	1	3.7	2	7.4	3	11.1	8	29.6	18	66.7
CENSUS DIVISION 9, PACIFIC	464	131	28.2	108	23.3	347	74.8	218	47.0	96	20.7	304	65.5	23	5.0	63	13.6	57	12.3	256	55.2	350	75.4
Alaska	14	5	35.7	3	21.4	10	71.4	6	42.9	2	14.3	9	64.3	1	7.1	1	7.1	1	7.1	3	21.4	9	64.3
California	296	75	25.3	64	21.6	217	73.3	140	47.3	64	21.6	193	65.2	14	4.7	41	13.9	34	11.5	182	61.5	216	73.0
Hawaii	21	6	28.6	3	14.3	10	47.6	6	28.6	3	14.3	11	52.4	3	14.3	4	19.0	3	14.3	9	42.9	15	71.4
Oregon	58	25	43.1	22	37.9	51	87.9	23	39.7	11	19.0	44	75.9	1	1.7	7	12.1	4	6.9	24	41.4	51	87.9
Washington	75	20	26.7	16	21.3	59	78.7	43	57.3	16	21.3	47	62.7	4	5.3	10	13.3	15	20.0	38	50.7	59	78.7

Table 7 (Continued)

These data include only hospital-based facilities and services as reported by responding hospitals in Section C of the 2012 AHA Annual Survey, beginning on page 215. All hospitals are represented with Community Hospitals listed separately under United States. No estimates have been made for nonresponding hospitals. Definitions of facilities and services are listed in the Glossary, page 201.

CLASSIFICATION	HOSPITALS REPORTING	OBSTETRICS INPATIENT CARE UNITS		OCCUPATIONAL HEALTH SERVICES		ONCOLOGY SERVICES		ORTHOPEDIC SERVICES		OTHER SPECIAL CARE UNITS		OUTPATIENT SURGERY		PAIN MANAGEMENT PROGRAM		PALLIATIVE CARE PROGRAM		PALLIATIVE CARE INPATIENT UNIT		PATIENT CONTROLLED ANALGESIA (PCA)		PATIENT EDUCATION CENTER	
	Number	Number	Percent	Number	Percent	Number	Percent	Number	Percent	Number	Percent	Number	Percent	Number	Percent	Number	Percent	Number	Percent	Number	Percent	Number	Percent
UNITED STATES	4,774	2,573	53.9	2,994	62.7	2,411	50.5	3,257	68.2	762	16.0	3,783	79.2	2,439	51.1	1,640	34.4	483	10.1	3,175	66.5	2,563	53.7
COMMUNITY HOSPITALS	4,054	2,542	62.7	2,772	68.4	2,325	57.4	3,067	75.7	716	17.7	3,585	88.4	2,258	55.7	1,539	38.0	419	10.3	2,966	73.2	2,332	57.5
CENSUS DIVISION 1, NEW ENGLAND	187	121	64.7	149	79.7	135	72.2	160	85.6	23	12.3	157	84.0	128	68.4	95	50.8	30	16.0	149	79.7	122	65.2
Connecticut	32	23	71.9	22	68.8	26	81.3	26	81.3	10	31.3	26	81.3	26	81.3	22	68.8	8	25.0	27	84.4	21	65.6
Maine	39	29	74.4	25	64.1	26	66.7	36	92.3	3	7.7	35	89.7	22	56.4	20	51.3	6	15.4	32	82.1	23	59.0
Massachusetts	68	39	57.4	59	86.8	48	70.6	57	83.8	5	7.4	54	79.4	50	73.5	25	36.8	8	11.8	50	73.5	48	70.6
New Hampshire	26	17	65.4	23	88.5	19	73.1	25	96.2	5	19.2	23	88.5	17	65.4	16	61.5	7	26.9	23	88.5	17	65.4
Rhode Island	9	5	55.6	9	100.0	7	77.8	6	66.7	0	0.0	8	88.9	7	77.8	4	44.4	0	0.0	7	77.8	7	77.8
Vermont	13	8	61.5	11	84.6	9	69.2	10	76.9	0	0.0	11	84.6	6	46.2	8	61.5	1	7.7	10	76.9	6	46.2
CENSUS DIVISION 2, MIDDLE ATLANTIC	420	243	57.9	305	72.6	291	69.3	339	80.7	82	19.5	351	83.6	305	72.6	220	52.4	79	18.8	312	74.3	272	64.8
New Jersey	72	45	62.5	47	65.3	54	75.0	57	79.2	11	15.3	57	79.2	54	75.0	44	61.1	16	22.2	53	73.6	50	69.4
New York	159	106	66.7	125	78.6	124	78.0	136	85.5	32	20.1	147	92.5	121	76.1	102	64.2	44	27.7	126	79.2	105	66.0
Pennsylvania	189	92	48.7	133	70.4	113	59.8	146	77.2	39	20.6	147	77.8	130	68.8	74	39.2	19	10.1	133	70.4	117	61.9
CENSUS DIVISION 3, SOUTH ATLANTIC	671	365	54.4	470	70.0	379	56.5	514	76.6	144	21.5	538	80.2	373	55.6	252	37.6	59	8.8	484	72.1	412	61.4
Delaware	7	4	57.1	4	57.1	4	57.1	5	71.4	2	28.6	5	71.4	3	42.9	3	42.9	1	14.3	5	71.4	4	57.1
District of Columbia	11	7	63.6	9	81.8	7	63.6	9	81.8	3	27.3	8	72.7	8	72.7	7	63.6	3	27.3	8	72.7	10	90.9
Florida	152	75	49.3	103	67.8	99	65.1	122	80.3	45	29.6	128	84.2	84	55.3	64	42.1	20	13.2	115	75.7	92	60.5
Georgia	107	56	52.3	66	61.7	49	45.8	73	68.2	17	15.9	81	75.7	54	50.5	27	25.2	7	6.5	67	62.6	58	54.2
Maryland	51	30	58.8	41	80.4	42	82.4	45	88.2	12	23.5	43	84.3	42	82.4	33	64.7	5	9.8	43	84.3	35	68.6
North Carolina	120	76	63.3	89	74.2	74	61.7	95	79.2	29	24.2	102	85.0	84	70.0	40	33.3	10	8.3	90	75.0	69	57.5
South Carolina	82	44	53.7	57	69.5	31	37.8	60	73.2	19	23.2	58	70.7	31	37.8	21	25.6	2	2.4	54	65.9	54	65.9
Virginia	80	44	55.0	67	83.8	50	62.5	64	80.0	15	18.8	68	85.0	49	61.3	39	48.8	8	10.0	66	82.5	55	68.8
West Virginia	61	29	47.5	34	55.7	23	37.7	41	67.2	2	3.3	45	73.8	18	29.5	18	29.5	3	4.9	36	59.0	35	57.4
CENSUS DIVISION 4, EAST NORTH CENTRAL	726	444	61.2	503	69.3	458	63.1	555	76.4	208	28.7	628	86.5	474	65.3	282	38.8	92	12.7	558	76.9	498	68.6
Illinois	159	102	64.2	105	66.0	109	68.6	128	80.5	19	11.9	146	91.8	110	69.2	65	40.9	16	10.1	130	81.8	100	62.9
Indiana	124	74	59.7	84	67.7	67	54.0	89	71.8	23	18.5	98	79.0	64	51.6	34	27.4	12	9.7	93	75.0	71	57.3
Michigan	135	76	56.3	103	76.3	92	68.1	107	79.3	29	21.5	116	85.9	86	63.7	58	43.0	19	14.1	105	77.8	86	63.7
Ohio	161	91	56.5	122	75.8	109	67.7	141	87.6	27	16.8	143	88.8	121	75.2	67	41.6	30	18.6	134	83.2	109	67.7
Wisconsin	147	101	68.7	89	60.5	81	55.1	90	61.2	110	74.8	125	85.0	93	63.3	58	39.5	15	10.2	96	65.3	132	89.8
CENSUS DIVISION 5, EAST SOUTH CENTRAL	398	188	47.2	192	48.2	152	38.2	222	55.8	64	16.1	297	74.6	127	31.9	78	19.6	24	6.0	207	52.0	182	45.7
Alabama	106	53	50.0	51	48.1	38	35.8	63	59.4	14	13.2	80	75.5	44	41.5	20	18.9	8	7.5	56	52.8	46	43.4
Kentucky	90	49	54.4	51	56.7	47	52.2	67	74.4	14	15.6	77	85.6	51	56.7	25	27.8	5	5.6	66	73.3	53	58.9
Mississippi	112	43	38.4	35	31.3	26	23.2	36	32.1	15	13.4	68	60.7	4	3.6	12	10.7	2	1.8	36	32.1	42	37.5
Tennessee	90	43	47.8	55	61.1	41	45.6	56	62.2	21	23.3	72	80.0	28	31.1	21	23.3	9	10.0	49	54.4	41	45.6
CENSUS DIVISION 6, WEST NORTH CENTRAL	670	353	52.7	433	64.6	297	44.3	397	59.3	76	11.3	566	84.5	283	42.2	201	30.0	53	7.9	422	63.0	318	47.5
Iowa	126	78	61.9	90	71.4	75	59.5	92	73.0	13	10.3	118	93.7	62	49.2	36	28.6	6	4.8	92	73.0	68	54.0
Kansas	151	68	45.0	80	53.0	41	27.2	65	43.0	12	7.9	120	79.5	57	37.7	28	18.5	8	5.3	81	53.6	53	35.1
Minnesota	106	76	71.7	81	76.4	52	49.1	69	65.1	9	8.5	101	95.3	41	38.7	41	38.7	11	10.4	72	67.9	52	49.1
Missouri	151	70	46.4	102	67.5	75	49.7	101	66.9	28	18.5	110	72.8	70	46.4	56	37.1	14	9.3	107	70.9	88	58.3
Nebraska	60	32	53.3	38	63.3	33	55.0	43	71.7	8	13.3	54	90.0	28	46.7	20	33.3	6	10.0	36	60.0	28	46.7
North Dakota	29	10	34.5	11	37.9	8	27.6	7	24.1	3	10.3	24	82.8	8	27.6	6	20.7	4	13.8	13	44.8	9	31.0
South Dakota	47	19	40.4	31	66.0	13	27.7	20	42.6	3	6.4	39	83.0	17	36.2	14	29.8	4	8.5	21	44.7	20	42.6
CENSUS DIVISION 7, WEST SOUTH CENTRAL	900	351	39.0	422	46.9	262	29.1	476	52.9	82	9.1	579	64.3	311	34.6	158	17.6	40	4.4	497	55.2	355	39.4
Arkansas	80	33	41.3	42	52.5	31	38.8	41	51.3	4	5.0	56	70.0	20	25.0	12	15.0	2	2.5	45	56.3	28	35.0
Louisiana	118	43	36.4	52	44.1	38	32.2	60	50.8	7	5.9	76	64.4	29	24.6	24	20.3	5	4.2	56	47.5	42	35.6
Oklahoma	129	52	40.3	51	39.5	27	20.9	68	52.7	11	8.5	93	72.1	46	35.7	24	18.6	10	7.8	65	50.4	37	28.7
Texas	573	223	38.9	277	48.3	166	29.0	307	53.6	60	10.5	354	61.8	216	37.7	98	17.1	23	4.0	331	57.8	248	43.3
CENSUS DIVISION 8, MOUNTAIN	338	204	60.4	198	58.6	157	46.4	229	67.8	24	7.1	266	78.7	178	52.7	108	32.0	38	11.2	217	64.2	159	47.0
Arizona	54	28	51.9	28	51.9	29	53.7	38	70.4	5	9.3	43	79.6	33	61.1	22	40.7	8	14.8	39	72.2	32	59.3
Colorado	68	48	70.6	50	73.5	46	67.6	54	79.4	11	16.2	63	92.6	40	58.8	31	45.6	5	7.4	54	79.4	32	47.1
Idaho	35	22	62.9	22	62.9	11	31.4	28	80.0	2	5.7	30	85.7	18	51.4	8	22.9	5	14.3	24	68.6	21	60.0
Montana	55	25	45.5	29	52.7	18	32.7	25	45.5	1	1.8	35	63.6	23	41.8	16	29.1	6	10.9	24	43.6	18	32.7
Nevada	34	12	35.3	19	55.9	13	38.2	21	61.8	1	2.9	19	55.9	13	38.2	9	26.5	4	11.8	16	47.1	14	41.2
New Mexico	30	22	73.3	14	46.7	13	43.3	20	66.7	0	0.0	26	86.7	11	36.7	6	20.0	5	16.7	20	66.7	9	30.0
Utah	35	28	80.0	20	57.1	16	45.7	24	68.6	3	8.6	29	82.9	25	71.4	10	28.6	3	8.6	24	68.6	22	62.9
Wyoming	27	19	70.4	16	59.3	11	40.7	19	70.4	1	3.7	21	77.8	15	55.6	6	22.2	2	7.4	16	59.3	11	40.7
CENSUS DIVISION 9, PACIFIC	464	304	65.5	322	69.4	280	60.3	365	78.7	59	12.7	401	86.4	260	56.0	246	53.0	68	14.7	329	70.9	245	52.8
Alaska	14	10	71.4	9	64.3	5	35.7	8	57.1	1	7.1	10	71.4	4	28.6	4	28.6	1	7.1	8	57.1	6	42.9
California	296	192	64.9	205	69.3	186	62.8	237	80.1	36	12.2	256	86.5	175	59.1	165	55.7	44	14.9	204	68.9	154	52.0
Hawaii	21	9	42.9	18	85.7	12	57.1	14	66.7	3	14.3	14	66.7	6	28.6	8	38.1	2	9.5	11	52.4	9	42.9
Oregon	58	50	86.2	36	62.1	35	60.3	47	81.0	5	8.6	55	94.8	35	60.3	30	51.7	9	15.5	51	87.9	34	58.6
Washington	75	43	57.3	54	72.0	42	56.0	59	78.7	14	18.7	66	88.0	40	53.3	39	52.0	12	16.0	55	73.3	42	56.0

Table 7 (Continued)

These data include only hospital-based facilities and services as reported by responding hospitals in Section C of the 2012 AHA Annual Survey, beginning on page 215. All hospitals are represented with Community Hospitals listed separately under United States. No estimates have been made for nonresponding hospitals. Definitions of facilities and services are listed in the Glossary, page 201.

CLASSIFICATION	HOSPITALS REPORTING	PATIENT REPRESENTATIVE SERVICES Number	PATIENT REPRESENTATIVE SERVICES Percent	PHYSICAL REHABILITATION INPATIENT CARE UNITS Number	PHYSICAL REHABILITATION INPATIENT CARE UNITS Percent	PRIMARY CARE DEPARTMENT Number	PRIMARY CARE DEPARTMENT Percent	PSYCHIATRIC INPATIENT CARE UNITS Number	PSYCHIATRIC INPATIENT CARE UNITS Percent	RETIREMENT HOUSING Number	RETIREMENT HOUSING Percent	ROBOTIC SURGERY Number	ROBOTIC SURGERY Percent	RURAL HEALTH CLINIC Number	RURAL HEALTH CLINIC Percent	SLEEP CENTER Number	SLEEP CENTER Percent	SOCIAL WORK SERVICES Number	SOCIAL WORK SERVICES Percent	SPORTS MEDICINE Number	SPORTS MEDICINE Percent	SUPPORT GROUPS Number	SUPPORT GROUPS Percent
UNITED STATES	4,774	3,149	66.0	1,450	30.4	1,841	38.6	1,645	34.5	141	3.0	1,107	23.2	990	20.7	2,218	46.5	4,020	84.2	1,829	38.3	2,942	61.6
COMMUNITY HOSPITALS	4,054	2,829	69.8	1,344	33.2	1,718	42.4	1,254	30.9	138	3.4	1,072	26.4	910	22.4	2,135	52.7	3,504	86.4	1,779	43.9	2,694	66.5
CENSUS DIVISION 1, NEW ENGLAND	187	144	77.0	47	25.1	108	57.8	97	51.9	7	3.7	55	29.4	25	13.4	106	56.7	179	95.7	103	55.1	162	86.6
Connecticut	32	27	84.4	10	31.3	20	62.5	25	78.1	2	6.3	20	62.5	0	0.0	23	71.9	31	96.9	17	53.1	31	96.9
Maine	39	29	74.4	13	33.3	31	79.5	12	30.8	3	7.7	3	7.7	15	38.5	22	56.4	38	97.4	16	41.0	35	89.7
Massachusetts	68	52	76.5	11	16.2	27	39.7	41	60.3	0	0.0	22	32.4	1	1.5	35	51.5	63	92.6	40	58.8	58	85.3
New Hampshire	26	21	80.8	7	26.9	19	73.1	8	30.8	1	3.8	6	23.1	5	19.2	16	61.5	26	100.0	19	73.1	22	84.6
Rhode Island	9	6	66.7	3	33.3	5	55.6	6	66.7	0	0.0	3	33.3	0	0.0	4	44.4	9	100.0	3	33.3	8	88.9
Vermont	13	9	69.2	3	23.1	6	46.2	5	38.5	1	7.7	1	7.7	4	30.8	6	46.2	12	92.3	8	61.5	8	61.5
CENSUS DIVISION 2, MIDDLE ATLANTIC	420	320	76.2	167	39.8	234	55.7	243	57.9	8	1.9	140	33.3	34	8.1	237	56.4	393	93.6	202	48.1	328	78.1
New Jersey	72	61	84.7	22	30.6	43	59.7	43	59.7	2	2.8	32	44.4	2	2.8	45	62.5	67	93.1	25	34.7	56	77.8
New York	159	133	83.6	68	42.8	115	72.3	101	63.5	3	1.9	54	34.0	20	12.6	84	52.8	153	96.2	91	57.2	134	84.3
Pennsylvania	189	126	66.7	77	40.7	76	40.2	99	52.4	3	1.6	54	28.6	12	6.3	108	57.1	173	91.5	86	45.5	138	73.0
CENSUS DIVISION 3, SOUTH ATLANTIC	671	483	72.0	220	32.8	256	38.2	243	36.2	6	0.9	203	30.3	99	14.8	351	52.3	581	86.6	280	41.7	457	68.1
Delaware	7	5	71.4	4	57.1	3	42.9	4	57.1	0	0.0	3	42.9	1	14.3	5	71.4	6	85.7	5	42.9	5	71.4
District of Columbia	11	9	81.8	3	27.3	6	54.5	9	81.8	0	0.0	6	54.5	0	0.0	7	63.6	11	100.0	7	63.6	8	72.7
Florida	152	105	69.1	41	27.0	52	34.2	45	29.6	0	0.0	65	42.8	19	12.5	68	44.7	120	78.9	73	48.0	109	71.7
Georgia	107	72	67.3	26	24.3	34	31.8	29	27.1	4	3.7	30	28.0	19	17.8	57	53.3	87	81.3	31	29.0	60	56.1
Maryland	51	45	88.2	16	31.4	24	47.1	32	62.7	0	0.0	20	39.2	0	0.0	35	68.6	49	96.1	23	45.1	44	86.3
North Carolina	120	86	71.7	34	28.3	49	40.8	51	42.5	1	0.8	39	32.5	17	14.2	69	57.5	107	89.2	54	45.0	82	68.3
South Carolina	82	53	64.6	58	70.7	20	24.4	26	31.7	0	0.0	11	13.4	17	20.7	36	43.9	74	90.2	27	32.9	50	61.0
Virginia	80	67	83.8	27	33.8	40	50.0	30	37.5	1	1.3	21	26.3	9	11.3	45	56.3	73	91.3	40	50.0	63	78.8
West Virginia	61	41	67.2	11	18.0	28	45.9	17	27.9	0	0.0	8	13.1	17	27.9	29	47.5	54	88.5	22	36.1	36	59.0
CENSUS DIVISION 4, EAST NORTH CENTRAL	726	561	77.3	253	34.8	346	47.7	278	38.3	26	3.6	193	26.6	130	17.9	448	61.7	664	91.5	380	52.3	555	76.4
Illinois	159	126	79.2	50	31.4	74	46.5	66	41.5	8	5.0	49	30.8	41	25.8	109	68.6	148	93.1	85	53.5	135	84.9
Indiana	124	88	71.0	37	29.8	45	36.3	45	36.3	3	2.4	26	21.0	10	8.1	72	58.1	101	81.5	46	37.1	94	75.8
Michigan	135	106	78.5	47	34.8	85	63.0	56	41.5	3	2.2	43	31.9	41	30.4	89	65.9	125	92.6	82	60.7	116	85.9
Ohio	161	129	80.1	49	30.4	81	50.3	70	43.5	3	1.9	48	29.8	16	9.9	106	65.8	153	95.0	92	57.1	120	74.5
Wisconsin	147	112	76.2	70	47.6	61	41.5	41	27.9	9	6.1	27	18.4	22	15.0	72	49.0	137	93.2	75	51.0	90	61.2
CENSUS DIVISION 5, EAST SOUTH CENTRAL	398	240	60.3	132	33.2	106	26.6	151	37.9	6	1.5	85	21.4	76	19.1	176	44.2	310	77.9	113	28.4	194	48.7
Alabama	106	51	48.1	25	23.6	20	18.9	46	43.4	3	2.8	24	22.6	14	13.2	47	44.3	67	63.2	36	34.0	51	48.1
Kentucky	90	67	74.4	29	32.2	39	43.3	32	35.6	2	2.2	17	18.9	30	33.3	55	61.1	78	86.7	27	30.0	57	63.3
Mississippi	112	64	57.1	52	46.4	24	21.4	44	39.3	0	0.0	20	17.9	27	24.1	26	23.2	99	88.4	20	17.9	38	33.9
Tennessee	90	58	64.4	26	28.9	23	25.6	29	32.2	1	1.1	24	26.7	5	5.6	48	53.3	66	73.3	30	33.3	48	53.3
CENSUS DIVISION 6, WEST NORTH CENTRAL	670	374	55.8	202	30.1	272	40.6	181	27.0	60	9.0	80	11.9	262	39.1	313	46.7	543	81.0	282	42.1	394	58.8
Iowa	126	73	57.9	29	23.0	66	52.4	38	30.2	18	14.3	16	12.7	44	34.9	68	54.0	108	85.7	58	46.0	95	75.4
Kansas	151	67	44.4	29	19.2	52	34.4	26	17.2	11	7.3	10	6.6	68	45.0	39	25.8	107	70.9	45	29.8	55	36.4
Minnesota	106	59	55.7	28	26.4	46	43.4	30	28.3	12	11.3	15	14.2	27	25.5	55	51.9	92	86.8	51	48.1	75	70.8
Missouri	151	111	73.5	86	57.0	56	37.1	61	40.4	1	0.7	22	14.6	60	39.7	91	60.3	135	89.4	69	45.7	91	60.3
Nebraska	60	30	50.0	16	26.7	21	35.0	13	21.7	2	3.3	12	20.0	28	46.7	32	53.3	47	78.3	26	43.3	35	58.3
North Dakota	29	14	48.3	7	24.1	13	44.8	8	27.6	5	17.2	2	6.9	15	51.7	10	34.5	26	89.7	16	55.2	15	51.7
South Dakota	47	20	42.6	7	14.9	18	38.3	5	10.6	11	23.4	3	6.4	20	42.6	18	38.3	28	59.6	17	36.2	28	59.6
CENSUS DIVISION 7, WEST SOUTH CENTRAL	900	497	55.2	228	25.3	189	21.0	219	24.3	22	1.3	136	15.1	177	19.7	283	31.4	668	74.2	200	22.2	375	41.7
Arkansas	80	42	52.5	20	25.0	17	21.3	31	38.8	2	2.5	13	16.3	18	22.5	36	45.0	61	76.3	24	30.0	37	46.3
Louisiana	118	55	46.6	39	33.1	31	26.3	45	38.1	3	2.5	18	15.3	26	22.0	27	22.9	84	71.2	22	18.6	46	39.0
Oklahoma	129	64	49.6	30	23.3	26	20.2	34	26.4	3	2.3	16	12.4	23	17.8	58	45.0	83	64.3	30	23.3	41	31.8
Texas	573	336	58.6	139	24.3	115	20.1	109	19.0	4	0.7	89	15.5	110	19.2	162	28.3	440	76.8	124	21.6	251	43.8
CENSUS DIVISION 8, MOUNTAIN	338	221	65.4	84	24.9	150	44.4	90	26.6	10	3.0	81	24.0	101	29.9	156	46.2	278	82.2	128	37.9	186	55.0
Arizona	54	41	75.9	17	31.5	14	25.9	18	33.3	0	0.0	21	38.9	9	16.7	16	29.6	48	88.9	17	31.5	37	68.5
Colorado	68	53	77.9	19	27.9	43	63.2	13	19.1	1	1.5	25	36.8	26	38.2	50	73.5	55	80.9	35	51.5	41	60.3
Idaho	35	25	71.4	8	22.9	17	48.6	10	28.6	0	0.0	7	20.0	16	45.7	17	48.6	27	77.1	15	42.9	17	48.6
Montana	55	26	47.3	9	16.4	30	54.5	8	14.5	7	12.7	9	16.4	32	58.2	19	34.5	45	81.8	24	43.6	25	45.5
Nevada	34	16	47.1	10	29.4	6	17.6	13	38.2	1	2.9	8	23.5	3	8.8	5	14.7	27	79.4	6	17.6	15	44.1
New Mexico	30	17	56.7	7	23.3	14	46.7	7	23.3	0	0.0	4	13.3	5	16.7	10	33.3	24	80.0	3	10.0	19	60.0
Utah	35	27	77.1	11	31.4	14	40.0	14	40.0	0	0.0	6	17.1	5	14.3	22	62.9	28	80.0	18	51.4	19	54.3
Wyoming	27	16	59.3	3	11.1	12	44.4	7	25.9	1	3.7	1	3.7	5	18.5	17	63.0	24	88.9	10	37.0	14	51.9
CENSUS DIVISION 9, PACIFIC	464	309	66.6	117	25.2	180	38.8	143	30.8	6	1.3	134	28.9	86	18.5	148	31.9	404	87.1	141	30.4	291	62.7
Alaska	14	7	50.0	2	14.3	4	28.6	6	42.9	0	0.0	2	14.3	2	14.3	9	64.3	13	92.9	3	21.4	6	42.9
California	296	192	64.9	82	27.7	99	33.4	95	32.1	3	1.0	89	30.1	41	13.9	70	23.6	263	88.9	77	26.0	179	60.5
Hawaii	21	11	52.4	5	23.8	7	33.3	8	38.1	0	0.0	4	9.5	4	19.0	4	19.0	18	85.7	6	28.6	9	42.9
Oregon	58	44	75.9	9	15.5	30	51.7	17	29.3	1	1.7	16	27.6	15	25.9	28	48.3	47	81.0	24	41.4	50	86.2
Washington	75	55	73.3	19	25.3	40	53.3	17	22.7	2	2.7	25	33.3	24	32.0	37	49.3	63	84.0	31	41.3	47	62.7

Table 7 (Continued)

These data include only hospital-based facilities and services as reported by responding hospitals in Section C of the 2012 AHA Annual Survey, beginning on page 215. All hospitals are represented with Community Hospitals listed separately under United States. No estimates have been made for nonresponding hospitals. Definitions of facilities and services are listed in the Glossary, page 201.

CLASSIFICATION	HOSPITALS REPORTING	SWING BED SERVICES Number	SWING BED SERVICES Percent	TEEN OUTREACH SERVICES Number	TEEN OUTREACH SERVICES Percent	TOBACCO TREATMENT/CESSATION PROGRAM Number	TOBACCO TREATMENT/CESSATION PROGRAM Percent	TRANSPORTATION TO HEALTH FACILITIES Number	TRANSPORTATION TO HEALTH FACILITIES Percent	URGENT CARE CENTER Number	URGENT CARE CENTER Percent	VIRTUAL COLONOSCOPY Number	VIRTUAL COLONOSCOPY Percent	VOLUNTEER SERVICES DEPARTMENT Number	VOLUNTEER SERVICES DEPARTMENT Percent	WOMEN'S HEALTH SERVICES Number	WOMEN'S HEALTH SERVICES Percent	WOUND MANAGEMENT SERVICES Number	WOUND MANAGEMENT SERVICES Percent
UNITED STATES	4,774	1,491	31.2	589	12.3	2,380	49.9	1,078	22.6	1,051	22.0	763	16.0	3,453	72.3	2,292	48.0	3,110	65.1
COMMUNITY HOSPITALS	4,054	1,436	35.4	564	13.9	2,183	53.8	927	22.9	990	24.4	736	18.2	3,214	79.3	2,186	53.9	2,851	70.3
CENSUS DIVISION 1, NEW ENGLAND	187	44	23.5	53	28.3	132	70.6	57	30.5	67	35.8	44	23.5	171	91.4	134	71.7	139	74.3
Connecticut	32	4	12.5	13	40.6	25	78.1	7	21.9	17	53.1	16	50.0	29	90.6	22	68.8	27	84.4
Maine	39	12	30.8	7	17.9	30	76.9	10	25.6	14	35.9	7	17.9	36	92.3	30	76.9	28	71.8
Massachusetts	68	5	7.4	21	30.9	40	58.8	27	39.7	24	35.3	14	20.6	61	89.7	45	66.2	52	76.5
New Hampshire	26	15	57.7	9	34.6	20	76.9	5	19.2	8	30.8	4	15.4	25	96.2	23	88.5	17	65.4
Rhode Island	9	1	11.1	2	22.2	6	66.7	4	44.4	2	22.2	1	11.1	8	88.9	6	66.7	6	66.7
Vermont	13	7	53.8	1	7.7	11	84.6	4	30.8	2	15.4	2	15.4	12	92.3	8	61.5	9	69.2
CENSUS DIVISION 2, MIDDLE ATLANTIC	420	68	16.2	106	25.2	282	67.1	139	33.1	109	26.0	96	22.9	372	88.6	284	67.6	309	73.6
New Jersey	72	7	9.7	26	36.1	44	61.1	40	55.6	22	30.6	17	23.6	62	86.1	52	72.2	62	86.1
New York	159	26	16.4	40	25.2	123	77.4	50	31.4	48	30.2	48	30.2	150	94.3	122	76.7	116	73.0
Pennsylvania	189	35	18.5	40	21.2	115	60.8	49	25.9	39	20.6	31	16.4	160	84.7	110	58.2	131	69.3
CENSUS DIVISION 3, SOUTH ATLANTIC	671	127	18.9	88	13.1	374	55.7	148	22.1	144	21.5	133	19.8	557	83.0	361	53.8	469	69.9
Delaware	7	0	0.0	4	57.1	4	57.1	3	42.9	2	28.6	1	14.3	5	71.4	4	57.1	5	71.4
District of Columbia	11	1	9.1	4	36.4	5	45.5	3	27.3	2	18.2	3	27.3	11	100.0	7	63.6	10	90.9
Florida	152	18	11.8	17	11.2	84	55.3	35	23.0	36	23.7	28	18.4	125	82.2	83	54.6	116	76.3
Georgia	107	27	25.2	11	10.3	47	43.9	21	19.6	20	18.7	13	12.1	80	74.8	53	49.5	70	65.4
Maryland	51	2	3.9	15	29.4	33	64.7	15	29.4	15	29.4	13	25.5	47	92.2	29	56.9	37	72.5
North Carolina	120	25	20.8	12	10.0	76	63.3	31	25.8	29	24.2	30	25.0	105	87.5	62	51.7	80	66.7
South Carolina	82	11	13.4	9	11.0	41	50.0	13	15.9	9	11.0	11	13.4	63	76.8	45	54.9	53	64.6
Virginia	80	19	23.8	10	12.5	48	60.0	16	20.0	19	23.8	23	28.8	72	90.0	45	56.3	61	76.3
West Virginia	61	24	39.3	6	9.8	36	59.0	11	18.0	12	19.7	11	18.0	49	80.3	33	54.1	37	60.7
CENSUS DIVISION 4, EAST NORTH CENTRAL	726	198	27.3	115	15.8	453	62.4	190	26.2	282	38.8	149	20.5	600	82.6	406	55.9	499	68.7
Illinois	159	47	29.6	30	18.9	88	55.3	47	29.6	52	32.7	44	27.7	138	86.8	92	57.9	111	69.8
Indiana	124	34	27.4	20	16.1	82	66.1	24	19.4	37	29.8	22	17.7	95	76.6	63	50.8	80	64.5
Michigan	135	22	16.3	23	17.0	96	71.1	38	28.1	51	37.8	26	19.3	120	88.9	83	61.5	101	74.8
Ohio	161	41	25.5	28	17.4	116	72.0	50	31.1	55	34.2	34	21.1	144	89.4	99	61.5	113	70.2
Wisconsin	147	54	36.7	14	9.5	71	48.3	31	21.1	87	59.2	23	15.6	103	70.1	69	46.9	94	63.9
CENSUS DIVISION 5, EAST SOUTH CENTRAL	398	142	35.7	33	8.3	158	39.7	61	15.3	54	13.6	41	10.3	229	57.5	150	37.7	198	49.7
Alabama	106	24	22.6	8	7.5	41	38.7	16	15.1	14	13.2	7	6.6	70	66.0	40	37.7	54	50.9
Kentucky	90	35	38.9	7	7.8	47	52.2	12	13.3	17	18.9	13	14.4	75	83.3	49	54.4	56	62.2
Mississippi	112	55	49.1	9	8.0	32	28.6	19	17.0	12	10.7	10	8.9	17	15.2	29	25.9	34	30.4
Tennessee	90	28	31.1	9	10.0	38	42.2	14	15.6	11	12.2	11	12.2	67	74.4	32	35.6	54	60.0
CENSUS DIVISION 6, WEST NORTH CENTRAL	670	407	60.7	58	8.7	316	47.2	162	24.2	118	17.6	83	12.4	430	64.2	244	36.4	410	61.2
Iowa	126	90	71.4	16	12.7	82	65.1	24	19.0	22	17.5	14	11.1	96	76.2	49	38.9	86	68.3
Kansas	151	100	66.2	6	4.0	47	31.1	32	21.2	16	10.6	18	11.9	74	49.0	41	27.2	84	55.6
Minnesota	106	63	59.4	12	11.3	55	51.9	21	19.8	37	34.9	17	16.0	78	73.6	44	41.5	69	65.1
Missouri	151	53	35.1	15	9.9	76	50.3	53	35.1	33	21.9	17	11.3	107	70.9	69	45.7	99	65.6
Nebraska	60	39	65.0	6	10.0	28	46.7	16	26.7	3	5.0	12	20.0	34	56.7	21	35.0	34	56.7
North Dakota	29	22	75.9	1	3.4	14	48.3	8	27.6	4	13.8	3	10.3	17	58.6	10	34.5	11	37.9
South Dakota	47	40	85.1	2	4.3	14	29.8	8	17.0	3	6.4	2	4.3	24	51.1	10	21.3	27	57.4
CENSUS DIVISION 7, WEST SOUTH CENTRAL	900	247	27.4	44	4.9	281	31.2	127	14.1	86	9.6	83	9.2	478	53.1	290	32.2	540	60.0
Arkansas	80	32	40.0	4	5.0	29	36.3	15	18.8	10	12.5	5	6.3	50	62.5	26	32.5	44	55.0
Louisiana	118	31	26.3	8	6.8	45	38.1	20	16.9	12	10.2	5	4.2	55	46.6	39	33.1	63	53.4
Oklahoma	129	56	43.4	4	3.1	48	37.2	24	18.6	16	12.4	13	10.1	83	64.3	43	33.3	71	55.0
Texas	573	128	22.3	28	4.9	159	27.7	68	11.9	48	8.4	60	10.5	290	50.6	182	31.8	362	63.2
CENSUS DIVISION 8, MOUNTAIN	338	150	44.4	36	10.7	173	51.2	72	21.3	82	24.3	54	16.0	243	71.9	176	52.1	215	63.6
Arizona	54	12	22.2	7	13.0	35	64.8	10	18.5	11	20.4	14	25.9	43	79.6	30	55.6	39	72.2
Colorado	68	28	41.2	9	13.2	34	50.0	9	13.2	14	20.6	9	13.2	55	80.9	46	67.6	55	80.9
Idaho	35	18	51.4	6	17.1	19	54.3	10	28.6	10	28.6	5	14.3	27	77.1	16	45.7	18	51.4
Montana	55	45	81.8	4	7.3	25	45.5	24	43.6	18	32.7	13	23.6	37	67.3	20	36.4	28	50.9
Nevada	34	5	14.7	0	0.0	13	38.2	6	17.6	5	14.7	1	2.9	17	50.0	14	41.2	20	58.8
New Mexico	30	9	30.0	2	6.7	15	50.0	3	10.0	8	26.7	2	6.7	19	63.3	14	46.7	18	60.0
Utah	35	12	34.3	6	17.1	16	45.7	4	11.4	7	20.0	4	11.4	27	77.1	23	65.7	24	68.6
Wyoming	27	21	77.8	2	7.4	16	59.3	6	22.2	9	33.3	6	22.2	18	66.7	13	48.1	13	48.1
CENSUS DIVISION 9, PACIFIC	464	108	23.3	56	12.1	211	45.5	122	26.3	109	23.5	80	17.2	373	80.4	247	53.2	331	71.3
Alaska	14	8	57.1	2	14.3	6	42.9	1	7.1	2	14.3	2	14.3	7	50.0	4	28.6	9	64.3
California	296	39	13.2	35	11.8	114	38.5	86	29.1	64	21.6	53	17.9	239	80.7	148	50.0	207	69.9
Hawaii	21	7	33.3	2	9.5	10	47.6	4	19.0	3	14.3	2	9.5	17	81.0	10	47.6	14	66.7
Oregon	58	28	48.3	5	8.6	41	70.7	17	29.3	19	32.8	12	20.7	51	87.9	40	69.0	50	86.2
Washington	75	26	34.7	12	16.0	40	53.3	14	18.7	21	28.0	11	14.7	59	78.7	45	60.0	51	68.0

Table 7 (Continued)

These data include only hospital-based facilities and services as reported by responding hospitals in Section C of the 2012 AHA Annual Survey, beginning on page 215. All hospitals are represented with Community Hospitals listed separately under United States. No estimates have been made for nonresponding hospitals. Definitions of facilities and services are listed in the Glossary, page 201.

Column groups: **GENERAL MEDICAL SURGICAL CARE** (Adult Units, Pediatric Units) · **INTENSIVE CARE UNITS** (Cardiac Units, Medical Surgical Units, Neonatal Units, Other Units, Pediatric Units) · **ACUTE LONG-TERM CARE UNITS** · **LONG-TERM CARE UNITS** (Skilled Nursing Care Units, Intermediate Nursing Care Units, Other Long-Term Care Units)

Classification	Hosp. Reporting	Adult No.	Adult %	Ped. No.	Ped. %	Cardiac No.	Cardiac %	Med/Surg No.	Med/Surg %	Neonatal No.	Neonatal %	Other No.	Other %	ICU Ped. No.	ICU Ped. %	Acute LT No.	Acute LT %	Skilled No.	Skilled %	Intermed. No.	Intermed. %	Other LT No.	Other LT %
UNITED STATES	4,774	4,000	83.8	1,996	41.8	1,324	27.7	2,961	62.0	962	20.2	549	11.5	434	9.1	386	8.1	1,139	23.9	393	8.2	266	5.6
COMMUNITY HOSPITALS	4,054	3,743	92.3	1,956	48.2	1,277	31.5	2,837	70.0	946	23.3	528	13.0	422	10.4	248	6.1	1,039	25.6	360	8.9	224	5.5
CENSUS DIVISION 1, NEW ENGLAND	187	155	82.9	102	54.5	52	27.8	143	76.5	30	16.0	16	8.6	16	8.6	8	4.3	31	16.6	19	10.2	8	4.3
Connecticut	32	25	78.1	17	53.1	12	37.5	25	78.1	11	34.4	3	9.4	2	6.3	1	3.1	4	12.5	1	3.1	0	0.0
Maine	39	35	89.7	22	56.4	6	15.4	32	82.1	3	7.7	5	12.8	3	7.7	1	2.6	12	30.8	8	20.5	0	0.0
Massachusetts	68	52	76.5	41	60.3	22	32.4	48	70.6	12	17.6	5	7.4	7	10.3	4	5.9	4	5.9	2	2.9	3	4.4
New Hampshire	26	23	88.5	15	57.7	6	23.1	21	80.8	1	7.7	2	7.7	1	3.8	1	3.8	8	30.8	7	26.9	0	0.0
Rhode Island	9	8	88.9	4	44.4	4	44.4	6	66.7	1	11.1	1	11.1	1	11.1	1	11.1	0	0.0	1	11.1	1	11.1
Vermont	13	12	92.3	3	23.1	2	15.4	11	84.6			1	7.7	1	7.7	0	0.0	3	23.1	0	0.0	0	0.0
CENSUS DIVISION 2, MIDDLE ATLANTIC	420	354	84.3	206	49.0	176	41.9	316	75.2	121	28.8	55	13.1	53	12.6	23	5.5	109	26.0	16	3.8	23	5.5
New Jersey	72	58	80.6	41	56.9	33	45.8	57	79.2	22	30.6	9	12.5	15	20.8	5	6.9	14	19.4	7	9.7	6	8.3
New York	159	149	93.7	94	59.1	84	52.8	135	84.9	54	34.0	23	14.5	28	17.6	9	5.7	50	31.4	5	3.1	13	8.2
Pennsylvania	189	147	77.8	71	37.6	59	31.2	124	65.6	45	23.8	23	12.2	10	5.3	9	4.8	45	23.8	4	2.1	4	2.1
CENSUS DIVISION 3, SOUTH ATLANTIC	671	562	83.8	285	42.5	223	33.2	480	71.5	148	22.1	103	15.4	71	10.6	76	11.3	171	25.5	67	10.0	56	8.3
Delaware	7	4	57.1	5	71.4	5	71.4	4	57.1	3	42.9	1	14.3	0	0.0	0	0.0	0	0.0	2	28.6	3	42.9
District of Columbia	11	7	63.6	3	27.3	6	54.5	7	63.6	6	54.5	1	9.1	2	18.2	0	0.0	2	18.2	0	0.0	0	0.0
Florida	152	133	87.5	54	35.5	67	44.1	121	79.6	44	28.9	26	17.1	27	17.8	14	9.2	21	13.8	14	9.2	7	4.6
Georgia	107	87	81.3	32	29.9	28	26.2	63	58.9	22	20.6	12	11.2	5	4.7	11	10.3	29	27.1	7	6.5	5	4.7
Maryland	51	43	84.3	30	58.8	20	39.2	43	84.3	14	27.5	5	9.8	5	9.8	4	7.8	13	25.5	2	3.9	3	5.9
North Carolina	120	104	86.7	53	44.2	32	26.7	88	73.3	26	21.7	15	12.5	13	10.8	10	8.3	33	27.5	14	11.7	2	1.7
South Carolina	82	65	79.3	49	59.8	25	30.5	56	68.3	10	12.2	32	39.0	6	7.3	28	34.1	33	40.2	11	13.4	29	35.4
Virginia	80	68	85.0	32	40.0	23	28.8	64	80.0	19	23.8	8	10.0	7	8.8	4	5.0	17	21.3	9	11.3	4	5.0
West Virginia	61	51	83.6	27	44.3	17	27.9	34	55.7	4	6.6	4	6.6	3	4.9	5	8.2	23	37.7	8	13.1	4	4.9
CENSUS DIVISION 4, EAST NORTH CENTRAL	726	622	85.7	371	51.1	223	30.7	482	66.4	128	17.6	124	17.1	72	9.9	46	6.3	143	19.7	39	5.4	38	5.2
Illinois	159	145	91.2	96	60.4	41	25.8	115	72.3	28	17.6	14	8.8	20	12.6	8	5.0	43	27.0	8	5.0	10	6.3
Indiana	124	94	75.8	56	45.2	24	19.4	72	58.1	21	16.9	7	5.6	8	6.5	9	7.3	18	14.5	11	8.9	2	1.6
Michigan	135	118	87.4	63	46.7	45	33.3	94	69.6	21	15.6	15	11.1	9	6.7	6	4.4	30	22.2	4	3.0	7	5.2
Ohio	161	139	86.3	59	36.6	51	31.7	126	78.3	29	18.0	17	10.6	11	6.8	10	6.2	30	18.6	11	6.8	11	6.8
Wisconsin	147	126	85.7	97	66.0	62	42.2	75	51.0	29	19.7	71	48.3	24	16.3	13	8.8	22	15.0	6	4.1	8	5.4
CENSUS DIVISION 5, EAST SOUTH CENTRAL	398	346	86.9	176	44.2	118	29.6	285	71.6	66	16.6	90	22.6	35	8.8	30	7.5	91	22.9	26	6.5	34	8.5
Alabama	106	87	82.1	34	32.1	30	28.3	65	61.3	17	16.0	17	16.0	7	6.6	12	11.3	14	13.2	8	7.5	4	3.8
Kentucky	90	77	85.6	42	46.7	28	31.1	64	71.1	20	22.2	16	17.8	9	10.0	12	13.3	32	35.6	9	10.0	9	10.0
Mississippi	112	107	95.5	73	65.2	39	34.8	104	92.9	15	13.4	46	41.1	12	10.7	0	0.0	24	21.4	0	0.0	18	16.1
Tennessee	90	75	83.3	27	30.0	21	23.3	52	57.8	14	15.6	11	12.2	7	7.8	6	6.7	21	23.3	9	10.0	3	3.3
CENSUS DIVISION 6, WEST NORTH CENTRAL	670	604	90.1	288	43.0	142	21.2	316	47.2	89	13.3	49	7.3	50	7.5	41	6.1	279	41.6	124	18.5	59	8.8
Iowa	126	119	94.4	60	47.6	21	16.7	67	53.2	19	15.1	9	7.1	11	8.7	7	5.6	56	44.4	40	31.7	15	11.9
Kansas	151	134	88.7	44	29.1	15	9.9	51	33.8	16	10.6	7	4.6	9	6.0	9	6.0	65	43.0	41	27.2	16	10.6
Minnesota	106	102	96.2	55	51.9	28	26.4	59	55.7	10	9.4	7	6.6	9	8.5	4	3.8	45	42.5	9	8.5	9	8.5
Missouri	151	120	79.5	79	52.3	43	28.5	83	55.0	20	13.2	17	11.3	8	5.3	15	9.9	40	26.5	14	9.3	9	6.0
Nebraska	60	56	93.3	20	33.3	16	26.7	23	38.3	15	25.0	3	5.0	5	8.3	2	3.3	32	53.3	7	11.7	6	10.0
North Dakota	29	27	93.1	11	37.9	8	27.6	13	44.8	6	20.7	2	6.9	5	17.2	3	10.3	13	44.8	3	10.3	2	6.9
South Dakota	47	46	97.9	19	40.4	11	23.4	20	42.6	3	6.4	4	8.5	3	6.4	1	2.1	28	59.6	10	21.3	8	17.0
CENSUS DIVISION 7, WEST SOUTH CENTRAL	900	649	72.1	255	28.3	148	16.4	403	44.8	155	17.2	49	5.4	55	6.1	119	13.2	102	11.3	24	2.7	17	1.9
Arkansas	80	62	77.5	21	26.3	24	30.0	37	46.3	12	15.0	4	5.0	2	2.5	9	11.3	14	17.5	3	3.8	1	1.3
Louisiana	118	83	70.3	47	39.8	21	17.8	59	50.0	26	22.0	7	5.9	14	11.9	17	14.4	21	17.8	4	3.4	3	2.5
Oklahoma	129	106	82.2	38	29.5	20	15.5	50	38.8	9	7.0	7	5.4	4	3.1	12	9.3	27	20.9	5	3.9	5	3.9
Texas	573	398	69.5	149	26.0	83	14.5	257	44.9	108	18.8	31	5.4	35	6.1	81	14.1	40	7.0	12	2.1	8	1.4
CENSUS DIVISION 8, MOUNTAIN	338	297	87.9	130	38.5	67	19.8	195	57.7	74	21.9	20	5.9	28	8.3	17	5.0	92	27.2	36	10.7	15	4.4
Arizona	54	44	81.5	15	27.8	18	33.3	36	66.7	12	22.2	2	3.7	6	11.1	2	3.7	6	11.1	1	1.9	1	1.9
Colorado	68	65	95.6	29	42.6	13	19.1	49	72.1	25	36.8	5	7.4	3	4.4	2	2.9	12	17.6	7	10.3	3	4.4
Idaho	35	32	91.4	14	40.0	6	17.1	17	48.6	7	20.0	3	8.6	2	5.7	2	5.7	11	31.4	4	11.4	1	2.9
Montana	55	53	96.4	20	36.4	10	18.2	21	38.2	6	10.9	3	5.5	4	7.3	5	9.1	33	60.0	11	20.0	4	7.3
Nevada	34	20	58.8	7	20.6	6	17.6	16	47.1	6	17.6	3	8.8	4	11.8	3	8.8	1	2.9	1	2.9	0	0.0
New Mexico	35	28	80.0	17	48.6	4	11.4	21	60.0	6	17.6	2	5.7	4	11.8	0	0.0	2	5.7	1	2.9	0	0.0
Utah	35	30	85.7	20	57.1	10	28.6	18	51.4	12	34.3	2	5.7	4	11.4	1	2.9	13	37.1	6	17.1	2	5.7
Wyoming	27	25	92.6	8	29.6	0	0.0	16	59.3	0	0.0	1	3.7	1	3.7	2	7.4	12	44.4	4	14.8	4	14.8
CENSUS DIVISION 9, PACIFIC	464	411	88.6	183	39.4	175	37.7	341	73.5	151	32.5	43	9.3	54	11.6	26	5.6	121	26.1	42	9.1	16	3.4
Alaska	14	12	85.7	3	21.4	3	21.4	7	50.0	1	7.1	3	21.4	1	7.1	0	0.0	7	50.0	5	35.7	1	7.1
California	296	259	87.5	118	39.9	130	43.9	228	77.0	122	41.2	27	9.1	42	14.2	22	7.4	85	28.7	16	5.4	12	4.1
Hawaii	21	16	76.2	4	19.0	7	33.3	12	57.1	3	14.3	2	9.5	2	9.5	3	14.3	10	47.6	9	42.9	2	9.5
Oregon	58	57	98.3	24	41.4	16	27.6	48	82.8	9	15.5	2	3.4	2	3.4	0	0.0	8	13.8	9	15.5	0	0.0
Washington	75	67	89.3	34	45.3	19	25.3	46	61.3	16	21.3	9	12.0	7	9.3	1	1.3	11	14.7	3	4.0	1	1.3

Table 7 (Continued)

These data include only hospital-based facilities and services as reported by responding hospitals in Section C of the 2012 AHA Annual Survey, beginning on page 215. All hospitals are represented with Community Hospitals listed separately under United States. No estimates have been made for nonresponding hospitals. Definitions of facilities and services are listed in the Glossary, page 201.

CARDIOLOGY AND CARDIAC SERVICES

CLASSIFICATION	HOSPITALS REPORTING	ADULT CARDIOLOGY SERVICES		PEDIATRIC CARDIOLOGY SERVICES		ADULT DIAGNOSTIC CATHETERIZATION		PEDIATRIC DIAGNOSTIC CATHETERIZATION		ADULT INTERVENTIONAL CARDIAC CATHETERIZATION		PEDIATRIC INTERVENTIONAL CARDIAC CATHETERIZATION		ADULT CARDIAC SURGERY		PEDIATRIC CARDIAC SURGERY		ADULT CARDIAC ELECTRO-PHYSIOLOGY		PEDIATRIC CARDIAC ELECTRO-PHYSIOLOGY		CARDIAC REHABILITATION	
		Number	Percent	Number	Percent	Number	Percent	Number	Percent	Number	Percent	Number	Percent	Number	Percent	Number	Percent	Number	Percent	Number	Percent	Number	Percent
UNITED STATES	4,774	2,297	48.1	406	8.5	1,790	37.5	204	4.3	1,528	32.0	188	3.9	1,117	23.4	184	3.9	1,309	27.4	208	4.4	2,479	51.9
COMMUNITY HOSPITALS	4,054	2,196	54.2	401	9.9	1,718	42.4	200	4.9	1,469	36.2	187	4.6	1,073	26.5	183	4.5	1,259	31.1	205	5.1	2,409	59.4
CENSUS DIVISION 1, NEW ENGLAND	187	117	62.6	17	9.1	73	39.0	10	5.3	55	29.4	10	5.3	41	21.9	9	4.8	59	31.6	9	4.8	129	69.0
Connecticut	32	24	75.0	3	9.4	16	50.0	2	6.3	15	46.9	2	6.3	13	40.6	2	6.3	13	40.6	2	6.3	22	68.8
Maine	39	19	48.7	4	10.3	11	28.2	1	2.6	6	15.4	1	2.6	4	10.3	1	2.6	8	20.5	2	5.1	29	74.4
Massachusetts	68	47	69.1	6	8.8	30	44.1	3	4.4	22	32.4	3	4.4	18	26.5	4	5.9	25	36.8	3	4.4	44	64.7
New Hampshire	26	15	57.7	2	7.7	8	30.8	2	7.7	6	23.1	1	3.8	3	11.5	1	3.8	7	26.9	1	3.8	19	73.1
Rhode Island	9	4	44.4	1	11.1	5	55.6	1	11.1	4	44.4	1	11.1	1	11.1	0	0.0	3	33.3	0	0.0	6	66.7
Vermont	13	8	61.5	1	7.7	3	23.1	1	7.7	2	15.4	2	15.4	2	15.4	1	7.7	3	23.1	0	0.0	9	69.2
CENSUS DIVISION 2, MIDDLE ATLANTIC	420	288	68.6	79	18.8	204	48.6	23	5.5	165	39.3	22	5.2	116	27.6	21	5.0	150	35.7	30	7.1	241	57.4
New Jersey	72	52	72.2	22	30.6	49	68.1	3	4.2	39	54.2	2	2.8	17	23.6	2	2.8	26	36.1	7	9.7	42	58.3
New York	159	121	76.1	36	22.6	68	42.8	14	8.8	53	33.3	14	8.8	36	22.6	11	6.9	59	37.1	16	10.1	89	56.0
Pennsylvania	189	115	60.8	21	11.1	87	46.0	6	3.2	73	38.6	6	3.2	63	33.3	8	4.2	65	34.4	7	3.7	110	58.2
CENSUS DIVISION 3, SOUTH ATLANTIC	671	390	58.1	60	8.9	325	48.4	28	4.2	255	38.0	26	3.9	162	24.1	27	4.0	231	34.4	28	4.2	362	53.9
Delaware	7	4	57.1	1	14.3	4	57.1	1	14.3	4	57.1	1	14.3	3	42.9	1	14.3	2	28.6	1	14.3	5	71.4
District of Columbia	11	7	63.6	2	18.2	5	45.5	1	9.1	4	36.4	1	9.1	3	27.3	1	9.1	2	18.2	1	9.1	5	45.5
Florida	152	108	71.1	17	11.2	91	59.9	11	7.2	80	52.6	10	6.6	57	37.5	11	7.2	71	46.7	9	5.9	72	47.4
Georgia	107	51	47.7	3	2.8	46	43.0	1	0.9	40	37.4	1	0.9	19	17.8	1	0.9	32	29.9	1	0.9	45	42.1
Maryland	51	39	76.5	6	11.8	35	68.6	2	3.9	24	47.1	2	3.9	10	19.6	2	3.9	29	56.9	3	5.9	33	64.7
North Carolina	120	70	58.3	13	10.8	54	45.0	5	4.2	37	30.8	5	4.2	26	21.7	5	4.2	38	31.7	7	5.8	76	63.3
South Carolina	82	35	42.7	5	6.1	31	37.8	1	1.2	18	22.0	1	1.2	19	23.2	1	1.2	15	18.3	1	1.2	41	50.0
Virginia	80	50	62.5	10	12.5	37	46.3	4	5.0	35	43.8	4	5.0	19	23.8	4	5.0	31	38.8	4	5.0	55	68.8
West Virginia	61	26	42.6	3	4.9	22	36.1	2	3.3	13	21.3	1	1.6	6	9.8	1	1.6	8	13.1	1	1.6	30	49.2
CENSUS DIVISION 4, EAST NORTH CENTRAL	726	406	55.9	69	9.5	321	44.2	27	3.7	279	38.4	26	3.6	212	29.2	30	4.1	254	35.0	32	4.4	504	69.4
Illinois	159	106	66.7	28	17.6	84	52.8	8	5.0	80	50.3	9	5.7	57	35.8	10	6.3	67	42.1	12	7.5	125	78.6
Indiana	124	58	46.8	9	7.3	46	37.1	4	3.2	42	33.9	3	2.4	32	25.8	4	3.2	34	27.4	4	3.2	75	60.5
Michigan	135	74	54.8	12	8.9	60	44.4	3	2.2	48	35.6	3	2.2	36	26.7	4	3.0	53	39.3	5	3.7	88	65.2
Ohio	161	109	67.7	12	7.5	82	50.9	8	5.0	63	39.1	7	4.3	54	33.5	7	4.3	59	36.6	7	4.3	105	65.2
Wisconsin	147	59	40.1	8	5.4	49	33.3	4	2.7	46	31.3	4	2.7	33	22.4	5	3.4	41	27.9	4	2.7	111	75.5
CENSUS DIVISION 5, EAST SOUTH CENTRAL	398	162	40.7	24	6.0	131	32.9	17	4.3	104	26.1	13	3.3	81	20.4	14	3.5	80	20.1	15	3.8	158	39.7
Alabama	106	40	37.7	4	3.8	38	35.8	5	4.7	33	31.1	3	2.8	25	23.6	3	2.8	27	25.5	3	2.8	37	34.9
Kentucky	90	49	54.4	5	5.6	37	41.1	2	2.2	28	31.1	2	2.2	21	23.3	3	3.3	17	18.9	3	3.3	53	58.9
Mississippi	90	28	31.1	4	4.4	19	21.1	1	1.1	15	16.7	1	1.1	14	15.6	1	1.1	12	13.4	3	3.3	23	20.5
Tennessee	112	45	40.2	11	9.8	37	33.3	9	8.0	28	25.0	7	6.3	21	18.8	7	6.3	24	26.7	6	6.7	45	50.0
CENSUS DIVISION 6, WEST NORTH CENTRAL	670	224	33.4	36	5.4	150	22.4	15	2.2	143	21.3	15	2.2	92	13.7	15	2.2	109	16.3	19	2.8	469	70.0
Iowa	126	43	34.1	4	3.2	27	21.4	2	1.6	27	21.4	2	1.6	13	10.3	1	0.7	22	17.5	3	2.4	108	85.7
Kansas	151	35	23.2	7	4.6	24	15.9	2	1.3	23	15.2	2	1.3	16	10.6	1	0.7	14	9.3	3	2.0	72	47.7
Minnesota	106	36	34.0	8	7.5	19	17.9	2	1.9	18	17.0	2	1.9	14	13.2	3	2.8	18	17.0	5	4.7	92	86.8
Missouri	151	73	48.3	8	5.3	55	36.4	4	2.6	52	34.4	4	2.6	35	23.2	6	4.0	39	25.8	5	3.3	91	60.3
Nebraska	60	21	35.0	4	6.7	13	21.7	1	1.7	13	21.7	1	1.7	6	10.0	1	1.7	10	16.7	1	1.7	45	75.0
North Dakota	29	6	20.7	2	6.9	4	13.8	2	6.9	4	13.8	2	6.9	4	13.8	2	6.9	3	10.3	1	3.4	19	65.5
South Dakota	47	10	21.3	3	6.4	8	17.0	2	4.3	6	12.8	2	4.3	4	8.5	1	2.1	3	6.4	1	2.1	42	89.4
CENSUS DIVISION 7, WEST SOUTH CENTRAL	900	317	35.2	38	4.2	266	29.6	28	3.1	239	26.6	26	2.9	192	21.3	22	2.4	183	20.3	23	2.6	276	30.7
Arkansas	80	31	38.8	3	3.8	23	28.8	1	1.3	22	27.5	2	2.5	17	21.3	1	1.3	13	16.3	2	2.5	32	40.0
Louisiana	118	47	39.8	11	9.3	41	34.7	7	5.9	37	31.4	7	5.9	27	22.9	4	3.4	30	25.4	6	5.1	33	28.0
Oklahoma	129	45	34.9	3	2.3	31	24.0	2	1.6	26	20.2	2	1.6	19	14.7	2	1.6	15	11.6	2	1.6	34	26.4
Texas	573	194	33.9	22	3.8	171	29.8	18	3.1	154	26.9	16	2.8	129	22.5	15	2.6	125	21.8	13	2.3	177	30.9
CENSUS DIVISION 8, MOUNTAIN	338	137	40.5	26	7.7	113	33.4	18	5.3	107	31.7	18	5.3	70	20.7	15	4.4	79	23.4	18	5.3	162	47.9
Arizona	54	30	55.6	4	7.4	26	48.1	3	3.7	27	50.0	3	3.7	18	33.3	3	5.6	21	38.9	3	5.6	27	50.0
Colorado	68	36	52.9	7	10.3	34	50.0	3	4.4	33	48.5	3	4.4	19	27.9	3	4.4	21	30.9	3	4.4	44	64.7
Idaho	35	14	40.0	3	8.6	11	31.4	2	5.7	9	25.7	2	5.7	5	14.3	1	2.9	5	14.3	1	2.9	11	31.4
Montana	55	10	18.2	2	3.6	8	14.5	1	1.8	8	14.5	1	1.8	5	9.1	1	1.8	6	10.9	1	1.8	28	50.9
Nevada	34	14	41.2	4	11.8	13	38.2	4	11.8	12	35.3	4	11.8	9	26.5	2	5.9	11	32.4	4	11.8	11	32.4
New Mexico	30	11	36.7	3	10.0	8	26.7	3	10.0	6	20.0	2	6.7	5	16.7	2	6.7	7	23.3	2	6.7	11	36.7
Utah	35	17	48.6	3	8.6	11	31.4	3	8.6	11	31.4	3	8.6	7	20.0	3	8.6	6	17.1	3	8.6	15	42.9
Wyoming	27	5	18.5	0	0.0	2	7.4	0	0.0	2	7.4	0	0.0	2	7.4	0	0.0	0	7.4	0	0.0	15	55.6
CENSUS DIVISION 9, PACIFIC	464	256	55.2	57	12.3	207	44.6	38	8.2	181	39.0	32	6.9	151	32.5	31	6.7	164	35.3	34	7.3	178	38.4
Alaska	14	5	35.7	3	21.4	3	21.4	1	7.1	3	21.4	2	14.3	1	7.1	1	7.1	1	7.1	1	7.1	5	35.7
California	296	177	59.8	38	12.8	144	48.6	23	7.8	124	41.9	21	7.1	110	37.2	21	7.1	115	38.9	22	7.4	111	37.5
Hawaii	21	10	47.6	1	4.8	7	33.3	2	9.5	6	28.6	1	4.8	6	28.6	0	0.0	7	33.3	1	4.8	4	19.0
Oregon	58	26	44.8	8	13.8	23	39.7	7	12.1	20	34.5	5	8.6	16	27.6	5	8.6	17	29.3	5	8.6	27	46.6
Washington	75	38	50.7	7	9.3	30	40.0	5	6.7	28	37.3	4	5.3	18	24.0	5	6.7	23	30.7	5	6.7	31	41.3

Table 7 (Continued)

These data include only hospital-based facilities and services as reported by responding hospitals in Section C of the 2012 AHA Annual Survey, beginning on page 215. All hospitals are represented with Community Hospitals listed separately under United States. No estimates have been made for nonresponding hospitals. Definitions of facilities and services are listed in the Glossary, page 201.

CLASSIFICATION	HOSPITALS REPORTING	EMERGENCY SERVICES								ENDOSCOPIC ULTRASOUND		ENDOSCOPIC SERVICES							
		EMERGENCY DEPARTMENT		PEDIATRIC EMERGENCY DEPARTMENT		FREESTANDING/ SATELLITE EMERGENCY DEPARTMENT		TRAUMA CENTER (CERTIFIED)				ABLATION OF BARRETT'S ESOPHAGUS		ESOPHAGEAL IMPEDANCE STUDY		ENDOSCOPIC RETROGRADE CHOLANGIO-PANCREATOGRAPHY		OPTICAL COLONOSCOPY	
		Number	Percent	Number	Percent	Number	Percent	Number	Percent	Number	Percent	Number	Percent	Number	Percent	Number	Percent	Number	Percent
UNITED STATES	4,774	3,930	82.3	636	13.3	323	6.8	1,674	35.1	1,518	31.8	1,067	22.4	1,011	21.2	1,929	40.4	2,872	60.2
COMMUNITY HOSPITALS	4,054	3,710	91.5	615	15.2	303	7.5	1,643	40.5	1,456	35.9	1,023	25.2	973	24.0	1,867	46.1	2,730	67.3
CENSUS DIVISION 1, NEW ENGLAND	187	152	81.3	36	19.3	18	9.6	58	31.0	72	38.5	53	28.3	54	28.9	99	52.9	132	70.6
Connecticut	32	25	78.1	6	18.8	5	15.6	10	31.3	17	53.1	16	50.0	16	50.0	24	75.0	24	75.0
Maine	39	35	89.7	6	15.4	5	12.8	13	33.3	11	28.2	7	17.9	10	25.6	9	23.1	30	76.9
Massachusetts	68	49	72.1	14	20.6	2	2.9	16	23.5	26	38.2	17	25.0	18	26.5	39	57.4	42	61.8
New Hampshire	26	23	88.5	8	30.8	6	23.1	14	53.8	11	42.3	9	34.6	6	23.1	14	53.8	19	73.1
Rhode Island	9	8	88.9	2	22.2	0	0.0	1	11.1	4	44.4	2	22.2	2	22.2	6	66.7	7	77.8
Vermont	13	12	92.3	1	7.7	0	0.0	4	30.8	3	23.1	2	15.4	2	15.4	7	53.8	10	76.9
CENSUS DIVISION 2, MIDDLE ATLANTIC	420	341	81.2	88	21.0	30	7.1	113	26.9	193	46.0	120	28.6	108	25.7	258	61.4	272	64.8
New Jersey	72	57	79.2	28	38.9	7	9.7	12	16.7	43	59.7	32	44.4	27	37.5	50	69.4	45	62.5
New York	159	143	89.9	41	25.8	10	6.3	66	41.5	81	50.9	51	32.1	38	23.9	107	67.3	115	72.3
Pennsylvania	189	141	74.6	19	10.1	13	6.9	35	18.5	69	36.5	37	19.6	43	22.8	101	53.4	112	59.3
CENSUS DIVISION 3, SOUTH ATLANTIC	671	547	81.5	95	14.2	54	8.0	149	22.2	243	36.2	176	26.2	196	29.2	340	50.7	451	67.2
Delaware	7	4	57.1	2	28.6	0	0.0	5	71.4	2	28.6	4	57.1	4	57.1	4	57.1	3	42.9
District of Columbia	11	8	72.7	2	18.2	2	18.2	6	54.5	7	63.6	4	36.4	5	45.5	5	45.5	6	54.5
Florida	152	128	84.2	33	21.7	12	7.9	24	15.8	71	46.7	52	34.2	52	34.2	97	63.8	119	78.3
Georgia	107	85	79.4	8	7.5	4	3.7	15	14.0	36	33.6	24	22.4	27	25.2	48	44.9	66	61.7
Maryland	51	42	82.4	14	27.5	6	11.8	10	19.6	26	51.0	14	27.5	16	31.4	31	60.8	37	72.5
North Carolina	120	102	85.0	11	9.2	12	10.0	20	16.7	39	32.5	32	26.7	35	29.2	57	47.5	92	76.7
South Carolina	82	59	72.0	3	3.7	3	3.7	19	23.2	21	25.6	16	19.5	15	18.3	29	35.4	34	41.5
Virginia	80	69	86.3	18	22.5	14	17.5	19	23.8	27	33.8	21	26.3	27	33.8	46	57.5	59	73.8
West Virginia	61	50	82.0	4	6.6	1	1.6	31	50.8	14	23.0	9	14.8	15	24.6	23	37.7	35	57.4
CENSUS DIVISION 4, EAST NORTH CENTRAL	726	610	84.0	92	12.7	77	10.6	267	36.8	265	36.5	207	28.5	181	24.9	325	44.8	473	65.2
Illinois	159	148	93.1	33	20.8	12	7.5	63	39.6	67	42.1	58	36.5	44	27.7	94	59.1	117	73.6
Indiana	124	88	71.0	9	7.3	7	5.6	14	11.3	39	31.5	28	22.6	21	16.9	45	36.3	78	62.9
Michigan	135	113	83.7	16	11.9	16	11.9	45	33.3	52	38.5	29	21.5	29	21.5	59	43.7	91	67.4
Ohio	161	137	85.1	25	15.5	33	20.5	44	27.3	64	39.8	49	30.4	47	29.2	77	47.8	102	63.4
Wisconsin	147	124	84.4	9	6.1	9	6.1	101	68.7	43	29.3	43	29.3	40	27.2	50	34.0	85	57.8
CENSUS DIVISION 5, EAST SOUTH CENTRAL	398	327	82.2	40	10.1	25	6.3	143	35.9	85	21.4	77	19.3	77	19.3	131	32.9	197	49.5
Alabama	106	88	83.0	10	9.4	4	3.8	38	35.8	20	18.9	18	17.0	18	17.0	36	34.0	56	52.8
Kentucky	90	78	86.7	5	5.6	8	8.9	17	18.9	26	28.9	21	23.3	20	22.2	42	46.7	51	56.7
Mississippi	112	88	78.6	11	9.8	9	8.0	75	67.0	13	11.6	16	14.3	16	14.3	23	20.5	39	34.8
Tennessee	90	73	81.1	14	15.6	4	4.4	13	14.4	26	28.9	22	24.4	23	25.6	30	33.3	51	56.7
CENSUS DIVISION 6, WEST NORTH CENTRAL	670	590	88.1	75	11.2	28	4.2	277	41.3	128	19.1	80	11.9	88	13.1	152	22.7	403	60.1
Iowa	126	119	94.4	14	11.1	3	2.4	91	72.2	29	23.0	11	8.7	17	13.5	22	17.5	83	65.9
Kansas	151	126	83.4	10	6.6	4	2.6	17	11.3	17	11.3	14	9.3	13	8.6	25	16.6	84	55.6
Minnesota	106	100	94.3	13	12.3	5	4.7	75	70.8	23	21.7	13	12.3	14	13.2	25	23.6	66	62.3
Missouri	151	117	77.5	21	13.9	8	5.3	31	20.5	29	19.2	27	17.9	23	15.2	58	38.4	80	53.0
Nebraska	60	55	91.7	7	11.7	4	6.7	28	46.7	21	35.0	10	16.7	12	20.0	12	20.0	42	70.0
North Dakota	29	27	93.1	5	17.2	3	10.3	15	51.7	2	6.9	2	6.9	3	10.3	4	13.8	19	65.5
South Dakota	47	46	97.9	5	10.6	1	2.1	20	42.6	7	14.9	3	6.4	6	12.8	6	12.8	29	61.7
CENSUS DIVISION 7, WEST SOUTH CENTRAL	900	671	74.6	88	9.8	48	5.3	343	38.1	204	22.7	140	15.6	108	12.0	272	30.2	430	47.8
Arkansas	80	62	77.5	5	6.3	3	3.8	41	51.3	19	23.8	10	12.5	13	16.3	18	22.5	45	56.3
Louisiana	118	73	61.9	14	11.9	3	2.5	16	13.6	34	28.8	19	16.1	18	15.3	36	30.5	55	46.6
Oklahoma	129	119	92.2	14	10.9	3	2.3	46	35.7	22	17.1	18	14.0	11	8.5	36	27.9	71	55.0
Texas	573	417	72.8	55	9.6	39	6.8	240	41.9	129	22.5	93	16.2	66	11.5	182	31.8	259	45.2
CENSUS DIVISION 8, MOUNTAIN	338	291	86.1	52	15.4	27	8.0	153	45.3	111	32.8	69	20.4	84	24.9	112	33.1	214	63.3
Arizona	54	42	77.8	10	18.5	8	14.8	21	38.9	31	57.4	18	33.3	17	31.5	28	51.9	34	63.0
Colorado	68	65	95.6	9	13.2	10	14.7	54	79.4	23	33.8	20	29.4	24	35.3	33	48.5	52	76.5
Idaho	35	31	88.6	6	17.1	1	2.9	6	17.1	11	31.4	7	20.0	6	17.1	9	25.7	24	68.6
Montana	55	52	94.5	9	16.4	0	0.0	30	54.5	8	14.5	3	5.5	6	10.9	7	12.7	28	50.9
Nevada	34	19	55.9	4	11.8	1	2.9	5	14.7	9	26.5	6	17.6	5	14.7	9	26.5	15	44.1
New Mexico	30	28	93.3	4	13.3	2	6.7	6	20.0	8	26.7	5	16.7	6	20.0	9	30.0	20	66.7
Utah	35	30	85.7	7	20.0	3	8.6	15	42.9	13	37.1	7	20.0	13	37.1	13	37.1	25	71.4
Wyoming	27	24	88.9	3	11.1	2	7.4	16	59.3	8	29.6	3	11.1	7	25.9	4	14.8	16	59.3
CENSUS DIVISION 9, PACIFIC	464	401	86.4	70	15.1	16	3.4	171	36.9	217	46.8	145	31.3	115	24.8	240	51.7	300	64.7
Alaska	14	12	85.7	0	0.0	0	0.0	2	14.3	3	21.4	1	7.1	0	0.0	2	14.3	9	64.3
California	296	246	83.1	45	15.2	8	2.7	70	23.6	143	48.3	103	34.8	82	27.7	181	61.1	182	61.5
Hawaii	21	17	81.0	2	9.5	0	0.0	6	28.6	8	38.1	5	23.8	3	14.3	7	33.3	7	33.3
Oregon	58	57	98.3	8	13.8	2	3.4	39	67.2	31	53.4	19	32.8	9	15.5	20	34.5	47	81.0
Washington	75	69	92.0	15	20.0	6	8.0	54	72.0	32	42.7	17	22.7	21	28.0	30	40.0	55	73.3

Table 7 (Continued)

These data include only hospital-based facilities and services as reported by responding hospitals in Section C of the 2012 AHA Annual Survey, beginning on page 215. All hospitals are represented with Community Hospitals listed separately under United States. No estimates have been made for nonresponding hospitals. Definitions of facilities and services are listed in the Glossary, page 201.

CLASSIFICATION	HOSPITALS REPORTING	PHYSICAL REHABILITATION SERVICES												PSYCHIATRIC SERVICES									
		ASSISTIVE TECHNOLOGY CENTER		ELECTRO-DIAGNOSTIC SERVICES		PHYSICAL REHABILITATION OUTPATIENT SERVICES		PROSTHETIC ORTHOTIC SERVICES		ROBOT ASSISTED WALKING THERAPY		SIMULATED REHABILITATION ENVIRONMENT		CHILD/ADOLESCENT SERVICES		CONSULTATION/LIAISON SERVICES		EDUCATION SERVICES		EMERGENCY SERVICES		GERIATRIC SERVICES	
		Number	Percent	Number	Percent	Number	Percent	Number	Percent	Number	Percent	Number	Percent	Number	Percent	Number	Percent	Number	Percent	Number	Percent	Number	Percent
UNITED STATES	4,774	800	16.8	1,132	23.7	3,455	72.4	879	18.4	190	4.0	1,181	24.7	857	18.0	1,526	32.0	1,158	24.3	1,569	32.9	1,442	30.2
COMMUNITY HOSPITALS	4,054	691	17.0	1,065	26.3	3,268	80.6	779	19.2	174	4.3	1,086	26.8	648	16.0	1,288	31.8	891	22.0	1,358	33.5	1,164	28.7
CENSUS DIVISION 1, NEW ENGLAND	187	43	23.0	56	29.9	157	84.0	44	23.5	14	7.5	59	31.6	66	35.3	103	55.1	76	40.6	95	50.8	80	42.8
Connecticut	32	11	34.4	12	37.5	25	78.1	13	40.6	5	15.6	16	50.0	17	53.1	25	78.1	20	62.5	25	78.1	18	56.3
Maine	39	5	12.8	8	20.5	33	84.6	5	12.8	1	2.6	10	25.6	11	28.2	13	33.3	9	23.1	10	25.6	10	25.6
Massachusetts	68	20	29.4	23	33.8	58	85.3	13	19.1	5	7.4	19	27.9	24	35.3	42	61.8	31	45.6	36	52.9	32	47.1
New Hampshire	26	3	11.5	6	23.1	24	92.3	7	26.9	2	7.7	7	26.9	8	30.8	12	46.2	9	34.6	11	42.3	10	38.5
Rhode Island	9	2	22.2	4	44.4	6	66.7	1	11.1	0	0.0	3	33.3	3	33.3	5	55.6	3	33.3	7	77.8	5	55.6
Vermont	13	2	15.4	3	23.1	11	84.6	5	38.5	1	7.7	4	30.8	3	23.1	6	46.2	4	30.8	6	46.2	5	38.5
CENSUS DIVISION 2, MIDDLE ATLANTIC	420	103	24.5	191	45.5	337	80.2	127	30.2	33	7.9	149	35.5	135	32.1	238	56.7	165	39.3	231	55.0	207	49.3
New Jersey	72	21	29.2	37	51.4	60	83.3	23	31.9	7	9.7	25	34.7	28	38.9	45	62.5	31	43.1	46	63.9	36	50.0
New York	159	39	24.5	74	46.5	137	86.2	61	38.4	11	6.9	60	37.7	61	38.4	104	65.4	73	45.9	96	60.4	89	56.0
Pennsylvania	189	43	22.8	80	42.3	140	74.1	43	22.8	15	7.9	64	33.9	46	24.3	89	47.1	61	32.3	89	47.1	82	43.4
CENSUS DIVISION 3, SOUTH ATLANTIC	671	122	18.2	182	27.1	502	74.8	185	27.6	38	5.7	188	28.0	118	17.6	234	34.9	177	26.4	256	38.2	206	30.7
Delaware	7	1	14.3	2	28.6	5	71.4	3	42.9	0	0.0	1	14.3	5	71.4	3	42.9	2	28.6	4	57.1	3	42.9
District of Columbia	11	5	45.5	5	45.5	9	81.8	4	36.4	3	27.3	5	45.5	4	36.4	7	63.6	4	36.4	8	72.7	6	54.5
Florida	152	43	28.3	41	27.0	126	82.9	37	24.3	11	7.2	46	30.3	24	15.8	56	36.8	34	22.4	55	36.2	43	28.3
Georgia	107	11	10.3	17	15.9	73	68.2	17	15.9	2	1.9	24	22.4	9	8.4	27	25.2	23	21.5	26	24.3	21	19.6
Maryland	51	13	25.5	26	51.0	41	80.4	19	37.3	2	3.9	18	35.3	19	37.3	36	70.6	24	47.1	36	70.6	29	56.9
North Carolina	120	25	20.8	37	30.8	98	81.7	22	18.3	7	5.8	40	33.3	20	16.7	38	31.7	35	29.2	47	39.2	42	35.0
South Carolina	82	6	7.3	9	11.0	39	47.6	50	61.0	5	6.1	13	15.9	12	14.6	21	25.6	16	19.5	23	28.0	20	24.4
Virginia	80	13	16.3	31	38.8	69	86.3	25	31.3	5	6.3	30	37.5	12	15.0	31	38.8	23	28.8	42	52.5	28	35.0
West Virginia	61	5	8.2	14	23.0	42	68.9	8	13.1	3	4.9	11	18.0	13	21.3	15	24.6	16	26.2	15	24.6	14	23.0
CENSUS DIVISION 4, EAST NORTH CENTRAL	726	124	17.1	235	32.4	587	80.9	163	22.5	23	3.2	258	35.5	162	22.3	296	40.8	233	32.1	286	39.4	257	35.4
Illinois	159	28	17.6	65	40.9	138	86.8	33	20.8	6	3.8	64	40.3	49	30.8	71	44.7	63	39.6	73	45.9	69	43.4
Indiana	124	19	15.3	30	24.2	91	73.4	21	16.9	3	2.4	35	28.2	26	21.0	33	26.6	31	25.0	38	30.6	37	29.8
Michigan	135	28	20.7	53	39.3	114	84.4	30	22.2	8	5.9	50	37.0	29	21.5	68	50.4	51	37.8	64	47.4	49	36.3
Ohio	161	30	18.6	57	35.4	123	76.4	39	24.2	4	2.5	56	34.8	24	14.9	67	41.6	48	29.8	62	38.5	55	34.2
Wisconsin	147	19	12.9	30	20.4	121	82.3	40	27.2	2	1.4	53	36.1	34	23.1	57	38.8	40	27.2	49	33.3	47	32.0
CENSUS DIVISION 5, EAST SOUTH CENTRAL	398	39	9.8	66	16.6	269	67.6	46	11.6	20	5.0	70	17.6	36	9.0	86	21.6	67	16.8	95	23.9	134	33.7
Alabama	106	12	11.3	15	14.2	70	66.0	17	16.0	7	6.6	18	17.0	11	10.4	27	25.5	24	22.6	30	28.3	41	38.7
Kentucky	90	8	8.9	20	22.2	67	74.4	9	10.0	5	5.6	14	15.6	7	7.8	22	24.4	14	15.6	23	25.6	18	20.0
Mississippi	112	5	4.5	12	10.7	61	54.5	8	7.1	2	1.8	18	16.1	8	7.1	17	15.2	14	12.5	16	14.3	46	41.1
Tennessee	90	14	15.6	19	21.1	71	78.9	12	13.3	6	6.7	20	22.2	10	11.1	20	22.2	15	16.7	26	28.9	29	32.2
CENSUS DIVISION 6, WEST NORTH CENTRAL	670	75	11.2	122	18.2	524	78.2	92	13.7	11	1.6	127	19.0	109	16.3	163	24.3	134	20.0	182	27.2	160	23.9
Iowa	126	21	16.7	22	17.5	103	81.7	13	10.3	1	0.8	27	21.4	27	21.4	33	26.2	32	25.4	42	33.3	33	26.2
Kansas	151	14	17.5	14	9.3	116	76.8	11	7.3	3	2.0	18	11.9	8	5.3	15	9.9	14	9.3	25	16.6	26	17.2
Minnesota	106	12	11.3	21	19.8	89	84.0	15	14.2	1	0.9	18	17.0	24	22.6	38	35.8	26	24.5	34	32.1	31	29.2
Missouri	151	14	9.3	32	21.2	109	72.2	33	21.9	5	3.3	43	28.5	28	18.5	54	35.8	42	27.8	55	36.4	50	33.1
Nebraska	60	8	13.3	15	25.0	49	81.7	11	18.3	1	1.7	11	18.3	10	16.7	10	16.7	9	15.0	10	16.7	9	15.0
North Dakota	29	7	24.1	8	27.6	22	75.9	4	13.8	0	0.0	3	10.3	7	24.1	5	17.2	6	20.7	7	24.1	7	24.1
South Dakota	47	2	4.3	10	21.3	36	76.6	5	10.6	0	0.0	7	14.9	5	10.6	8	17.0	5	10.6	9	19.1	4	8.5
CENSUS DIVISION 7, WEST SOUTH CENTRAL	900	154	17.1	99	11.0	526	58.4	87	9.7	26	2.9	173	19.2	88	9.8	161	17.9	126	14.0	166	18.4	200	22.2
Arkansas	80	14	17.5	14	17.5	53	66.3	7	8.8	3	3.8	11	13.8	12	15.0	18	22.5	11	13.8	20	25.0	26	32.5
Louisiana	118	15	12.7	15	12.7	53	44.9	11	9.3	1	0.8	23	19.5	11	9.3	21	17.8	18	15.3	26	22.0	38	32.2
Oklahoma	129	20	15.5	16	12.4	82	63.6	16	12.4	0	0.0	23	17.8	10	7.8	28	21.7	17	13.2	28	21.7	26	20.2
Texas	573	105	18.3	59	10.3	338	59.0	53	9.2	22	3.8	116	20.2	55	9.6	94	16.4	80	14.0	92	16.1	110	19.2
CENSUS DIVISION 8, MOUNTAIN	338	62	18.3	58	17.2	231	68.3	45	13.3	13	3.8	62	18.3	61	18.0	89	26.3	75	22.2	114	33.7	90	26.6
Arizona	54	9	16.7	17	31.5	32	59.3	7	13.0	2	3.7	13	24.1	13	24.1	21	38.9	16	29.6	19	35.2	19	35.2
Colorado	68	11	16.2	16	23.5	56	82.4	11	16.2	4	5.9	19	27.9	11	16.2	17	25.0	13	19.1	20	29.4	13	19.1
Idaho	35	7	20.0	4	11.4	22	62.9	4	11.4	0	0.0	7	20.0	5	14.3	11	31.4	10	28.6	11	31.4	6	17.1
Montana	55	8	14.5	7	12.7	40	72.7	4	7.3	0	0.0	5	9.1	6	10.9	11	20.0	7	12.7	19	34.5	11	20.0
Nevada	34	3	8.8	3	8.8	19	55.9	3	8.8	3	8.8	5	14.7	8	23.5	5	14.7	6	17.6	11	32.4	11	32.4
New Mexico	30	10	33.3	4	13.3	26	86.7	3	10.0	2	6.7	4	13.3	8	26.7	7	23.3	8	26.7	9	30.0	12	40.0
Utah	35	12	34.3	7	20.0	22	62.9	9	25.7	2	5.7	6	17.1	7	20.0	11	31.4	10	28.6	15	42.9	10	28.6
Wyoming	27	2	7.4	0	0.0	14	51.9	4	14.8	0	0.0	3	11.1	5	18.5	6	22.2	5	18.5	10	37.0	8	29.6
CENSUS DIVISION 9, PACIFIC	464	78	16.8	123	26.5	322	69.4	90	19.4	12	2.6	95	20.5	82	17.7	156	33.6	105	22.6	144	31.0	108	23.3
Alaska	14	2	14.3	2	14.3	11	78.6	3	21.4	0	0.0	1	7.1	1	7.1	6	42.9	4	28.6	6	42.9	5	35.7
California	296	43	14.5	72	24.3	196	66.2	55	18.6	6	2.0	63	21.3	50	16.9	103	34.8	70	23.6	86	29.1	76	25.7
Hawaii	21	5	23.8	3	14.3	13	61.9	5	23.8	1	4.8	4	19.0	3	14.3	4	19.0	5	23.8	5	23.8	5	23.8
Oregon	58	11	19.0	19	32.8	48	82.8	8	13.8	2	3.4	6	10.3	9	15.5	20	34.5	9	15.5	24	41.4	7	12.1
Washington	75	17	22.7	27	36.0	54	72.0	19	25.3	3	4.0	21	28.0	14	18.7	23	30.7	17	22.7	23	30.7	15	20.0

Table 7 (Continued)

These data include only hospital-based facilities and services as reported by responding hospitals in Section C of the 2012 AHA Annual Survey, beginning on page 215. All hospitals are represented with Community Hospitals listed separately under United States. No estimates have been made for nonresponding hospitals. Definitions of facilities and services are listed in the Glossary, page 201.

CLASSIFICATION	HOSPITALS REPORTING	PSYCHIATRIC SERVICES — OUTPATIENT SERVICES Number	Percent	PARTIAL HOSPITALIZATION PROGRAM Number	Percent	RESIDENTIAL TREATMENT Number	Percent	CT SCANNER Number	Percent	RADIOLOGY, DIAGNOSTIC — DIAGNOSTIC RADIOISOTOPE FACILITY Number	Percent	ELECTRON BEAM COMPUTED TOMOGRAPHY (EBCT) Number	Percent	FULL-FIELD DIGITAL MAMMOGRAPHY (FFDM) Number	Percent	MAGNETIC RESONANCE IMAGING (MRI) Number	Percent	INTRAOPERATIVE MAGNETIC IMAGING Number	Percent	MAGNETO-ENCEPHALO-GRAPHY Number	Percent	MULTI-SLICE SPIRAL COMPUTED TOMOGRAPHY (<64 SLICE CT) Number	Percent
UNITED STATES	4,774	1,309	27.4	739	15.5	303	6.3	3,922	82.2	2,643	55.4	356	7.5	2,448	51.3	3,046	63.8	220	4.6	129	2.7	2,776	58.1
COMMUNITY HOSPITALS	4,054	1,049	25.9	556	13.7	164	4.0	3,704	91.4	2,550	62.9	335	8.3	2,393	59.0	2,895	71.4	204	5.0	122	3.0	2,652	65.4
CENSUS DIVISION 1, NEW ENGLAND	187	96	51.3	60	32.1	11	5.9	155	82.9	128	68.4	9	4.8	124	66.3	121	64.7	11	5.9	7	3.7	115	61.5
Connecticut	32	23	71.9	17	53.1	5	15.6	26	81.3	22	68.8	4	12.5	22	68.8	25	78.1	4	12.5	0	0.0	22	68.8
Maine	39	14	35.9	7	17.9	0	0.0	35	89.7	30	76.9	0	0.0	24	61.5	24	61.5	2	5.1	0	0.0	20	51.3
Massachusetts	68	36	52.9	23	33.8	5	7.4	53	77.9	48	70.6	5	7.4	45	66.2	41	60.3	5	7.4	5	7.4	42	61.8
New Hampshire	26	9	34.6	6	23.1	0	0.0	22	84.6	13	50.0	0	0.0	18	69.2	15	57.7	0	0.0	2	7.7	17	65.4
Rhode Island	9	6	66.7	4	44.4	0	0.0	7	77.8	6	66.7	0	0.0	7	77.8	7	77.8	0	0.0	0	0.0	7	77.8
Vermont	13	8	61.5	3	23.1	1	7.7	12	92.3	9	69.2	0	0.0	8	61.5	9	69.2	0	0.0	0	0.0	7	53.8
CENSUS DIVISION 2, MIDDLE ATLANTIC	420	173	41.2	92	21.9	48	11.4	360	85.7	302	71.9	62	14.8	265	63.1	313	74.5	24	5.7	15	3.6	264	62.9
New Jersey	72	32	44.4	29	40.3	13	18.1	58	80.6	52	72.2	16	22.2	46	63.9	55	76.4	8	11.1	6	8.3	51	70.8
New York	159	88	55.3	34	21.4	23	14.5	150	94.3	122	76.7	21	13.2	111	69.8	128	80.5	7	4.4	6	3.8	106	66.7
Pennsylvania	189	53	28.0	29	15.3	12	6.3	152	80.4	128	67.7	25	13.2	108	57.1	130	68.8	9	4.8	3	1.6	107	56.6
CENSUS DIVISION 3, SOUTH ATLANTIC	671	173	25.8	112	16.7	42	6.3	558	83.2	438	65.3	61	9.1	388	57.8	479	71.4	23	3.4	17	2.5	448	66.8
Delaware	7	4	57.1	3	42.9	0	0.0	5	71.4	4	57.1	2	28.6	4	57.1	5	71.4	1	14.3	0	0.0	4	57.1
District of Columbia	11	5	45.5	4	36.4	1	9.1	8	72.7	7	63.6	1	9.1	6	54.5	8	72.7	0	0.0	0	0.0	7	63.6
Florida	152	35	23.0	16	10.5	8	5.3	133	87.5	103	67.8	26	17.1	93	61.2	121	79.6	7	4.6	8	5.3	114	75.0
Georgia	107	24	22.4	18	16.8	8	7.5	92	86.0	65	60.7	3	2.8	65	60.7	77	72.0	5	4.7	3	2.8	65	60.7
Maryland	51	30	58.8	24	47.1	5	9.8	43	84.3	37	72.5	4	7.8	31	60.8	38	74.5	2	3.9	1	2.0	38	74.5
North Carolina	120	30	25.0	14	11.7	6	5.0	100	83.3	79	65.8	11	9.2	70	58.3	89	74.2	4	3.3	2	1.7	82	68.3
South Carolina	82	16	19.5	10	12.2	5	6.1	59	72.0	49	59.8	5	6.1	43	52.4	49	59.8	1	1.2	1	1.2	50	61.0
Virginia	80	21	26.3	16	20.0	6	7.5	69	86.3	56	70.0	7	8.8	48	60.0	60	75.0	3	3.8	2	2.5	54	67.5
West Virginia	61	8	13.1	7	11.5	3	4.9	49	80.3	38	62.3	2	3.3	28	45.9	32	52.5	0	0.0	0	0.0	34	55.7
CENSUS DIVISION 4, EAST NORTH CENTRAL	726	247	34.0	153	21.1	61	8.4	625	86.1	482	66.4	66	9.1	462	63.6	501	69.0	53	7.3	23	3.2	445	61.3
Illinois	159	72	45.3	48	30.2	13	8.2	150	94.3	110	69.2	7	4.4	118	74.2	114	71.7	6	3.8	5	3.1	107	67.3
Indiana	124	33	26.6	23	18.5	14	11.3	97	78.2	70	56.5	11	8.9	68	54.8	88	71.0	6	4.8	7	5.6	71	57.3
Michigan	135	46	34.1	24	17.8	6	4.4	115	85.2	101	74.8	9	6.7	88	65.2	84	62.2	6	4.4	3	2.2	85	63.0
Ohio	161	51	31.7	33	20.5	15	9.3	142	88.2	119	73.9	23	14.3	107	66.5	128	79.5	11	6.8	6	3.7	113	70.2
Wisconsin	147	45	30.6	25	17.0	13	8.8	121	82.3	82	55.8	16	10.9	81	55.1	87	59.2	24	16.3	2	1.4	69	46.9
CENSUS DIVISION 5, EAST SOUTH CENTRAL	398	75	18.8	46	11.6	22	5.5	325	81.7	217	54.5	24	6.0	163	41.0	253	63.6	20	5.0	11	2.8	213	53.5
Alabama	106	27	25.5	14	13.2	7	6.6	88	83.0	58	54.7	5	4.7	40	37.7	69	65.1	3	2.8	3	2.8	61	57.5
Kentucky	90	14	15.6	8	8.9	2	2.2	78	86.7	54	60.0	3	3.3	49	54.4	72	80.0	4	4.4	3	3.3	57	63.3
Mississippi	112	16	14.3	10	8.9	6	5.4	85	75.9	52	46.4	8	7.1	29	25.9	51	45.5	6	5.4	1	0.9	42	37.5
Tennessee	90	18	20.0	14	15.6	7	7.8	74	82.2	53	58.9	8	8.9	45	50.0	61	67.8	7	7.8	4	4.4	53	58.9
CENSUS DIVISION 6, WEST NORTH CENTRAL	670	164	24.5	66	9.9	30	4.5	574	85.7	253	37.8	24	3.6	323	48.2	377	56.3	15	2.2	6	0.9	387	57.8
Iowa	126	30	23.8	13	10.3	5	4.0	115	91.3	46	36.5	5	4.0	75	59.5	72	57.1	0	0.0	2	1.6	84	66.7
Kansas	151	14	9.3	6	4.0	4	2.6	121	80.1	50	33.1	3	2.0	43	28.5	55	36.4	2	1.3	1	0.7	78	51.7
Minnesota	106	37	34.9	14	13.2	6	5.7	99	93.4	44	41.5	5	4.7	63	59.4	73	68.9	5	4.7	2	1.9	56	52.8
Missouri	151	55	36.4	16	10.6	11	7.3	119	78.8	73	48.3	7	4.6	71	47.0	111	73.5	5	3.3	0	0.0	90	59.6
Nebraska	60	16	26.7	9	15.0	4	6.7	56	93.3	22	36.7	4	6.7	39	65.0	38	63.3	2	3.3	1	1.7	40	66.7
North Dakota	29	8	27.6	6	20.7	0	0.0	23	79.3	7	24.1	0	0.0	14	48.3	10	34.5	1	3.4	0	0.0	16	55.2
South Dakota	47	4	8.5	2	4.3	0	0.0	41	87.2	11	23.4	0	0.0	18	38.3	18	38.3	0	0.0	0	0.0	23	48.9
CENSUS DIVISION 7, WEST SOUTH CENTRAL	900	157	17.4	82	9.1	40	4.4	634	70.4	347	38.6	38	4.2	303	33.7	457	50.8	26	2.9	15	1.7	416	46.2
Arkansas	80	18	22.5	8	10.0	8	10.0	61	76.3	33	41.3	2	2.5	27	33.8	47	58.8	1	1.3	1	1.3	41	51.3
Louisiana	118	27	22.9	16	13.6	5	4.2	75	63.6	47	39.8	11	9.3	52	44.1	55	46.6	3	2.5	3	2.5	46	39.0
Oklahoma	129	27	20.9	8	6.2	13	10.1	102	79.1	48	37.2	5	3.9	52	40.3	74	57.4	2	1.6	2	1.6	64	49.6
Texas	573	85	14.8	50	8.7	14	2.4	396	69.1	219	38.2	20	3.5	172	30.0	281	49.0	20	3.5	9	1.6	265	46.2
CENSUS DIVISION 8, MOUNTAIN	338	92	27.2	53	15.7	21	6.2	285	84.3	172	50.9	23	6.8	170	50.3	221	65.4	17	5.0	14	4.1	195	57.7
Arizona	54	20	37.0	9	16.7	3	5.6	43	79.6	34	63.0	5	9.3	24	44.4	42	77.8	3	5.6	2	3.7	34	63.0
Colorado	68	18	26.5	8	11.8	3	4.4	65	95.6	45	66.2	4	5.9	41	60.3	57	83.8	5	7.4	2	2.9	46	67.6
Idaho	35	9	25.7	3	8.6	3	8.6	32	91.4	17	48.6	0	0.0	16	45.7	24	68.6	1	2.9	1	2.9	22	62.9
Montana	55	10	18.2	8	14.5	2	3.6	43	78.2	19	34.5	2	3.6	22	40.0	22	40.0	2	3.6	2	3.6	25	45.5
Nevada	34	11	32.4	7	20.6	3	8.8	20	58.8	16	47.1	3	8.8	13	38.2	19	55.9	2	5.9	2	5.9	15	44.1
New Mexico	30	9	30.0	2	6.7	1	3.3	28	93.3	13	43.3	2	6.7	19	63.3	18	60.0	1	3.3	3	10.0	19	63.3
Utah	35	9	25.7	9	25.7	4	11.4	30	85.7	18	51.4	6	17.1	20	57.1	22	62.9	2	5.7	2	5.7	21	60.0
Wyoming	27	6	22.2	7	25.9	2	7.4	24	88.9	10	37.0	1	3.7	15	55.6	17	63.0	1	3.7	0	0.0	13	48.1
CENSUS DIVISION 9, PACIFIC	464	132	28.4	75	16.2	28	6.0	406	87.5	304	65.5	49	10.6	250	53.9	324	69.8	31	6.7	21	4.5	293	63.1
Alaska	14	7	50.0	2	14.3	2	14.3	11	78.6	6	42.9	0	0.0	7	50.0	8	57.1	0	0.0	0	0.0	8	57.1
California	296	88	29.7	53	17.9	14	4.7	256	86.5	201	67.9	36	12.2	147	49.7	207	69.9	23	7.8	16	5.4	183	61.8
Hawaii	21	4	19.0	3	14.3	2	9.5	14	66.7	10	47.6	3	14.3	10	47.6	11	52.4	0	0.0	1	4.8	5	23.8
Oregon	58	11	19.0	7	12.1	2	3.4	56	96.6	39	67.2	4	6.9	44	75.9	43	74.1	6	10.3	2	3.4	44	75.9
Washington	75	22	29.3	10	13.3	8	10.7	69	92.0	48	64.0	6	8.0	42	56.0	55	73.3	2	2.7	2	2.7	53	70.7

Table 7 (Continued)

These data include only hospital-based facilities and services as reported by responding hospitals in Section C of the 2012 AHA Annual Survey, beginning on page 215. All hospitals are represented with Community Hospitals listed separately under United States. No estimates have been made for nonresponding hospitals. Definitions of facilities and services are listed in the Glossary, page 201.

| | | RADIOLOGY, DIAGNOSTIC | | | | | | | | | | RADIOLOGY, THERAPEUTIC | | | | | | | | | |
| | | MULTI-SLICE SPIRAL COMPUTED TOMOGRAPHY (64+ SLICE CT) | | POSITRON EMISSION TOMOGRAPHY (PET) | | POSITRON EMISSION TOMOGRAPHY/CT (PET/CT) | | SINGLE PHOTON EMISSION COMPUTERIZED TOMOGRAPHY (SPECT) | | ULTRASOUND | | IMAGE-GUIDED RADIATION THERAPY (IGRT) | | INTENSITY-MODULATED RADIATION THERAPY (IMRT) | | PROTON BEAM THERAPY | | SHAPED BEAM RADIATION SYSTEM | | STEREOTACTIC RADIOSURGERY | |
CLASSIFICATION	HOSPITALS REPORTING	Number	Percent	Number	Percent	Number	Percent	Number	Percent	Number	Percent	Number	Percent	Number	Percent	Number	Percent	Number	Percent	Number	Percent
UNITED STATES	4,774	2,045	42.8	778	16.3	1,015	21.3	1,743	36.5	3,790	79.4	965	20.2	1,097	23.0	96	2.0	875	18.3	816	17.1
COMMUNITY HOSPITALS	4,054	1,956	48.2	736	18.2	967	23.9	1,687	41.6	3,576	88.2	935	23.1	1,065	26.3	84	2.1	854	21.1	798	19.7
CENSUS DIVISION 1, NEW ENGLAND	187	100	53.5	43	23.0	53	28.3	100	53.5	160	85.6	56	29.9	61	32.6	3	1.6	52	27.8	50	26.7
Connecticut	32	20	62.5	15	46.9	19	59.4	23	71.9	27	84.4	19	59.4	18	56.3	3	3.1	16	50.0	16	50.0
Maine	39	19	48.7	3	7.7	6	15.4	18	46.2	34	87.2	4	10.3	6	15.4	0	0.0	5	12.8	4	10.3
Massachusetts	68	40	58.8	15	22.1	18	26.5	35	51.5	57	83.8	24	35.3	27	39.7	2	2.9	25	36.8	23	33.8
New Hampshire	26	12	46.2	5	19.2	5	19.2	13	50.0	23	88.5	5	19.2	6	23.1	0	0.0	4	15.4	5	19.2
Rhode Island	9	2	22.2	2	22.2	2	22.2	4	44.4	7	77.8	2	22.2	2	22.2	0	0.0	1	11.1	1	11.1
Vermont	13	7	53.8	3	23.1	3	23.1	7	53.8	12	92.3	2	15.4	2	15.4	0	0.0	1	7.7	1	7.7
CENSUS DIVISION 2, MIDDLE ATLANTIC	420	237	56.4	99	23.6	124	29.5	225	53.6	359	85.5	134	31.9	165	39.3	11	2.6	130	31.0	113	26.9
New Jersey	72	36	50.0	18	25.0	25	34.7	40	55.6	60	83.3	31	43.1	37	51.4	0	0.0	33	45.8	21	29.2
New York	159	100	62.9	37	23.3	44	27.7	83	52.2	150	94.3	48	30.2	62	39.0	5	3.1	48	30.2	40	29.2
Pennsylvania	189	101	53.4	44	23.3	55	29.1	102	54.0	149	78.8	55	29.1	66	34.9	6	3.2	49	25.9	52	27.5
CENSUS DIVISION 3, SOUTH ATLANTIC	671	338	50.4	126	18.8	176	26.2	306	45.6	558	83.2	178	26.5	196	29.2	12	1.8	165	24.6	142	21.2
Delaware	7	4	57.1	3	42.9	5	71.4	4	57.1	5	71.4	4	42.9	4	57.1	0	0.0	3	42.9	3	42.9
District of Columbia	11	5	45.5	4	36.4	5	45.5	6	54.5	9	81.8	4	36.4	5	45.5	0	0.0	5	45.5	4	36.4
Florida	152	93	61.2	40	26.3	53	34.9	64	42.1	129	84.9	44	28.9	46	30.3	2	1.3	43	28.3	46	30.3
Georgia	107	46	43.0	20	18.7	28	26.2	32	29.9	91	85.0	25	23.4	25	23.4	2	1.9	22	20.6	23	21.5
Maryland	51	34	66.7	11	21.6	14	27.5	33	64.7	44	86.3	21	41.2	21	41.2	2	3.9	17	33.3	13	25.5
North Carolina	120	57	47.5	16	13.3	29	24.2	68	56.7	103	85.8	36	30.0	39	32.5	6	5.0	34	28.3	21	17.5
South Carolina	82	30	36.6	4	4.9	9	11.0	24	29.3	60	73.2	8	9.8	15	18.3	0	0.0	9	11.0	7	8.5
Virginia	80	45	56.3	16	20.0	23	28.8	51	63.8	68	85.0	29	36.3	32	40.0	0	0.0	23	28.8	17	21.3
West Virginia	61	24	39.3	12	19.7	10	16.4	24	39.3	49	80.3	8	13.1	10	16.4	0	0.0	9	14.8	8	13.1
CENSUS DIVISION 4, EAST NORTH CENTRAL	726	381	52.5	169	23.3	219	30.2	337	46.4	611	84.2	195	26.9	217	29.9	16	2.2	177	24.4	147	20.2
Illinois	159	105	66.0	27	17.0	41	25.8	70	44.0	142	89.3	48	30.2	55	34.6	4	2.5	43	27.0	33	20.8
Indiana	124	52	41.9	23	18.5	34	27.4	46	37.1	98	79.0	34	27.4	38	30.6	4	3.2	30	24.2	21	16.9
Michigan	135	85	63.0	27	20.0	41	30.4	69	51.1	119	88.1	38	28.1	42	31.1	2	1.5	36	26.7	37	27.4
Ohio	161	80	49.7	54	33.5	59	36.6	86	53.4	140	87.0	43	26.7	45	28.0	4	2.5	38	23.6	34	21.1
Wisconsin	147	59	40.1	38	25.9	44	29.9	66	44.9	112	76.2	32	21.8	37	25.2	2	1.4	30	20.4	22	15.0
CENSUS DIVISION 5, EAST SOUTH CENTRAL	398	137	34.4	57	14.3	74	18.6	137	34.4	320	80.4	58	14.6	70	17.6	6	1.5	49	12.3	49	12.3
Alabama	106	38	35.8	19	17.9	25	23.6	31	29.2	85	80.2	15	14.2	16	15.1	2	1.9	11	10.4	11	10.4
Kentucky	90	38	42.2	11	12.2	18	20.0	37	41.1	80	88.9	15	16.7	19	21.1	1	1.1	13	14.4	15	16.7
Mississippi	112	26	23.2	14	12.5	12	10.7	33	29.5	83	74.1	12	10.7	10	8.9	1	0.9	7	6.3	5	4.5
Tennessee	90	35	38.9	13	14.4	19	21.1	36	40.0	72	80.0	16	17.8	25	27.8	2	2.2	18	20.0	18	20.0
CENSUS DIVISION 6, WEST NORTH CENTRAL	670	197	29.4	68	10.1	100	14.9	171	25.5	520	77.6	92	13.7	108	16.1	12	1.8	76	11.3	73	10.9
Iowa	126	34	27.0	12	9.5	14	11.1	37	29.4	113	89.7	12	9.5	15	11.9	0	0.0	13	10.3	12	9.5
Kansas	151	26	17.2	8	5.3	12	7.9	26	17.2	97	64.2	10	6.6	15	9.9	4	2.6	12	7.9	8	5.3
Minnesota	106	47	44.3	11	10.4	19	17.9	28	26.4	92	86.8	17	16.0	18	17.0	1	0.9	11	10.4	13	12.3
Missouri	151	60	39.7	19	12.6	34	22.5	52	34.4	119	78.8	29	19.2	35	23.2	4	2.6	20	13.2	20	13.2
Nebraska	60	18	30.0	11	18.3	14	23.3	16	26.7	48	80.0	15	25.0	13	21.7	2	3.3	10	16.7	13	21.7
North Dakota	29	3	10.3	4	13.8	4	13.8	4	13.8	16	55.2	2	6.9	3	10.3	1	3.4	2	6.9	2	6.9
South Dakota	47	9	19.1	5	10.6	3	6.4	8	17.0	35	74.5	7	14.9	9	19.1	1	2.1	7	14.9	5	10.6
CENSUS DIVISION 7, WEST SOUTH CENTRAL	900	275	30.6	67	7.4	90	10.0	190	21.1	587	65.2	81	9.0	95	10.6	9	1.0	72	8.0	94	10.4
Arkansas	80	26	32.5	7	8.8	8	10.0	16	20.0	58	72.5	7	8.8	6	7.5	1	1.3	4	5.0	9	11.3
Louisiana	118	39	33.1	10	8.5	17	14.4	23	19.5	76	64.4	16	13.6	15	12.7	2	1.7	12	10.2	15	12.7
Oklahoma	129	39	30.2	13	10.1	20	15.5	23	17.8	92	71.3	18	14.0	19	14.7	1	0.8	17	13.2	12	9.3
Texas	573	171	29.8	37	6.5	45	7.9	128	22.3	361	63.0	40	7.0	55	9.6	5	0.9	39	6.8	58	10.1
CENSUS DIVISION 8, MOUNTAIN	338	158	46.7	58	17.2	63	18.6	97	28.7	276	81.7	61	18.0	64	18.9	14	3.8	55	16.3	54	16.0
Arizona	54	32	59.3	16	29.6	16	29.6	25	46.3	43	79.6	10	18.5	11	20.4	2	3.7	11	20.4	10	18.5
Colorado	68	44	64.7	15	22.1	17	25.0	21	30.9	63	92.6	16	23.5	17	25.0	3	4.4	17	25.0	18	26.5
Idaho	35	12	34.3	4	11.4	5	14.3	9	25.7	29	82.9	6	17.1	6	17.1	1	2.9	5	14.3	4	11.4
Montana	55	19	34.5	6	10.9	7	12.7	11	20.0	41	74.5	8	14.5	8	14.5	3	5.5	6	10.9	6	10.9
Nevada	34	10	29.4	2	5.9	2	5.9	7	20.6	20	58.8	4	11.8	4	11.8	1	2.9	3	8.8	5	14.7
New Mexico	30	16	53.3	4	13.3	6	20.0	10	33.3	26	86.7	4	13.3	7	23.3	2	6.7	5	16.7	5	16.7
Utah	35	17	48.6	8	22.9	10	28.6	9	25.7	30	85.7	8	22.9	7	20.0	1	2.9	6	17.1	4	11.4
Wyoming	27	8	29.6	3	11.1	0	0.0	5	18.5	24	88.9	4	14.8	4	14.8	0	0.0	2	7.4	2	7.4
CENSUS DIVISION 9, PACIFIC	464	222	47.8	91	19.6	116	25.0	180	38.8	399	86.0	110	23.7	121	26.1	14	3.0	99	21.3	94	20.3
Alaska	14	5	35.7	0	0.0	0	0.0	2	14.3	12	85.7	0	0.0	2	14.3	0	0.0	1	7.1	1	7.1
California	296	150	50.7	64	21.6	79	26.7	121	40.9	253	85.5	71	24.0	78	26.4	11	3.7	62	20.9	69	23.3
Hawaii	21	10	47.6	2	9.5	4	19.0	3	14.3	14	66.7	2	9.5	2	9.5	0	0.0	1	4.8	1	4.8
Oregon	58	28	48.3	9	15.5	12	20.7	28	48.3	56	96.6	15	25.9	15	25.9	3	5.2	13	22.4	9	15.5
Washington	75	29	38.7	17	22.7	21	28.0	26	34.7	64	85.3	22	29.3	22	29.3	0	0.0	21	28.0	14	18.7

Table 7 (Continued)

These data include only hospital-based facilities and services as reported by responding hospitals in Section C of the 2012 AHA Annual Survey, beginning on page 215. All hospitals are represented with Community Hospitals listed separately under United States. No estimates have been made for nonresponding hospitals. Definitions of facilities and services are listed in the Glossary, page 201.

CLASSIFICATION	HOSPITALS REPORTING	BONE MARROW Number	Percent	HEART Number	Percent	KIDNEY Number	Percent	TRANSPLANT LIVER Number	Percent	LUNG Number	Percent	TISSUE Number	Percent	OTHER Number	Percent
UNITED STATES	4,774	206	4.4	136	2.8	223	4.7	125	2.6	73	1.5	350	7.3	253	5.3
COMMUNITY HOSPITALS	4,054	204	5.0	131	3.2	221	5.5	124	3.1	72	1.8	335	8.3	248	6.1
CENSUS DIVISION 1, NEW ENGLAND	187	12	6.4	6	3.2	17	9.1	7	3.7	3	1.6	20	10.7	17	9.1
Connecticut	32	1	3.1	2	6.3	3	9.4	2	6.3	0	0.0	3	9.4	4	12.5
Maine	39	0	0.0	0	0.0	2	5.1	0	0.0	0	0.0	1	2.6	1	2.6
Massachusetts	68	9	13.2	4	5.9	9	13.2	5	7.4	3	4.4	12	17.6	8	11.8
New Hampshire	26	1	3.8	0	0.0	1	3.8	0	0.0	0	0.0	2	7.7	2	7.7
Rhode Island	9	0	0.0	0	0.0	1	11.1	0	0.0	0	0.0	0	0.0	1	11.1
Vermont	13	1	7.7	0	0.0	1	7.7	0	0.0	0	0.0	2	15.4	1	7.7
CENSUS DIVISION 2, MIDDLE ATLANTIC	420	28	6.7	16	3.8	35	8.3	19	4.5	8	1.9	48	11.4	42	10.0
New Jersey	72	2	2.8	2	2.8	5	6.9	2	2.8	1	1.4	4	5.6	5	6.9
New York	159	12	7.5	5	3.1	13	8.2	6	3.8	1	0.6	21	13.2	18	11.3
Pennsylvania	189	14	7.4	9	4.8	17	9.0	11	5.8	6	3.2	23	12.2	19	10.1
CENSUS DIVISION 3, SOUTH ATLANTIC	671	37	5.5	27	4.0	30	4.5	19	2.8	15	2.2	55	8.2	41	6.1
Delaware	7	2	28.6	1	14.3	2	28.6	1	14.3	1	14.3	0	0.0	0	0.0
District of Columbia	11	2	18.2	2	18.2	2	18.2	1	9.1	0	0.0	0	0.0	3	27.3
Florida	152	12	7.9	8	5.3	7	4.6	6	3.9	5	3.3	14	9.2	6	3.9
Georgia	107	4	3.7	4	3.7	4	3.7	3	2.8	2	1.9	8	7.5	5	4.7
Maryland	51	3	5.9	2	3.9	2	3.9	2	3.9	2	3.9	5	9.8	6	11.8
North Carolina	120	4	3.3	4	3.3	5	4.2	1	0.8	2	1.7	5	4.2	9	7.5
South Carolina	82	4	4.9	1	1.2	1	1.2	1	1.2	1	1.2	7	8.5	4	4.9
Virginia	80	5	6.3	5	6.3	6	7.5	2	2.5	2	2.5	10	12.5	7	8.8
West Virginia	61	1	1.6	0	0.0	1	1.6	0	0.0	0	0.0	4	6.6	1	1.6
CENSUS DIVISION 4, EAST NORTH CENTRAL	726	34	4.7	24	3.3	35	4.8	21	2.9	14	1.9	71	9.8	33	4.5
Illinois	159	10	6.3	6	3.8	9	5.7	6	3.8	2	1.3	15	9.4	11	6.9
Indiana	124	2	1.6	3	2.4	3	2.4	1	0.8	1	0.8	8	6.5	2	1.6
Michigan	135	8	5.9	6	4.4	10	7.4	6	4.4	4	3.0	24	17.8	9	6.7
Ohio	161	10	6.2	5	3.1	9	5.6	5	3.1	3	1.9	18	11.2	6	3.7
Wisconsin	147	4	2.7	4	2.7	4	2.7	3	2.0	4	2.7	6	4.1	5	3.4
CENSUS DIVISION 5, EAST SOUTH CENTRAL	398	16	4.0	9	2.3	10	2.5	5	1.3	4	1.0	18	4.5	15	3.8
Alabama	106	2	1.9	1	0.9	1	0.9	1	0.9	1	0.9	4	3.8	3	2.8
Kentucky	90	5	5.6	3	3.3	3	3.3	2	2.2	2	2.2	5	5.6	4	4.4
Mississippi	112	1	0.9	1	0.9	1	0.9	0	0.0	0	0.0	2	1.8	0	0.0
Tennessee	90	8	8.9	4	4.4	5	5.6	2	2.2	1	1.1	7	7.8	8	8.9
CENSUS DIVISION 6, WEST NORTH CENTRAL	670	14	2.1	8	1.2	21	3.1	10	1.5	4	0.6	34	5.1	26	3.9
Iowa	126	1	0.8	1	0.8	3	2.4	1	0.8	1	0.8	4	3.2	6	4.8
Kansas	151	2	1.3	0	0.0	3	1.3	1	0.7	1	0.7	2	1.3	3	2.0
Minnesota	106	3	2.8	2	1.9	3	2.8	1	0.9	1	0.9	9	8.5	2	1.9
Missouri	151	5	3.3	4	2.6	8	5.3	6	4.0	2	1.3	11	7.3	9	6.0
Nebraska	60	2	3.3	1	1.7	1	1.7	1	1.7	0	0.0	3	6.7	3	5.0
North Dakota	29	0	0.0	0	0.0	0	0.0	0	0.0	0	0.0	1	3.4	1	3.4
South Dakota	47	1	2.1	0	0.0	2	4.3	0	0.0	0	0.0	3	6.4	2	4.3
CENSUS DIVISION 7, WEST SOUTH CENTRAL	900	22	2.4	16	1.8	34	3.8	18	2.0	11	1.2	36	4.0	28	3.1
Arkansas	80	3	3.8	2	2.5	3	3.8	1	1.3	0	0.0	2	2.5	1	1.3
Louisiana	118	3	2.5	1	0.8	2	1.7	1	0.8	1	0.8	8	6.8	2	1.7
Oklahoma	129	3	2.3	1	0.8	5	3.9	2	1.6	1	0.8	4	3.1	3	2.3
Texas	573	13	2.3	12	2.1	24	4.2	14	2.4	9	1.6	22	3.8	22	3.8
CENSUS DIVISION 8, MOUNTAIN	338	15	4.4	10	3.0	15	4.4	10	3.0	5	1.5	22	6.5	14	4.1
Arizona	54	4	7.4	3	5.6	4	7.4	3	5.6	2	3.7	6	11.1	4	7.4
Colorado	68	4	5.9	2	2.9	4	5.9	3	4.4	1	1.5	6	8.8	3	4.4
Idaho	35	1	2.9	0	0.0	0	0.0	0	0.0	0	0.0	2	5.7	1	2.9
Montana	55	2	3.6	1	1.8	1	1.8	1	1.8	1	1.8	3	5.5	1	1.8
Nevada	34	0	0.0	0	0.0	1	2.9	0	0.0	0	0.0	1	2.9	0	0.0
New Mexico	30	1	3.3	0	0.0	2	6.7	0	0.0	0	0.0	1	3.3	2	6.7
Utah	35	3	8.6	4	11.4	3	8.6	3	8.6	1	2.9	3	8.6	3	8.6
Wyoming	27	0	0.0	0	0.0	0	0.0	0	0.0	0	0.0	0	0.0	0	0.0
CENSUS DIVISION 9, PACIFIC	464	30	6.5	20	4.3	26	5.6	16	3.4	9	1.9	46	9.9	37	8.0
Alaska	14	0	0.0	0	0.0	0	0.0	0	0.0	0	0.0	0	0.0	0	0.0
California	296	21	7.1	15	5.1	19	6.4	12	4.1	8	2.7	36	12.2	26	8.8
Hawaii	21	1	4.8	0	0.0	0	0.0	0	0.0	0	0.0	0	0.0	2	9.5
Oregon	58	3	5.2	2	3.4	2	3.4	1	1.7	0	0.0	4	6.9	5	8.6
Washington	75	5	6.7	3	4.0	5	6.7	3	4.0	1	1.3	6	8.0	4	5.3

Table 8

Metropolitan Statistical Areas

Metropolitan Statistical Areas (MSAs) definitions announced by the U.S. Office of Management and Budget (OMB) effective June 6, 2003 were added with the 2006 edition.

According to the OMB, an MSA is a geographical designation that represents an integrated social and economic unit with a large population nucleus. Under these standards, an area qualifies for recognition as an MSA if there is a city within the area of at least 50,000 with a total metropolitan population of at least 100,000. MSAs are defined as entire counties. In addition to the county containing the main city, an MSA also includes additional counties having strong economic and social ties to the central county. Such counties must have a specified level of commuting to the central counties and must meet certain standards regarding metropolitan character, such as population density.

When an MSA encompasses two or more central cities, up to three cities may be specified in the MSA title. They will be listed in order of population size. When a single central city exists, the MSA is named for that particular city. A MSA may extend beyond a single state.

An MSA containing a single core with a population of 2.5 million or more may be subdivided to form smaller groupings of counties referred to as Metropolitan Divisions. Where they exist the Metropolitan Divisions are shown in this table rather than the entire MSA.

TABLE 8

U.S. CENSUS DIVISION 1, NEW ENGLAND

U.S. Community Hospitals
(Nonfederal, short-term general and other special hospitals)

2012 Utilization, Personnel and Finances

CLASSIFICATION	Hospitals	Beds	Admissions	Inpatient Days	Adjusted Inpatient Days	Average Daily Census	Adjusted Average Daily Census	Average Stay (days)	Surgical Operations	NEWBORNS Bassinets	NEWBORNS Births	OUTPATIENT VISITS Emergency	OUTPATIENT VISITS Total
UNITED STATES	4,999	800,566	34,422,071	185,423,035	362,159,266	507,292	990,999	5.4	26,811,231	55,987	3,715,479	133,221,030	674,971,331
Nonmetropolitan	1,980	132,450	4,000,957	25,115,368	70,833,735	68,747	193,921	6.3	4,071,289	10,624	446,664	23,768,413	125,342,725
Metropolitan.	3,019	668,116	30,421,114	160,307,667	291,325,531	438,545	797,078	5.3	22,739,942	45,363	3,268,815	109,452,617	549,628,606
CENSUS DIVISION 1, NEW ENGLAND	207	34,399	1,608,353	8,482,806	19,727,217	23,200	53,966	5.3	1,378,706	2,424	146,147	7,131,256	47,887,435
Nonmetropolitan	58	3,765	143,467	855,133	2,885,660	2,350	7,943	6.0	169,787	377	13,443	1,041,242	7,739,416
Metropolitan.	149	30,634	1,464,886	7,627,673	16,841,557	20,850	46,023	5.2	1,208,919	2,047	132,704	6,090,014	40,148,019
Connecticut	34	8,120	378,130	2,053,559	4,103,348	5,613	11,211	5.4	315,571	514	35,891	1,643,476	8,986,230
Nonmetropolitan	5	351	19,333	88,420	228,672	243	625	4.6	19,868	43	2,158	149,840	745,188
Metropolitan.	29	7,769	358,797	1,965,139	3,874,676	5,370	10,586	5.5	295,703	471	33,733	1,493,636	8,241,042
Bridgeport-Stamford-Norwalk	6	1,874	90,267	478,169	958,429	1,306	2,618	5.3	66,226	165	10,956	371,928	2,197,021
Hartford-West Hartford-East Hartford	12	2,928	139,169	816,039	1,597,726	2,229	4,365	5.9	119,930	128	12,102	531,737	3,554,692
New Haven-Milford	9	2,527	104,983	558,152	1,039,876	1,527	2,842	5.3	89,414	146	8,261	433,946	1,773,583
Norwich-New London	2	440	24,378	112,779	278,645	308	761	4.6	20,133	32	2,414	156,025	715,746
Maine	37	3,523	142,159	783,992	2,073,986	2,140	5,666	5.5	160,307	293	11,224	790,258	6,177,495
Nonmetropolitan	22	1,281	42,091	272,790	852,185	744	2,328	6.5	49,882	134	3,899	386,520	2,472,219
Metropolitan.	15	2,242	100,068	511,202	1,221,801	1,396	3,338	5.1	110,425	159	7,325	403,738	3,705,276
Bangor	4	491	28,173	127,770	267,839	350	731	4.5	30,363	20	1,726	82,603	595,100
Lewiston-Auburn	2	361	15,729	71,816	185,629	196	507	4.6	12,018	35	1,331	76,887	1,101,337
Portland-South Portland-Biddeford.	9	1,390	56,166	311,616	768,333	850	2,100	5.5	68,044	104	4,268	244,248	2,008,839
Massachusetts	83	16,233	802,312	4,130,110	9,308,103	11,293	25,438	5.1	619,144	1,099	70,702	3,164,871	22,514,418
Nonmetropolitan	2	44	2,011	6,878	48,890	19	133	3.4	2,372	10	264	25,017	110,407
Metropolitan.	81	16,189	800,301	4,123,232	9,259,213	11,274	25,305	5.2	616,772	1,089	70,438	3,139,854	22,404,011
Barnstable Town	3	414	22,469	103,055	260,001	282	711	4.6	14,425	18	1,320	130,285	943,870
Boston-Cambridge-Quincy.	50	10,728	536,887	2,798,306	6,319,821	7,650	17,274	5.2	414,617	717	47,765	1,854,666	14,349,522
Pittsfield.	3	313	16,408	73,900	206,938	202	565	4.5	15,352	26	1,087	95,378	658,209
Providence-New Bedford-Fall River	4	1,185	58,578	279,673	574,251	765	1,570	4.8	39,832	67	4,634	296,732	1,556,962
Springfield	12	1,932	78,462	452,828	947,439	1,238	2,589	5.8	61,461	114	7,131	337,269	2,284,137
Worcester.	9	1,617	87,497	415,470	950,763	1,137	2,596	4.7	71,085	147	8,501	425,524	2,611,311
New Hampshire	28	2,831	119,814	627,784	1,771,229	1,727	4,899	5.2	124,321	267	12,035	652,190	4,983,127
Nonmetropolitan	17	1,297	53,224	300,797	950,462	835	2,657	5.7	62,581	112	4,294	259,014	2,807,737
Metropolitan.	11	1,534	66,590	326,987	820,767	892	2,242	4.9	61,740	155	7,741	393,176	2,175,390
Manchester-Nashua	5	847	38,293	182,176	478,237	497	1,306	4.8	30,708	96	4,537	183,963	1,195,340
Rockingham County-Strafford County	6	687	28,297	144,811	342,530	395	936	5.1	31,032	59	3,204	209,213	980,050
Rhode Island	11	2,461	117,051	580,207	1,209,620	1,587	3,307	5.0	99,656	142	11,045	578,431	2,183,753
Metropolitan.	11	2,461	117,051	580,207	1,209,620	1,587	3,307	5.0	99,656	142	11,045	578,431	2,183,753
Providence-New Bedford-Fall River	11	2,461	117,051	580,207	1,209,620	1,587	3,307	5.0	99,656	142	11,045	578,431	2,183,753
Vermont	14	1,231	48,887	307,154	1,260,931	840	3,445	6.3	59,707	109	5,250	302,030	3,042,412
Nonmetropolitan	12	792	26,808	186,248	805,451	509	2,200	6.9	35,084	78	2,828	220,851	1,603,865
Metropolitan.	2	439	22,079	120,906	455,480	331	1,245	5.5	24,623	31	2,422	81,179	1,438,547
Burlington-South Burlington	2	439	22,079	120,906	455,480	331	1,245	5.5	24,623	31	2,422	81,179	1,438,547

2012 Utilization, Personnel and Finances

	FULL-TIME EQUIVALENT PERSONNEL				FULL-TIME EQUIV. TRAINEES			EXPENSES						
								LABOR				TOTAL		
Physicians and Dentists	Registered Nurses	Licensed Practical Nurses	Other Salaried Personnel	Total Personnel	Medical and Dental Residents	Other Trainees	Total Trainees	Payroll (in thousands)	Employee Benefits (in thousands)	Total (in thousands)	Percent of Total	Amount (in thousands)	Adjusted per Admission	Adjusted per Inpatient Day
114,479	1,351,164	82,268	3,183,037	4,730,948	102,904	7,230	110,134	$296,335,931	$81,153,797	$377,489,736	49.9	$756,916,757	$11,220.70	$2,090.01
15,188	160,970	24,883	469,925	670,966	1,935	276	2,211	35,636,252	9,721,437	45,357,688	52.4	86,549,339	7,649.75	1,221.87
99,291	1,190,194	57,385	2,713,112	4,059,982	100,969	6,954	107,923	260,699,679	71,432,359	332,132,048	49.5	670,367,418	11,940.32	2,301.09
12,938	67,046	2,497	196,510	278,991	9,287	1,277	10,564	19,205,847	5,150,662	24,356,505	51.5	47,321,636	12,289.80	2,398.80
1,593	7,663	518	24,289	34,063	457	22	479	2,339,482	643,047	2,982,528	56.0	5,325,146	10,536.00	1,845.38
11,345	59,383	1,979	172,221	244,928	8,830	1,255	10,085	16,866,365	4,507,615	21,373,977	50.9	41,996,491	12,554.79	2,493.62
1,039	14,597	370	38,334	54,340	1,591	106	1,697	3,964,949	1,201,256	5,166,206	52.7	9,795,239	12,753.54	2,387.13
54	614	42	1,768	2,478	1	0	1	209,458	59,435	268,893	53.1	505,996	9,970.17	2,212.76
985	13,983	328	36,566	51,862	1,590	106	1,696	3,755,490	1,141,821	4,897,313	52.7	9,289,243	12,950.47	2,397.42
275	2,875	37	8,171	11,358	392	12	404	947,120	294,365	1,241,485	52.9	2,345,302	12,826.02	2,447.03
505	5,235	123	15,219	21,082	162	41	203	1,515,921	457,693	1,973,615	54.4	3,627,575	13,256.36	2,270.46
130	5,115	141	10,972	16,358	1,020	31	1,051	1,032,595	315,839	1,348,435	49.0	2,753,897	13,741.73	2,648.29
75	758	27	2,204	3,064	16	22	38	259,854	73,923	333,778	59.3	562,469	9,315.01	2,018.58
1,521	7,171	262	20,271	29,225	337	7	344	1,909,870	489,955	2,399,825	54.3	4,421,718	11,678.63	2,131.99
454	2,642	131	8,221	11,448	27	5	32	674,323	172,844	847,169	55.2	1,535,543	11,133.66	1,801.89
1,067	4,529	131	12,050	17,777	310	2	312	1,235,547	317,111	1,552,656	53.8	2,886,174	11,990.90	2,362.23
279	1,235	30	2,963	4,507	41	2	43	303,006	80,993	383,998	51.9	739,565	11,982.01	2,761.23
199	575	34	1,773	2,581	21	0	21	207,836	39,865	247,701	54.4	455,357	11,261.75	2,453.05
589	2,719	67	7,314	10,689	248	0	248	724,705	196,253	920,957	54.5	1,691,252	12,207.68	2,201.20
7,750	32,608	1,222	99,531	141,111	5,873	1,060	6,933	9,403,023	2,355,418	11,758,439	48.8	24,080,576	12,687.49	2,587.06
40	79		339	462	0	0	0	44,385	8,580	52,965	62.1	85,325	5,732.28	1,745.24
7,710	32,529	1,218	99,192	140,649	5,873	1,060	6,933	9,358,638	2,346,838	11,705,474	48.8	23,995,251	12,742.47	2,591.50
52	560	14	1,709	2,335	0	2	2	227,467	76,953	304,420	54.3	560,535	9,595.25	2,155.90
6,097	23,536	800	72,368	102,801	4,814	998	5,812	6,826,488	1,668,114	8,494,600	47.3	17,954,151	14,144.61	2,840.93
80	608	52	1,875	2,615	76	5	81	200,429	51,635	252,063	60.0	419,874	8,937.86	2,028.98
51	1,939	61	4,830	6,881	9	1	10	498,511	128,503	627,015	58.4	1,074,032	8,863.77	1,870.32
478	2,997	141	8,793	12,409	379	4	383	726,773	169,578	896,352	51.6	1,735,902	9,777.42	1,832.20
952	2,889	150	9,617	13,608	595	50	645	878,970	252,054	1,131,024	50.3	2,250,757	10,735.42	2,367.32
1,175	5,997	344	18,882	26,398	438	13	451	1,742,303	494,985	2,237,287	55.6	4,024,998	11,876.90	2,272.43
810	3,099	205	9,798	13,912	418	13	431	1,008,063	285,362	1,293,423	57.9	2,233,615	13,505.96	2,350.03
365	2,898	139	9,084	12,486	20	0	20	734,240	209,623	943,864	52.7	1,791,383	10,324.20	2,182.57
291	1,626	82	5,084	7,083	11	0	11	402,705	119,988	522,693	53.4	977,957	9,633.43	2,044.92
74	1,272	57	4,000	5,403	9	0	9	331,535	89,635	421,171	51.8	813,426	11,298.21	2,374.76
710	4,045	100	11,205	16,060	731	3	734	1,317,059	365,068	1,682,126	54.8	3,067,815	12,433.49	2,536.18
710	4,045	100	11,205	16,060	731	3	734	1,317,059	365,068	1,682,126	54.8	3,067,815	12,433.49	2,536.18
710	4,045	100	11,205	16,060	731	3	734	1,317,059	365,068	1,682,126	54.8	3,067,815	12,433.49	2,536.18
743	2,628	199	8,287	11,857	317	88	405	868,643	243,979	1,112,622	57.6	1,931,291	8,769.98	1,531.64
235	1,229	136	4,163	5,763	11	4	15	403,253	116,825	520,078	53.9	964,667	7,067.72	1,197.67
508	1,399	63	4,124	6,094	306	84	390	465,390	127,154	592,544	61.3	966,624	11,544.95	2,122.21
508	1,399	63	4,124	6,094	306	84	390	465,390	127,154	592,544	61.3	966,624	11,544.95	2,122.21

MSAs

TABLE 8

U.S. CENSUS DIVISION 2, MIDDLE ATLANTIC

U.S. Community Hospitals
(Nonfederal, short-term general and other special hospitals)

2012 Utilization, Personnel and Finances

MSAs

CLASSIFICATION	Hospitals	Beds	Admissions	Inpatient Days	Adjusted Inpatient Days	Average Daily Census	Adjusted Average Daily Census	Average Stay (days)	Surgical Operations	NEWBORNS Bassinets	Births	OUTPATIENT VISITS Emergency	Total
UNITED STATES	4,999	800,566	34,422,071	185,423,035	362,159,266	507,292	990,999	5.4	26,811,231	55,987	3,715,479	133,221,030	674,971,331
Nonmetropolitan	1,980	132,450	4,000,957	25,115,368	70,833,735	68,747	193,921	6.3	4,071,289	10,624	446,664	23,768,413	125,342,725
Metropolitan	3,019	668,116	30,421,114	160,307,667	291,325,531	438,545	797,078	5.3	22,739,942	45,363	3,268,815	109,452,617	549,628,606
CENSUS DIVISION 2, MIDDLE ATLANTIC.	447	117,624	5,183,982	31,440,731	56,730,915	85,976	155,137	6.1	4,008,706	6,401	468,787	18,321,971	111,261,973
Nonmetropolitan	85	10,652	334,663	2,415,048	6,452,292	6,609	17,646	7.2	368,744	676	29,400	1,738,876	12,739,323
Metropolitan	362	106,972	4,849,319	29,025,683	50,278,623	79,367	137,491	6.0	3,639,962	5,725	439,387	16,583,095	98,522,650
New Jersey	77	21,162	1,047,545	5,370,619	8,461,664	14,679	23,130	5.1	624,801	1,409	101,599	3,703,899	15,587,498
Metropolitan	77	21,162	1,047,545	5,370,619	8,461,664	14,679	23,130	5.1	624,801	1,409	101,599	3,703,899	15,587,498
Allentown-Bethlehem-Easton	2	251	10,872	46,263	103,440	127	283	4.3	16,437	12	866	43,566	173,631
Atlantic City	4	842	43,309	209,537	346,995	572	949	4.8	18,148	56	3,558	180,350	420,093
Camden	10	2,803	145,584	695,898	1,084,418	1,902	2,963	4.8	80,350	145	12,163	566,473	1,517,865
Edison.	17	4,931	244,932	1,272,170	1,919,219	3,478	5,245	5.2	133,172	398	25,539	808,968	2,637,688
New York-White Plains-Wayne. . .	13	4,327	240,484	1,036,029	1,560,239	2,831	4,265	4.3	137,885	302	23,806	759,320	5,384,660
Newark-Union	19	5,843	263,392	1,597,840	2,533,519	4,368	6,928	6.1	164,774	341	26,833	944,322	3,425,285
Ocean City	1	180	9,271	34,370	63,335	94	173	3.7	4,306	16	533	47,206	167,428
Trenton-Ewing	6	1,346	61,833	326,047	585,370	890	1,600	5.3	47,344	91	5,019	225,318	1,434,376
Vineland-Millville-Bridgeton	2	372	18,926	98,404	178,125	269	486	5.2	15,125	24	2,016	87,175	309,878
Wilmington	3	267	8,942	54,061	87,004	148	238	6.0	7,260	24	1,266	41,201	116,594
New York	178	57,148	2,444,350	16,783,079	30,426,945	45,921	83,252	6.9	1,925,307	3,117	232,967	8,379,030	56,643,838
Nonmetropolitan	38	4,860	139,517	1,215,166	3,383,441	3,327	9,261	8.7	158,557	294	13,936	750,628	5,835,783
Metropolitan	140	52,288	2,304,833	15,567,913	27,043,504	42,594	73,991	6.8	1,766,750	2,823	219,031	7,628,402	50,808,055
Albany-Schenectady-Troy	9	2,401	107,545	710,856	1,389,677	1,942	3,799	6.6	91,332	112	8,180	371,379	2,645,164
Binghamton	2	610	27,493	145,099	388,776	397	1,062	5.3	33,917	46	2,795	105,578	2,113,755
Buffalo-Niagara Falls.	10	4,440	151,837	1,404,162	2,302,931	3,837	6,293	9.2	155,931	219	13,442	489,354	3,637,862
Elmira	2	456	15,803	116,365	220,920	319	604	7.4	11,549	20	1,187	93,661	483,867
Glens Falls	1	300	15,702	77,831	135,510	213	370	5.0	15,085	22	1,393	53,110	823,658
Ithaca	1	193	6,344	29,635	100,883	81	276	4.7	7,415	19	900	31,946	201,283
Kingston	3	295	13,601	72,543	118,761	198	325	5.3	7,468	13	466	47,207	171,703
Nassau-Suffolk	24	8,760	408,595	2,725,541	4,387,068	7,498	12,063	6.7	315,615	485	36,528	1,129,592	5,693,231
New York-White Plains-Wayne. . .	60	27,495	1,244,364	8,258,503	13,907,353	22,568	38,015	6.6	861,452	1,393	123,458	4,225,766	24,328,239
Poughkeepsie-Newburgh-Middle-town	7	1,460	68,530	364,319	608,350	995	1,664	5.3	54,258	99	7,168	263,958	1,065,488
Rochester.	10	3,007	122,164	861,112	1,907,708	2,353	5,214	7.0	114,879	192	11,669	432,947	6,194,213
Syracuse	6	1,895	86,128	538,723	958,604	1,474	2,620	6.3	68,747	131	8,237	254,528	2,176,256
Utica-Rome	5	976	36,627	263,224	616,963	719	1,686	7.2	29,102	72	3,608	129,376	1,273,336
Pennsylvania	192	39,314	1,692,087	9,287,033	17,842,306	25,376	48,755	5.5	1,458,598	1,875	134,221	6,239,042	39,030,637
Nonmetropolitan	47	5,792	195,146	1,199,882	3,068,851	3,282	8,385	6.1	210,187	382	15,464	988,248	6,903,540
Metropolitan	145	33,522	1,496,941	8,087,151	14,773,455	22,094	40,370	5.4	1,248,411	1,493	118,757	5,250,794	32,127,097
Allentown-Bethlehem-Easton	9	2,279	108,841	605,732	1,126,645	1,654	3,077	5.6	68,490	87	8,841	382,815	2,176,469
Altoona	4	530	22,713	119,643	249,491	327	681	5.3	26,825	30	1,582	86,630	542,471
Erie	6	1,202	41,058	228,282	392,904	624	1,074	5.6	32,629	73	3,239	164,705	598,111
Harrisburg-Carlisle	9	1,770	80,585	440,608	774,772	1,203	2,116	5.5	70,796	74	7,080	297,921	2,024,006
Johnstown	3	624	25,453	148,646	277,281	406	757	5.1	26,998	14	1,351	78,927	551,620
Lancaster	4	1,041	47,290	222,855	449,477	609	1,228	4.7	52,357	84	5,921	176,443	1,905,843
Lebanon	1	164	8,139	40,537	102,368	111	280	5.0	9,273	19	847	54,272	276,694
Philadelphia	46	12,204	595,281	3,038,608	5,123,724	8,299	14,002	5.1	454,646	568	48,328	1,938,148	10,097,660
Pittsburgh.	36	8,876	367,585	2,146,565	3,932,109	5,867	10,747	5.8	357,514	304	23,511	1,209,317	8,298,202
Reading.	3	959	39,294	222,341	420,756	608	1,150	5.7	23,785	56	4,384	173,929	1,170,570
Scranton--Wilkes-Barre	12	1,803	75,862	403,988	784,039	1,104	2,143	5.3	52,064	55	5,668	318,726	2,021,095
State College	2	285	12,916	61,567	131,032	168	358	4.8	11,542	5	1,340	50,796	243,422
Williamsport	3	388	13,390	105,235	272,915	287	745	7.9	18,748	22	1,195	75,965	275,724
York-Hanover	4	848	38,846	202,921	449,029	555	1,228	5.2	22,378	73	4,172	149,522	1,276,267
Youngstown-Warren-Boardman . .	3	549	19,688	99,623	286,913	272	784	5.1	20,366	29	1,298	92,678	668,943

TABLE 8

U.S. CENSUS DIVISION 2, MIDDLE ATLANTIC

U.S. Community Hospitals
(Nonfederal, short-term general and other special hospitals)

2012 Utilization, Personnel and Finances

FULL-TIME EQUIVALENT PERSONNEL					FULL-TIME EQUIV. TRAINEES			EXPENSES						
								LABOR				TOTAL		
Physicians and Dentists	Registered Nurses	Licensed Practical Nurses	Other Salaried Personnel	Total Personnel	Medical and Dental Residents	Other Trainees	Total Trainees	Payroll (in thousands)	Employee Benefits (in thousands)	Total (in thousands)	Percent of Total	Amount (in thousands)	Adjusted per Admission	Adjusted per Inpatient Day
114,479	1,351,164	82,268	3,183,037	4,730,948	102,904	7,230	110,134	$296,335,931	$81,153,797	$377,489,736	49.9	$756,916,757	$11,220.70	$2,090.01
15,188	160,970	24,883	469,925	670,966	1,935	276	2,211	35,636,252	9,721,437	45,357,688	52.4	86,549,339	7,649.75	1,221.87
99,291	1,190,194	57,385	2,713,112	4,059,982	100,969	6,954	107,923	260,699,679	71,432,359	332,132,048	49.5	670,367,418	11,940.32	2,301.09
24,443	194,980	10,364	508,530	738,317	28,871	1,016	29,887	49,007,632	14,408,862	63,416,499	53.2	119,193,201	12,760.79	2,101.03
1,602	12,207	2,066	39,226	55,101	568	21	589	2,892,308	797,242	3,689,552	52.5	7,026,289	7,779.91	1,088.96
22,841	182,773	8,298	469,304	683,216	28,303	995	29,298	46,115,324	13,611,620	59,726,947	53.2	112,166,912	13,293.94	2,230.91
2,449	34,535	907	82,158	120,049	2,526	59	2,585	8,286,040	2,104,227	10,390,269	52.5	19,790,865	11,973.29	2,338.89
2,449	34,535	907	82,158	120,049	2,526	59	2,585	8,286,040	2,104,227	10,390,269	52.5	19,790,865	11,973.29	2,338.89
26	431	29	1,239	1,725	22	1	23	88,123	22,674	110,796	51.3	216,178	8,948.16	2,089.89
98	1,729	27	3,667	5,521	41	2	43	360,594	117,142	477,736	53.8	888,584	12,423.58	2,560.80
332	4,743	115	10,411	15,601	112	7	119	999,549	262,285	1,261,834	47.2	2,672,154	11,887.81	2,464.14
364	8,212	218	17,897	26,691	430	9	439	1,871,498	475,544	2,347,043	52.1	4,506,233	12,148.47	2,347.95
692	7,253	131	18,645	26,721	560	30	590	1,906,856	460,005	2,366,862	52.6	4,497,810	12,358.29	2,882.77
707	9,109	236	22,173	32,225	1,190	4	1,194	2,332,669	561,360	2,894,029	55.5	5,217,546	12,590.48	2,059.41
0	230	3	655	888	0	2	2	49,320	19,334	68,654	60.8	112,831	6,604.51	1,781.50
225	2,036	84	5,779	8,124	102	4	106	472,469	122,263	594,732	49.7	1,196,264	10,470.58	2,043.60
0	486	30	1,073	1,589	65	0	65	141,916	47,180	189,096	56.7	333,497	9,330.67	1,872.26
5	306	34	619	964	4	0	4	63,047	16,440	79,487	53.1	149,767	9,306.32	1,721.38
14,386	92,139	5,802	266,227	378,554	17,837	404	18,241	26,944,762	8,587,460	35,532,226	57.2	62,122,861	14,129.32	2,041.71
795	4,680	970	17,701	24,146	79	1	80	1,352,813	349,929	1,702,743	58.4	2,913,431	7,423.23	861.09
13,591	87,459	4,832	248,526	354,408	17,758	403	18,161	25,591,949	8,237,531	33,829,483	57.1	59,209,430	14,786.61	2,189.41
247	4,348	245	11,809	16,649	461	1	462	882,758	180,227	1,062,984	50.1	2,122,565	10,454.18	1,527.38
96	1,071	146	3,698	5,011	86	0	86	299,878	87,273	387,150	51.3	754,718	9,789.07	1,941.27
402	6,543	436	14,509	21,890	93	80	173	1,404,833	560,411	1,965,245	57.6	3,411,490	13,658.36	1,481.37
48	680	64	1,814	2,606	25	1	26	124,139	36,655	160,794	50.6	317,543	10,716.21	1,437.36
57	754	31	1,706	2,548	35	4	39	139,000	38,664	177,664	59.0	301,000	11,010.32	2,221.24
10	338	2	806	1,156	1	0	1	60,308	22,344	82,652	50.9	162,428	7,521.21	1,610.06
4	397	24	1,084	1,509	5	1	6	78,716	21,972	100,688	51.2	196,773	8,952.77	1,656.88
4,043	15,322	474	46,831	66,670	4,112	31	4,143	4,592,591	1,399,617	5,992,208	59.0	10,154,955	15,490.88	2,314.75
7,441	45,093	2,315	134,383	189,232	11,802	276	12,078	15,105,769	5,001,324	20,107,095	57.3	35,096,502	16,585.38	2,523.59
79	2,180	63	4,851	7,173	28	3	31	484,288	174,037	658,325	50.2	1,311,592	11,499.85	2,155.98
956	5,811	501	15,273	22,541	656	6	662	1,314,592	354,463	1,669,055	57.2	2,887,414	10,928.23	1,513.55
102	3,575	347	7,741	11,765	419	0	419	800,828	276,319	1,077,147	59.5	1,810,631	12,433.95	1,888.82
106	1,347	184	4,021	5,658	35	0	35	304,250	84,226	388,476	57.0	681,818	8,711.66	1,105.12
7,608	68,306	3,655	160,145	239,714	8,508	553	9,061	13,776,830	3,717,175	17,494,004	46.9	37,279,476	11,327.95	2,089.39
807	7,527	1,096	21,525	30,955	489	20	509	1,539,496	447,314	1,986,809	48.3	4,112,859	8,054.05	1,340.19
6,801	60,779	2,559	138,620	208,759	8,019	533	8,552	12,237,335	3,269,861	15,507,195	46.8	33,166,618	11,929.27	2,245.01
612	4,566	129	9,857	15,164	485	70	555	795,770	201,536	997,307	46.3	2,155,893	10,996.14	1,913.55
34	882	71	1,767	2,754	25	0	25	170,124	50,365	220,488	53.7	410,864	8,041.02	1,646.81
141	1,628	98	3,322	5,189	87	16	103	248,178	65,292	313,471	44.9	698,026	9,769.16	1,776.58
871	3,336	295	10,193	14,695	694	133	827	760,401	208,723	969,122	49.0	1,977,795	13,662.48	2,552.74
15	955	96	2,527	3,593	82	0	82	162,781	46,189	208,971	52.2	399,953	8,135.74	1,442.41
191	1,809	120	5,088	7,208	59	5	64	445,400	152,018	597,418	52.2	1,143,569	11,690.43	2,544.22
26	248	29	935	1,238	0	0	0	57,705	16,061	73,765	44.3	166,388	8,095.53	1,625.39
3,404	24,547	504	52,802	81,257	4,854	221	5,075	5,614,258	1,453,575	7,067,835	49.0	14,422,979	14,185.88	2,814.94
1,104	15,593	490	34,024	51,211	1,352	83	1,435	2,480,926	644,276	3,125,201	40.9	7,633,463	10,860.70	1,941.32
258	1,460	143	4,656	6,517	90	2	92	351,734	95,370	447,103	49.5	902,660	12,018.64	2,145.33
51	2,499	299	5,479	8,328	69	1	70	446,504	111,788	558,293	42.4	1,316,751	8,623.13	1,679.45
2	390	23	1,043	1,458	0	0	0	121,161	32,652	153,813	52.1	295,262	10,554.51	2,253.36
12	554	93	1,166	1,825	28	0	28	107,513	26,895	134,408	44.1	304,594	10,217.18	1,116.08
57	1,627	110	4,006	5,800	194	0	194	355,008	122,658	477,666	49.0	974,668	11,151.04	2,170.61
23	685	59	1,755	2,522	0	2	2	119,872	42,462	162,334	44.6	363,754	6,403.44	1,267.82

MSAs

TABLE 8

U.S. CENSUS DIVISION 3, SOUTH ATLANTIC

U.S. Community Hospitals
(Nonfederal, short-term general and other special hospitals)

2012 Utilization, Personnel and Finances

CLASSIFICATION	Hospitals	Beds	Admissions	Inpatient Days	Adjusted Inpatient Days	Average Daily Census	Adjusted Average Daily Census	Average Stay (days)	Surgical Operations	NEWBORNS		OUTPATIENT VISITS	
										Bassinets	Births	Emergency	Total
UNITED STATES	4,999	800,566	34,422,071	185,423,035	362,159,266	507,292	990,999	5.4	26,811,231	55,987	3,715,479	133,221,030	674,971,331
Nonmetropolitan	1,980	132,450	4,000,957	25,115,368	70,833,735	68,747	193,921	6.3	4,071,289	10,624	446,664	23,768,413	125,342,725
Metropolitan	3,019	668,116	30,421,114	160,307,667	291,325,531	438,545	797,078	5.3	22,739,942	45,363	3,268,815	109,452,617	549,628,606
CENSUS DIVISION 3, SOUTH ATLANTIC	766	156,937	6,928,298	37,724,388	70,506,190	103,120	192,757	5.4	5,198,453	10,242	690,305	26,665,515	101,520,652
Nonmetropolitan	240	23,039	790,288	4,855,874	11,964,682	13,273	32,729	6.1	742,573	1,696	74,637	4,633,140	17,188,438
Metropolitan	526	133,898	6,138,010	32,868,514	58,541,508	89,847	160,028	5.4	4,455,880	8,546	615,668	22,032,375	84,332,214
Delaware	7	1,998	104,803	526,678	992,431	1,439	2,713	5.0	96,406	88	11,358	437,706	2,091,304
Nonmetropolitan	2	253	14,059	55,611	125,722	152	344	4.0	16,329	23	1,753	87,866	611,380
Metropolitan	5	1,745	90,744	471,067	866,709	1,287	2,369	5.2	80,077	65	9,605	349,840	1,479,924
Dover	1	316	17,307	90,473	201,979	247	552	5.2	13,508	13	2,236	83,467	565,884
Wilmington	4	1,429	73,437	380,594	664,730	1,040	1,817	5.2	66,569	52	7,369	266,373	914,040
District of Columbia	11	3,617	132,539	933,177	1,517,018	2,549	4,147	7.0	105,785	220	13,783	499,154	2,460,221
Metropolitan	11	3,617	132,539	933,177	1,517,018	2,549	4,147	7.0	105,785	220	13,783	499,154	2,460,221
Washington-Arlington-Alexandria	11	3,617	132,539	933,177	1,517,018	2,549	4,147	7.0	105,785	220	13,783	499,154	2,460,221
Florida	216	53,785	2,472,181	12,372,261	20,795,147	33,825	56,856	5.0	1,411,315	2,794	196,681	8,126,914	23,494,285
Nonmetropolitan	30	1,990	97,374	417,224	935,620	1,141	2,559	4.3	62,632	105	4,804	448,178	1,341,605
Metropolitan	186	51,795	2,374,807	11,955,037	19,859,527	32,684	54,297	5.0	1,348,683	2,689	191,877	7,678,736	22,152,680
Cape Coral-Fort Myers	4	1,563	80,119	412,287	751,516	1,127	2,053	5.1	40,576	129	6,374	184,189	486,359
Deltona-Daytona Beach-Ormond Beach	5	1,236	56,947	270,591	496,622	740	1,357	4.8	36,239	59	4,036	301,625	698,201
Fort Lauderdale-Pompano Beach-Deerfield Beach	20	5,724	242,696	1,220,739	2,010,416	3,337	5,494	5.0	119,910	252	21,481	892,692	2,294,655
Fort Walton Beach-Crestview-Destin	3	424	21,070	90,614	148,912	248	408	4.3	11,020	32	1,567	89,597	233,568
Gainesville	3	1,435	66,431	377,117	555,514	1,031	1,518	5.7	52,400	49	5,587	103,783	879,887
Jacksonville	13	3,964	188,778	980,162	1,662,155	2,678	4,546	5.2	132,451	294	17,206	605,633	1,891,332
Lakeland	5	1,744	74,568	333,388	603,350	912	1,650	4.5	38,175	52	5,793	288,669	624,003
Miami-Miami Beach-Kendall	26	7,590	312,790	1,675,717	2,753,812	4,581	7,528	5.4	160,209	357	25,615	963,541	3,080,212
Naples-Marco Island	2	754	34,212	149,431	230,677	409	631	4.4	14,398	36	2,961	106,213	339,384
North Port-Bradenton-Sarasota	8	1,865	77,539	383,893	640,385	1,050	1,753	5.0	44,183	59	4,456	259,346	931,444
Ocala	3	721	37,743	170,646	275,972	467	755	4.5	19,400	26	2,550	140,820	253,374
Orlando-Kissimmee	11	5,642	296,752	1,478,771	2,367,548	4,041	6,469	5.0	164,035	428	28,928	1,009,332	2,468,282
Palm Bay-Melbourne-Titusville	7	1,371	58,631	314,595	525,366	860	1,437	5.4	35,873	88	4,734	160,181	666,151
Palm Coast	1	99	6,752	26,701	67,221	73	184	4.0	5,933	0	0	40,119	63,149
Panama City-Lynn Haven	4	554	29,383	145,868	249,468	398	682	5.0	18,765	28	2,740	116,606	300,137
Pensacola-Ferry Pass-Brent	7	1,429	66,219	310,376	571,682	848	1,564	4.7	40,795	69	6,571	283,066	967,825
Port St. Lucie-Fort Pierce	3	846	45,615	206,104	352,740	564	965	4.5	29,704	50	3,940	138,675	236,394
Punta Gorda	3	636	26,770	134,014	210,426	367	575	5.0	20,594	8	827	56,857	144,925
Sebastian-Vero Beach	3	450	20,815	103,577	158,285	283	432	5.0	12,446	22	1,057	65,848	195,328
Tallahassee	4	792	41,403	204,836	361,939	559	990	4.9	22,041	62	4,475	104,345	656,584
Tampa-St. Petersburg-Clearwater	37	9,230	407,811	2,105,541	3,414,259	5,759	9,337	5.2	240,873	407	27,745	1,319,077	3,314,723
West Palm Beach-Boca Raton-Boynton Beach	14	3,726	181,763	860,069	1,451,262	2,352	3,969	4.7	88,663	182	13,234	448,522	1,426,763
Georgia	148	24,657	953,817	5,970,497	11,802,725	16,332	32,297	6.3	732,200	1,881	119,564	4,153,101	15,034,217
Nonmetropolitan	62	5,870	141,134	1,296,214	3,192,949	3,551	8,759	9.2	148,509	377	17,844	917,333	3,134,890
Metropolitan	86	18,787	812,683	4,674,283	8,609,776	12,781	23,538	5.8	583,691	1,504	101,720	3,235,768	11,899,327
Albany	3	567	22,604	124,243	228,180	341	625	5.5	15,491	42	1,419	146,164	817,096
Athens-Clarke County	2	508	27,435	117,373	229,382	321	627	4.3	23,018	52	3,543	98,296	413,450
Atlanta-Sandy Springs-Marietta	44	9,911	442,639	2,580,090	4,637,289	7,054	12,679	5.8	306,737	832	64,574	1,743,803	6,024,228
Augusta-Richmond County	8	1,565	63,081	367,481	634,645	1,003	1,735	5.8	62,401	120	6,180	282,724	1,084,921
Brunswick	1	366	11,736	133,130	284,463	364	777	11.3	9,742	9	1,301	50,980	190,528
Chattanooga	1	185	6,191	61,301	131,060	168	359	9.9	5,223	15	749	23,314	101,518
Columbus	5	1,139	38,532	221,406	401,769	606	1,099	5.7	24,151	31	2,208	100,630	382,961
Dalton	2	263	12,268	43,856	98,453	120	269	3.6	4,645	40	1,780	85,855	283,374
Gainesville	1	513	26,974	114,788	203,652	314	556	4.3	17,575	64	3,553	103,993	341,148
Hinesville-Fort Stewart	1	133	2,253	8,742	18,690	24	51	3.9	717	6	536	6,950	30,264
Macon	5	1,072	48,101	259,373	439,423	710	1,202	5.4	25,567	96	3,454	121,150	530,954
Rome	3	574	25,877	134,417	254,208	368	695	5.2	19,207	30	2,200	110,355	340,063
Savannah	5	1,223	51,202	383,883	650,911	890	1,778	6.4	40,855	71	5,849	194,519	792,268
Valdosta	3	492	18,114	111,470	238,081	305	650	6.2	14,489	62	2,228	84,407	274,793
Warner Robins	2	276	15,676	70,730	159,570	193	436	4.5	13,873	34	2,146	82,628	291,761

TABLE 8

U.S. CENSUS DIVISION 3, SOUTH ATLANTIC

U.S. Community Hospitals
(Nonfederal, short-term general and other special hospitals)

2012 Utilization, Personnel and Finances

FULL-TIME EQUIVALENT PERSONNEL					FULL-TIME EQUIV. TRAINEES			EXPENSES						
								LABOR				TOTAL		
Physicians and Dentists	Registered Nurses	Licensed Practical Nurses	Other Salaried Personnel	Total Personnel	Medical and Dental Residents	Other Trainees	Total Trainees	Payroll (in thousands)	Employee Benefits (in thousands)	Total (in thousands)	Percent of Total	Amount (in thousands)	Adjusted per Admission	Adjusted per Inpatient Day
114,479	1,351,164	82,268	3,183,037	4,730,948	102,904	7,230	110,134	$296,335,931	$81,153,797	$377,489,736	49.9	$756,916,757	$11,220.70	$2,090.01
15,188	160,970	24,883	469,925	670,966	1,935	276	2,211	35,636,252	9,721,437	45,357,688	52.4	86,549,339	7,649.75	1,221.87
99,291	1,190,194	57,385	2,713,112	4,059,982	100,969	6,954	107,923	260,699,679	71,432,359	332,132,048	49.5	670,367,418	11,940.32	2,301.09
15,871	262,733	14,441	576,734	869,779	16,751	669	17,420	50,866,182	12,696,661	63,562,844	47.8	132,934,775	10,228.36	1,885.43
1,689	28,233	3,785	74,007	107,714	216	27	243	5,544,722	1,422,076	6,966,796	51.3	13,567,955	6,989.12	1,134.00
14,182	234,500	10,656	502,727	762,065	16,535	642	17,177	45,321,460	11,274,585	56,596,048	47.4	119,366,821	10,797.16	2,039.01
656	5,082	202	12,081	18,021	356	3	359	1,135,392	359,204	1,494,595	56.1	2,662,273	13,383.90	2,682.58
52	698	11	1,595	2,356	0	0	0	131,696	48,072	179,768	49.3	364,419	11,392.36	2,898.61
604	4,384	191	10,486	15,665	356	3	359	1,003,695	311,132	1,314,827	57.2	2,297,854	13,765.54	2,651.24
42	721	46	1,982	2,791	0	0	0	175,939	51,866	227,805	52.6	432,778	11,201.14	2,142.69
562	3,663	145	8,504	12,874	356	3	359	827,756	259,266	1,087,022	58.3	1,865,076	14,537.85	2,805.76
1,416	6,305	267	15,071	23,059	1,545	25	1,570	1,712,717	346,071	2,058,786	52.3	3,937,621	18,061.24	2,595.63
1,416	6,305	267	15,071	23,059	1,545	25	1,570	1,712,717	346,071	2,058,786	52.3	3,937,621	18,061.24	2,595.63
1,416	6,305	267	15,071	23,059	1,545	25	1,570	1,712,717	346,071	2,058,786	52.3	3,937,621	18,061.24	2,595.63
3,970	83,919	3,936	169,980	261,805	4,953	187	5,140	15,308,776	3,724,517	19,033,293	46.6	40,816,430	9,713.88	1,962.79
178	2,622	348	6,576	9,724	26	3	29	702,100	113,959	816,060	61.8	1,320,479	6,286.08	1,411.34
3,792	81,297	3,588	163,404	252,081	4,927	184	5,111	14,606,676	3,610,557	18,217,233	46.1	39,495,952	9,894.26	1,988.77
217	2,830	174	6,842	10,063	524	35	559	609,524	189,267	798,791	51.6	1,548,223	10,557.48	2,060.13
151	1,913	123	5,163	7,350	35	0	35	371,350	108,059	479,409	51.0	939,980	8,928.29	1,892.75
596	7,935	284	14,399	23,214	256	4	260	1,416,751	316,746	1,733,497	47.1	3,676,878	8,964.28	1,828.91
22	541	35	984	1,582	11	0	11	80,435	18,272	98,707	46.4	212,616	6,073.02	1,427.80
14	2,658	82	5,700	8,454	515	4	519	468,580	123,820	592,400	42.3	1,401,107	14,121.78	2,522.18
480	6,632	161	11,837	19,110	565	42	607	1,034,645	323,832	1,358,477	42.2	3,215,737	9,859.20	1,934.68
27	2,444	144	5,412	8,027	9	0	9	403,204	85,941	489,143	51.0	958,194	7,092.59	1,588.12
546	11,773	532	24,639	37,490	1,576	29	1,605	2,409,004	560,242	2,969,248	46.1	6,443,043	12,459.79	2,339.68
4	1,181	52	1,944	3,181	1	0	1	175,386	34,344	209,731	46.8	448,549	8,497.18	1,944.49
35	2,869	182	5,082	8,168	56	2	58	417,580	103,388	520,968	47.2	1,103,838	8,314.03	1,723.71
24	1,310	55	2,319	3,708	16	1	17	201,479	46,965	248,444	46.9	530,206	8,651.62	1,921.23
571	12,303	369	24,492	37,735	475	5	480	1,942,255	510,154	2,452,408	42.1	5,821,121	12,317.88	2,458.71
60	1,433	67	4,445	6,005	16	12	28	366,878	90,334	457,213	55.8	819,123	8,037.95	1,559.15
41	177	1	565	784	0	0	0	38,456	11,941	50,397	47.5	106,164	6,245.32	1,579.33
16	777	89	1,404	2,286	0	0	0	147,650	33,086	180,737	44.1	409,760	7,689.83	1,642.54
75	2,102	93	4,102	6,372	59	7	66	316,781	53,801	370,582	37.6	985,492	8,002.44	1,723.85
92	1,090	68	2,834	4,084	21	0	21	247,425	60,136	307,561	50.3	611,493	7,791.60	1,733.55
15	741	56	1,393	2,205	20	0	20	132,948	27,765	160,712	44.3	363,027	8,622.76	1,725.20
51	633	32	1,365	2,081	0	0	0	119,882	26,944	146,826	54.2	270,755	8,124.70	1,710.56
102	1,378	107	2,885	4,472	57	0	57	253,681	67,038	320,719	52.3	613,285	8,197.03	1,694.44
560	14,042	657	27,065	42,324	607	41	648	2,511,878	592,096	3,103,975	47.3	6,564,281	9,864.91	1,922.61
93	4,535	225	8,533	13,386	108	2	110	940,904	226,385	1,167,288	47.6	2,453,079	7,959.06	1,690.31
1,642	36,320	3,168	82,690	123,820	1,156	73	1,229	6,879,634	1,766,117	8,645,752	48.9	17,663,915	9,488.27	1,496.60
351	5,536	1,224	15,420	22,531	46	5	51	1,027,801	284,508	1,312,310	50.9	2,580,086	7,265.70	808.06
1,291	30,784	1,944	67,270	101,289	1,110	68	1,178	5,851,833	1,481,609	7,333,442	48.6	15,083,829	10,012.14	1,751.94
95	1,055	51	2,472	3,673	78	5	83	228,023	62,513	290,535	50.7	572,612	13,818.52	2,509.47
24	912	37	2,401	3,374	6	0	6	200,072	60,994	261,067	49.9	522,931	9,766.01	2,279.74
691	16,945	864	36,390	54,890	529	49	578	3,155,208	761,609	3,916,817	48.5	8,073,234	9,936.31	1,740.94
20	2,603	238	5,145	8,006	8	0	8	486,533	117,959	604,493	44.9	1,345,548	12,198.87	2,120.16
74	346	47	1,039	1,506	0	0	0	112,436	30,657	143,093	53.7	266,582	10,630.55	937.14
22	234	25	649	930	11	1	12	45,628	15,382	61,011	54.9	111,146	8,397.28	848.06
131	1,332	82	2,974	4,519	52	3	55	260,280	65,279	325,559	48.8	667,572	9,147.58	1,661.58
3	342	40	761	1,146	0	0	0	84,223	22,013	106,235	49.1	216,511	6,554.97	2,199.13
94	738	23	1,728	2,583	119	5	124	192,540	52,208	244,748	47.2	518,110	10,826.45	2,544.10
12	117	13	328	470	6	1	7	18,180	6,129	24,309	54.9	44,285	9,193.46	2,369.44
13	1,758	92	3,674	5,537	126	0	126	314,197	90,521	404,718	48.9	828,365	10,336.08	1,885.12
73	896	104	2,249	3,322	36	0	36	190,097	49,847	239,945	50.7	473,099	9,391.17	1,861.07
20	1,996	138	4,427	6,581	131	4	135	359,174	75,929	435,102	48.8	891,677	9,923.29	1,369.89
17	820	77	1,739	2,653	0	0	0	115,286	43,682	158,968	48.3	328,902	9,135.14	1,381.47
2	690	113	1,294	2,099	8	0	8	89,956	26,886	116,842	52.3	223,255	6,307.35	1,399.10

Table continues

MSAs

TABLE 8

U.S. CENSUS DIVISION 3, SOUTH ATLANTIC
CONTINUED

U.S. Community Hospitals
(Nonfederal, short-term general and other special hospitals)

2012 Utilization, Personnel and Finances

CLASSIFICATION	Hospitals	Beds	Admissions	Inpatient Days	Adjusted Inpatient Days	Average Daily Census	Adjusted Average Daily Census	Average Stay (days)	Surgical Operations	NEWBORNS Bassinets	Births	OUTPATIENT VISITS Emergency	Total
Maryland.	50	12,271	659,128	3,230,567	5,556,376	8,842	15,201	4.9	542,080	928	67,554	2,552,154	9,796,328
Nonmetropolitan	6	407	26,638	99,781	235,791	274	645	3.7	37,640	46	2,531	202,625	980,232
Metropolitan.	44	11,864	632,490	3,130,786	5,320,585	8,568	14,556	4.9	504,440	882	65,023	2,349,529	8,816,096
Baltimore-Towson.	24	7,550	399,335	2,059,916	3,408,886	5,629	9,315	5.2	339,096	437	33,805	1,372,914	5,606,276
Bethesda-Gaithersburg-Frederick . .	7	1,780	111,374	488,268	825,440	1,335	2,257	4.4	68,060	224	18,936	318,629	1,134,589
Cumberland	1	371	13,932	91,009	183,001	249	500	6.5	10,054	20	993	57,146	527,275
Hagerstown-Martinsburg.	1	272	15,533	66,865	128,402	183	351	4.3	8,799	41	1,976	77,151	204,459
Salisbury	3	546	23,778	132,483	267,059	362	730	5.6	19,029	28	2,037	94,025	562,386
Washington-Arlington-Alexandria. .	7	1,226	62,192	268,451	451,883	745	1,250	4.3	51,853	120	6,593	384,065	614,901
Wilmington	1	119	6,346	23,794	55,914	65	153	3.7	7,549	12	683	45,599	166,210
North Carolina	118	22,708	1,027,640	5,726,216	12,048,286	15,643	32,923	5.6	831,275	1,699	114,140	4,636,192	19,730,853
Nonmetropolitan	57	6,201	241,933	1,311,905	3,315,067	3,583	9,057	5.4	203,382	585	24,223	1,560,978	5,136,580
Metropolitan.	61	16,507	785,707	4,414,311	8,733,219	12,060	23,866	5.6	627,893	1,114	89,917	3,075,214	14,594,273
Asheville	6	1,237	57,484	292,489	570,956	798	1,559	5.1	52,701	58	5,037	180,529	1,366,172
Burlington.	1	218	11,703	48,485	127,761	132	349	4.1	10,156	21	1,263	57,252	180,365
Charlotte-Gastonia-Concord.	13	3,595	178,452	953,126	1,932,579	2,606	5,282	5.3	134,771	297	23,946	788,302	3,051,434
Durham	6	1,979	93,761	593,891	1,177,456	1,623	3,218	6.3	84,402	63	8,798	243,615	2,425,572
Fayetteville	1	666	34,002	213,905	352,239	584	962	6.3	15,543	44	4,403	132,647	575,851
Goldsboro	1	274	10,927	48,872	118,910	134	325	4.5	12,659	30	1,468	60,502	154,091
Greensboro-High Point.	6	1,859	75,005	441,747	909,097	1,206	2,484	5.9	46,659	111	9,121	332,898	1,278,723
Greenville.	1	875	46,920	258,492	364,036	706	995	5.5	20,441	42	3,725	114,826	384,572
Hickory-Lenoir-Morganton	5	880	34,366	196,947	420,695	538	1,151	5.7	29,442	62	3,728	169,886	545,130
Jacksonville	1	144	8,018	29,994	81,837	82	224	3.7	5,429	23	1,863	63,772	137,766
Raleigh-Cary.	6	1,835	91,283	504,999	1,124,578	1,379	3,073	5.5	98,577	156	14,347	418,784	2,412,783
Rocky Mount.	3	396	17,821	98,039	191,484	268	524	5.5	11,454	34	1,649	90,789	244,388
Wilmington	4	888	42,761	235,964	492,616	645	1,345	5.5	33,398	48	4,249	176,146	532,129
Winston-Salem	7	1,661	83,204	497,361	868,975	1,359	2,375	6.0	72,261	125	6,320	245,266	1,305,297
South Carolina	67	12,539	506,072	2,861,439	5,209,566	7,814	14,234	5.7	507,171	874	53,353	1,435,010	6,549,778
Nonmetropolitan	24	2,917	98,065	558,195	1,225,089	1,524	3,349	5.7	99,014	235	9,561	326,642	1,211,403
Metropolitan.	43	9,622	408,007	2,303,244	3,984,477	6,290	10,885	5.6	408,157	639	43,792	1,108,368	5,338,375
Anderson.	2	428	20,269	108,807	180,467	297	493	5.4	15,911	28	1,942	61,749	699,014
Augusta-Richmond County	2	293	12,721	65,813	108,401	179	296	5.2	10,499	18	1,140	55,755	151,410
Charleston-North Charleston	7	1,874	86,867	450,830	791,705	1,231	2,163	5.2	81,621	137	9,488	246,842	1,513,963
Charlotte-Gastonia-Concord.	2	330	15,848	81,962	125,175	224	342	5.2	15,515	37	1,934	66,101	167,262
Columbia	7	2,126	89,767	527,843	924,518	1,442	2,527	5.9	73,516	115	9,559	145,890	776,110
Florence	6	1,245	45,773	268,597	426,123	733	1,163	5.9	56,614	58	3,557	54,954	203,703
Greenville.	10	1,554	69,627	399,611	709,187	1,092	1,937	5.7	77,557	111	8,526	203,552	899,939
Myrtle Beach-Conway-North Myrtle Beach.	3	801	27,972	181,441	368,085	496	1,006	6.5	26,879	54	2,575	87,850	248,331
Spartanburg	3	701	34,046	176,602	274,199	482	749	5.2	39,386	57	3,697	126,360	546,140
Sumter	1	270	5,117	41,738	76,617	114	209	8.2	10,659	24	1,374	59,315	132,503
Virginia.	94	18,150	796,004	4,516,303	9,006,658	12,343	24,614	5.7	660,662	1,339	93,114	3,600,733	15,553,341
Nonmetropolitan	30	2,638	85,347	574,383	1,385,278	1,568	3,785	6.7	87,795	160	7,093	551,028	2,239,197
Metropolitan.	64	15,512	710,657	3,941,920	7,621,380	10,775	20,829	5.5	572,867	1,179	86,021	3,049,705	13,314,144
Blacksburg-Christiansburg-Radford	4	328	15,678	62,468	151,532	171	414	4.0	18,641	32	2,103	92,225	245,167
Charlottesville	3	754	40,768	215,778	427,027	589	1,166	5.3	73,922	42	3,329	114,229	2,165,613
Danville.	1	151	8,385	37,895	78,311	104	215	4.5	5,517	20	1,177	22,175	108,952
Harrisonburg.	1	238	14,034	53,874	129,506	147	354	3.8	17,431	22	1,725	75,475	371,436
Kingsport-Bristol-Bristol	2	141	7,691	32,444	81,951	89	224	4.2	8,468	16	783	40,695	121,886
Lynchburg	2	1,205	32,929	329,010	596,624	899	1,630	10.0	17,282	39	2,536	115,075	509,450
Richmond.	14	3,606	154,065	853,801	1,474,309	2,334	4,031	5.5	98,276	197	13,205	500,185	1,954,128
Roanoke	3	1,177	60,296	344,318	587,827	942	1,608	5.7	42,817	67	4,905	250,660	649,203
Virginia Beach-Norfolk-Newport News	16	3,586	160,272	944,174	2,004,924	2,580	5,479	5.9	130,963	283	18,676	894,768	4,107,991
Washington-Arlington-Alexandria. .	17	3,851	192,252	948,237	1,873,299	2,592	5,118	4.9	148,694	445	35,279	874,172	2,646,754
Winchester	1	475	24,287	119,921	216,070	328	590	4.9	10,856	16	2,303	70,046	433,564
West Virginia.	55	7,212	276,114	1,587,250	3,577,983	4,333	9,772	5.7	311,559	419	20,758	1,224,551	6,810,325
Nonmetropolitan	29	2,763	85,738	542,561	1,549,166	1,480	4,231	6.3	87,272	165	6,828	538,490	2,533,151
Metropolitan.	26	4,449	190,376	1,044,689	2,028,817	2,853	5,541	5.5	224,287	254	13,930	686,061	4,277,174
Charleston	7	1,277	52,774	290,233	555,359	793	1,517	5.5	92,839	69	3,828	159,171	986,891
Cumberland	1	25	799	3,285	15,499	9	42	4.1	1,282	0	0	12,764	49,439
Hagerstown-Martinsburg.	2	207	8,521	43,675	113,979	119	311	5.1	8,312	21	931	57,946	246,464
Huntington-Ashland.	3	730	45,362	197,548	344,933	540	942	4.4	31,690	55	2,952	129,677	734,207
Morgantown	4	792	38,397	217,683	340,320	595	929	5.7	35,704	10	2,373	87,856	869,769
Parkersburg-Marietta-Vienna	2	478	16,351	88,564	155,383	242	425	5.4	17,423	25	1,563	69,598	322,355
Washington-Arlington-Alexandria. .	1	25	1,606	4,785	19,141	13	52	3.0	2,920	10	280	28,914	75,634
Weirton-Steubenville	1	168	6,017	31,948	85,113	87	233	5.3	6,148	21	393	38,181	185,959
Wheeling	4	703	20,074	152,929	328,042	417	896	7.6	27,720	43	1,610	92,592	762,161
Winchester.	1	44	475	14,039	71,048	38	194	29.6	249	0	0	9,362	44,295

TABLE 8

U.S. CENSUS DIVISION 3, SOUTH ATLANTIC CONITNUED

U.S. Community Hospitals
(Nonfederal, short-term general and other special hospitals)

2012 Utilization, Personnel and Finances

| | FULL-TIME EQUIVALENT PERSONNEL | | | | | FULL-TIME EQUIV. TRAINEES | | | EXPENSES | | | | | | |
| | | | | | | | | | LABOR | | | | TOTAL | | |
Physicians and Dentists	Registered Nurses	Licensed Practical Nurses	Other Salaried Personnel	Total Personnel	Medical and Dental Residents	Other Trainees	Total Trainees	Payroll (in thousands)	Employee Benefits (in thousands)	Total (in thousands)	Percent of Total	Amount (in thousands)	Adjusted per Admission	Adjusted per Inpatient Day
2,826	23,768	625	60,582	87,801	1,695	95	1,790	5,336,514	1,293,887	6,630,404	48.0	13,808,394	11,856.76	2,485.14
45	904	21	2,450	3,420	3	11	14	212,795	53,708	266,504	51.9	513,713	8,180.40	2,178.68
2,781	22,864	604	58,132	84,381	1,692	84	1,776	5,123,719	1,240,179	6,363,900	47.9	13,294,681	12,066.30	2,498.73
2,426	15,879	334	40,872	59,511	1,584	73	1,657	3,516,792	858,614	4,375,407	46.3	9,441,633	13,655.50	2,769.71
142	2,996	91	6,956	10,185	72	7	79	707,897	170,639	878,536	52.7	1,667,352	9,005.31	2,019.96
36	496	23	1,348	1,903	0	0	0	109,711	33,736	143,447	46.9	305,799	10,915.93	1,671.02
7	618	16	1,283	1,924	0	0	0	115,284	31,385	146,669	51.9	282,643	9,475.75	2,201.23
53	765	67	2,148	3,033	0	0	0	176,852	43,898	220,750	50.2	440,140	9,478.62	1,648.10
80	1,887	65	4,889	6,921	36	1	37	438,064	91,483	529,548	51.8	1,022,585	9,642.93	2,262.94
37	223	8	636	904	0	3	3	59,119	10,424	69,543	51.7	134,531	9,021.04	2,406.03
1,864	46,407	1,648	103,934	153,853	3,184	125	3,309	8,812,862	2,231,592	11,044,455	48.7	22,659,692	10,392.65	1,880.74
421	9,303	648	23,732	34,104	18	1	19	1,667,337	438,948	2,106,283	51.0	4,132,348	6,741.97	1,246.54
1,443	37,104	1,000	80,202	119,749	3,166	124	3,290	7,145,525	1,792,644	8,938,172	48.2	18,527,344	11,820.22	2,121.48
133	2,783	53	6,345	9,314	0	11	11	556,011	119,454	675,464	54.3	1,244,393	10,562.80	2,179.49
29	451	3	1,269	1,752	0	0	0	85,532	22,299	107,830	44.1	244,503	7,928.62	1,913.75
387	7,916	167	17,180	25,650	303	12	315	1,569,557	380,168	1,949,726	43.6	4,473,419	12,199.46	2,314.74
53	6,131	91	12,230	18,505	1,669	14	1,683	1,193,377	296,990	1,490,369	47.0	3,170,966	17,168.11	2,693.07
140	1,246	125	3,264	4,775	2	0	2	304,790	74,046	378,836	57.4	660,080	11,789.04	1,873.95
0	507	13	1,075	1,595	0	0	0	76,473	24,804	101,277	53.3	189,928	7,143.92	1,597.24
341	3,256	166	7,662	11,425	58	0	58	618,470	187,604	806,074	53.2	1,516,232	9,805.74	1,667.84
0	2,223	2	4,603	6,828	373	21	394	346,677	111,717	458,394	46.6	982,934	14,875.36	2,700.10
105	1,227	36	3,346	4,714	24	0	24	279,557	72,496	352,053	49.1	716,895	9,557.45	1,704.07
0	360	15	676	1,051	0	0	0	53,119	15,327	68,446	50.2	136,259	6,228.42	1,665.01
242	4,700	57	9,285	14,284	0	15	15	944,170	203,984	1,148,154	52.8	2,176,491	10,680.38	1,935.38
2	721	37	1,549	2,309	0	0	0	124,890	31,853	156,744	50.1	312,909	8,429.65	1,634.12
6	1,512	40	3,544	5,102	63	0	63	286,414	80,098	366,512	47.6	769,742	9,450.36	1,562.56
5	4,071	195	8,174	12,445	674	51	725	706,488	171,805	878,293	45.4	1,932,594	13,340.47	2,223.99
1,419	20,262	888	43,379	65,948	1,253	0	1,253	3,513,074	920,934	4,434,008	45.6	9,729,645	10,436.77	1,867.65
205	3,431	277	8,306	12,219	30	0	30	637,882	177,639	815,522	47.8	1,706,321	7,945.25	1,392.81
1,214	16,831	611	35,073	53,729	1,223	0	1,223	2,875,192	743,295	3,618,486	45.1	8,023,324	11,182.54	2,013.65
101	837	57	2,507	3,502	52	0	52	168,284	45,573	213,857	49.9	429,000	12,316.26	2,377.17
12	375	17	619	1,023	0	0	0	58,210	12,388	70,598	44.9	157,074	7,534.99	1,449.01
19	4,006	105	7,222	11,352	658	0	658	696,312	181,719	878,032	43.8	2,004,289	12,815.39	2,531.61
0	482	11	1,082	1,575	0	0	0	73,696	17,207	90,904	41.6	218,389	8,700.05	1,744.67
135	3,828	170	8,111	12,244	238	0	238	675,935	175,746	851,681	49.1	1,734,361	10,990.74	1,875.96
54	1,748	115	3,379	5,296	25	0	25	274,621	66,716	341,337	45.2	755,894	9,914.67	1,773.89
765	2,827	50	5,629	9,271	190	0	190	466,211	117,641	583,851	41.5	1,407,767	10,646.99	1,985.04
5	981	53	1,845	2,884	0	0	0	145,832	41,830	187,661	46.4	404,255	7,802.20	1,098.27
123	1,291	24	3,662	5,100	60	0	60	239,964	63,564	303,528	42.3	716,729	13,564.13	2,613.90
0	456	9	1,017	1,482	0	0	0	76,127	20,911	97,037	49.6	195,566	20,820.35	2,552.51
1,475	30,194	2,411	62,743	96,823	1,949	138	2,087	6,260,259	1,496,027	7,756,282	47.0	16,505,378	10,163.32	1,832.58
153	2,946	607	7,615	11,321	34	5	39	600,578	146,133	746,708	49.2	1,517,023	6,958.21	1,095.10
1,322	27,248	1,804	55,128	85,502	1,915	133	2,048	5,659,681	1,349,894	7,009,574	46.8	14,988,356	10,660.31	1,966.62
9	577	45	1,107	1,738	5	0	5	106,493	24,036	130,528	47.1	277,299	7,286.60	1,829.97
64	2,117	147	5,061	7,389	732	34	766	494,139	106,315	600,454	45.6	1,317,661	15,343.76	3,085.66
22	278	20	731	1,051	6	0	6	55,502	15,241	70,743	50.5	139,951	8,076.58	1,787.12
71	607	87	1,556	2,321	0	0	0	136,321	31,589	167,910	51.8	324,055	9,605.62	2,502.24
1	234	35	574	844	0	0	0	38,789	7,518	46,307	38.6	120,086	5,914.99	1,465.34
103	920	180	3,418	4,621	19	8	27	276,173	77,804	353,977	57.8	612,118	10,472.87	1,025.97
193	6,205	419	11,266	18,083	772	74	846	1,249,147	326,928	1,576,074	47.7	3,301,809	12,267.81	2,239.56
434	2,373	145	4,763	7,715	239	1	240	558,503	119,056	677,559	50.8	1,333,564	12,639.22	2,268.63
131	6,081	452	12,914	19,578	5	9	14	1,234,175	305,373	1,539,547	44.1	3,488,264	9,763.53	1,739.85
287	6,956	223	12,159	19,625	129	7	136	1,362,301	296,118	1,658,420	45.8	3,622,539	9,620.06	1,933.77
7	900	51	1,579	2,537	8	0	8	148,138	39,916	188,055	41.7	451,010	10,306.44	2,087.33
603	10,476	1,296	26,274	38,649	660	23	683	1,906,954	558,313	2,465,269	47.9	5,151,428	8,376.16	1,439.76
284	2,793	649	8,313	12,039	59	2	61	564,532	159,109	723,641	50.5	1,433,566	6,083.89	925.38
319	7,683	647	17,961	26,610	601	21	622	1,342,422	399,204	1,741,628	46.8	3,717,861	9,799.89	1,832.53
128	2,461	205	5,105	7,899	175	0	175	387,876	116,153	504,029	45.0	1,120,900	11,048.68	2,018.33
0	46	9	146	201	0	0	0	7,011	1,695	8,707	38.7	22,515	5,972.17	1,452.68
2	320	17	662	1,001	0	0	0	60,906	14,768	75,674	49.5	152,756	7,763.59	1,340.22
31	1,395	146	2,863	4,435	0	0	0	245,600	100,883	346,483	48.3	717,790	8,855.37	2,080.95
40	1,681	110	4,255	6,086	337	21	358	320,658	90,059	410,717	46.3	887,707	14,019.37	2,608.45
19	446	11	1,406	1,882	18	0	18	83,362	20,696	104,058	42.0	247,667	8,301.77	1,593.91
0	75	8	179	262	0	0	0	17,234	4,265	21,499	51.8	41,466	6,454.88	2,166.35
8	240	12	595	855	0	0	0	38,331	11,363	49,694	54.3	91,592	5,713.76	1,076.12
87	993	118	2,630	3,828	71	0	71	173,669	37,714	211,384	51.0	414,171	7,474.26	1,262.56
4	26	11	120	161	0	0	0	7,775	1,608	9,383	44.1	21,298	8,859.43	299.77

CLASSIFICATION	Hospitals	Beds	Admissions	Inpatient Days	Adjusted Inpatient Days	Average Daily Census	Adjusted Average Daily Census	Average Stay (days)	Surgical Operations	NEWBORNS Bassinets	NEWBORNS Births	OUTPATIENT VISITS Emergency	OUTPATIENT VISITS Total
UNITED STATES	4,999	800,566	34,422,071	185,423,035	362,159,266	507,292	990,999	5.4	26,811,231	55,987	3,715,479	133,221,030	674,971,331
Nonmetropolitan	1,980	132,450	4,000,957	25,115,368	70,833,735	68,747	193,921	6.3	4,071,289	10,624	446,664	23,768,413	125,342,725
Metropolitan	3,019	668,116	30,421,114	160,307,667	291,325,531	438,545	797,078	5.3	22,739,942	45,363	3,268,815	109,452,617	549,628,606
CENSUS DIVISION 4, EAST NORTH CENTRAL	776	121,997	5,477,164	27,190,027	58,508,725	74,355	159,969	5.0	4,685,851	9,532	524,244	22,161,580	136,939,750
Nonmetropolitan	273	17,643	624,805	3,224,485	11,131,810	8,844	30,474	5.2	691,784	1,779	66,809	3,996,400	24,965,194
Metropolitan	503	104,354	4,852,359	23,965,542	47,376,915	65,511	129,495	4.9	3,994,067	7,753	457,435	18,165,180	111,974,556
Illinois	188	32,662	1,484,155	7,190,230	14,788,624	19,659	40,420	4.8	1,105,492	2,609	150,234	5,422,193	33,116,861
Nonmetropolitan	64	3,957	143,097	670,414	2,095,842	1,837	5,727	4.7	141,618	305	13,141	836,560	5,517,505
Metropolitan	124	28,705	1,341,058	6,519,816	12,692,782	17,822	34,693	4.9	963,874	2,304	137,093	4,585,633	27,599,356
Bloomington-Normal	2	353	15,911	60,526	116,976	165	319	3.8	11,283	39	2,516	64,948	490,669
Champaign-Urbana	4	586	29,284	147,597	287,064	404	785	5.0	22,685	66	3,548	112,078	604,824
Chicago-Naperville-Joliet	75	20,061	963,581	4,692,124	8,833,740	12,826	24,147	4.9	640,505	1,564	97,842	3,107,417	18,871,166
Danville	2	226	7,302	48,457	121,324	132	333	6.6	3,830	26	663	44,632	222,420
Davenport-Moline-Rock Island	5	552	22,362	106,768	276,151	292	754	4.8	17,630	73	2,388	108,787	553,338
Decatur	2	420	19,556	84,053	227,547	230	622	4.3	16,599	36	1,597	82,093	467,342
Kankakee-Bradley	2	468	17,844	80,354	186,191	220	509	4.5	16,887	34	1,420	75,187	560,224
Lake County-Kenosha County	5	901	53,661	207,846	425,902	568	1,164	3.9	40,104	106	6,714	203,732	787,154
Peoria	7	1,290	61,344	312,438	603,358	854	1,649	5.1	67,785	79	5,233	206,526	1,837,207
Rockford	4	907	40,727	202,442	361,655	553	988	5.0	37,303	83	4,449	164,252	1,112,366
Springfield	3	953	45,393	237,805	411,919	650	1,126	5.2	34,903	54	3,582	123,255	729,014
St. Louis	13	1,988	64,093	339,406	840,955	928	2,297	5.3	54,360	144	7,141	292,726	1,363,632
Indiana	124	17,556	731,046	3,739,056	8,071,440	10,222	22,069	5.1	642,625	1,481	73,460	3,207,214	17,918,304
Nonmetropolitan	40	2,261	86,163	413,696	1,445,629	1,130	3,954	4.8	108,462	281	11,656	667,071	3,820,396
Metropolitan	84	15,295	644,883	3,325,360	6,625,811	9,092	18,115	5.2	534,163	1,200	61,804	2,540,143	14,097,908
Anderson	2	210	8,533	40,444	128,986	110	352	4.7	14,349	12	464	55,079	314,476
Bloomington	3	350	15,032	63,333	148,018	173	405	4.2	13,006	19	2,039	73,626	331,497
Cincinnati-Middletown	1	78	4,141	15,096	42,337	41	116	3.6	6,432	11	497	19,050	142,764
Columbus	1	198	9,359	36,714	83,660	100	229	3.9	11,107	20	1,226	41,675	236,771
Elkhart-Goshen	2	392	18,701	70,304	152,257	192	416	3.8	12,558	66	2,804	96,400	573,086
Evansville	7	1,275	50,304	279,926	559,248	765	1,529	5.6	37,555	62	4,720	179,593	991,887
Fort Wayne	9	1,633	65,533	356,515	681,036	975	1,861	5.4	76,887	124	7,110	215,895	1,044,905
Gary	11	2,518	109,503	607,436	1,114,403	1,663	3,050	5.5	68,389	215	6,961	422,557	1,840,224
Indianapolis	24	5,050	205,128	1,098,538	2,188,738	3,004	5,984	5.4	160,054	387	21,010	827,697	5,638,414
Kokomo	4	360	11,910	57,306	160,332	157	438	4.8	17,981	37	988	55,906	332,102
Lafayette	3	512	21,157	103,575	226,338	283	619	4.9	15,677	35	1,914	110,204	464,539
Louisville	6	661	33,722	167,444	344,856	457	942	5.0	30,656	38	2,858	116,163	659,891
Michigan City-La Porte	2	375	14,071	71,431	149,645	195	409	5.1	12,017	35	1,213	54,029	265,480
Muncie	1	346	17,454	85,349	146,797	233	401	4.9	6,188	24	1,666	61,594	328,683
South Bend-Mishawaka	3	744	35,247	158,921	248,059	435	678	4.5	22,745	59	3,830	105,161	334,848
Terre Haute	5	593	25,088	113,028	251,101	309	686	4.5	28,562	56	2,504	105,514	598,341
Michigan	151	25,100	1,182,541	6,037,474	12,941,178	16,516	35,417	5.1	1,003,548	1,669	106,525	4,781,685	32,819,446
Nonmetropolitan	58	4,102	139,056	797,433	2,773,472	2,197	7,631	5.7	174,289	349	13,664	876,775	6,221,740
Metropolitan	93	20,998	1,043,485	5,240,041	10,167,706	14,319	27,786	5.0	829,259	1,320	92,861	3,904,910	26,597,356
Ann Arbor	5	1,598	83,945	449,713	892,927	1,229	2,440	5.4	82,564	56	7,477	199,958	3,338,419
Battle Creek	3	322	13,919	61,204	167,876	167	459	4.4	10,598	26	1,570	69,365	393,353
Bay City	2	364	15,999	84,460	136,880	231	374	5.3	10,107	14	897	44,384	363,396
Detroit-Livonia-Dearborn	20	5,208	261,762	1,326,521	2,562,873	3,625	7,005	5.1	176,807	310	20,211	1,054,981	5,618,124
Flint	4	1,204	61,395	301,908	546,288	826	1,492	4.9	44,552	89	5,281	225,884	1,440,312
Grand Rapids-Wyoming	8	1,851	96,825	430,363	828,683	1,175	2,263	4.4	98,099	144	12,148	362,453	3,253,799
Holland-Grand Haven	3	226	10,774	39,232	99,169	107	272	3.6	9,179	52	1,170	128,809	617,905
Jackson	2	347	19,056	92,865	213,493	254	583	4.9	11,978	11	1,669	79,191	579,280
Kalamazoo-Portage	5	895	43,229	204,792	395,732	560	1,081	4.7	35,740	70	5,254	198,971	1,401,835
Lansing-East Lansing	5	1,030	49,903	236,312	508,836	645	1,391	4.7	45,348	41	5,477	203,423	1,209,379
Monroe	1	179	9,856	41,007	96,015	112	262	4.2	8,130	13	856	48,658	177,453
Muskegon-Norton Shores	4	452	18,967	82,307	218,341	226	597	4.3	20,715	26	2,135	106,324	920,598
Niles-Benton Harbor	3	471	17,764	123,732	194,870	338	533	7.0	10,762	35	544	80,241	378,742
Saginaw-Saginaw Township North	4	1,119	43,004	299,708	466,265	818	1,275	7.0	22,032	31	3,064	136,359	652,261
South Bend-Mishawaka	1	25	836	2,767	13,392	8	37	3.3	570	0	0	10,128	107,264
Warren-Farmington Hills-Troy	23	5,707	296,251	1,463,150	2,826,066	3,998	7,722	4.9	242,078	402	25,108	955,781	6,145,586

MSAs

TABLE 8

U.S. CENSUS DIVISION 4, EAST NORTH CENTRAL

U.S. Community Hospitals
(Nonfederal, short-term general and other special hospitals)

2012 Utilization, Personnel and Finances

FULL-TIME EQUIVALENT PERSONNEL					FULL-TIME EQUIV. TRAINEES			EXPENSES						
								LABOR				TOTAL		
Physicians and Dentists	Registered Nurses	Licensed Practical Nurses	Other Salaried Personnel	Total Personnel	Medical and Dental Residents	Other Trainees	Total Trainees	Payroll (in thousands)	Employee Benefits (in thousands)	Total (in thousands)	Percent of Total	Amount (in thousands)	Adjusted per Admission	Adjusted per Inpatient Day
114,479	1,351,164	82,268	3,183,037	4,730,948	102,904	7,230	110,134	$296,335,931	$81,153,797	$377,489,736	49.9	$756,916,757	$11,220.70	$2,090.01
15,188	160,970	24,883	469,925	670,966	1,935	276	2,211	35,636,252	9,721,437	45,357,688	52.4	86,549,339	7,649.75	1,221.87
99,291	1,190,194	57,385	2,713,112	4,059,982	100,969	6,954	107,923	260,699,679	71,432,359	332,132,048	49.5	670,367,418	11,940.32	2,301.09
21,586	226,315	10,287	543,532	801,720	21,184	1,292	22,476	49,458,738	13,282,554	62,741,292	48.8	128,508,223	10,925.75	2,196.39
2,856	27,056	3,014	82,534	115,460	203	68	271	6,452,969	1,906,794	8,359,763	52.2	16,007,133	7,804.81	1,437.96
18,730	199,259	7,273	460,998	686,260	20,981	1,224	22,205	43,005,768	11,375,760	54,381,529	48.3	112,501,090	11,584.89	2,374.60
5,350	56,718	2,025	134,506	198,599	6,244	254	6,498	12,200,448	3,332,345	15,532,791	48.7	31,914,764	10,403.72	2,158.06
544	5,806	794	17,427	24,571	43	3	46	1,290,713	408,517	1,699,228	52.2	3,254,912	7,331.81	1,553.03
4,806	50,912	1,231	117,079	174,028	6,201	251	6,452	10,909,735	2,923,828	13,833,563	48.3	28,659,853	10,923.51	2,257.96
97	531	10	1,198	1,836	2	0	2	121,378	31,742	153,120	49.3	310,608	10,081.08	2,655.32
18	1,209	35	2,107	3,369	27	0	27	172,310	45,362	217,673	40.4	539,150	10,342.82	1,878.15
3,801	36,906	769	83,594	125,070	5,624	224	5,848	8,101,194	2,166,103	10,267,299	48.5	21,149,992	11,518.93	2,394.23
7	228	19	691	945	0	0	0	45,611	11,860	57,471	47.2	121,720	7,057.88	1,003.26
37	869	26	2,020	2,952	0	0	0	144,517	33,860	178,377	43.3	412,088	7,480.68	1,492.26
73	542	89	2,258	2,962	15	0	15	159,333	41,643	200,976	46.3	433,634	7,866.81	1,905.69
41	659	20	1,683	2,403	12	0	12	131,197	32,124	163,321	46.5	351,268	8,520.33	1,886.60
51	1,618	32	3,602	5,303	1	0	1	350,142	97,129	447,271	47.1	949,523	8,884.26	2,229.44
376	2,741	48	5,981	9,146	240	8	248	597,240	137,187	734,427	51.1	1,436,761	12,034.39	2,381.28
249	1,664	23	4,064	6,000	0	17	17	361,588	111,907	473,495	51.8	914,137	12,203.13	2,527.65
1	1,526	81	4,276	5,884	270	0	270	315,141	93,140	408,281	41.6	980,985	12,254.81	2,381.50
55	2,419	79	5,605	8,158	10	2	12	410,084	121,770	531,852	50.2	1,059,985	6,850.46	1,260.45
2,094	30,808	1,898	72,899	107,699	1,180	193	1,373	6,576,139	1,814,157	8,390,297	46.8	17,926,527	10,991.88	2,220.98
548	3,926	526	12,176	17,176	6	42	48	934,781	259,744	1,194,525	51.5	2,320,518	7,423.90	1,605.20
1,546	26,882	1,372	60,723	90,523	1,174	151	1,325	5,641,358	1,554,413	7,195,772	46.1	15,606,009	11,837.85	2,355.34
15	356	26	757	1,154	0	0	0	82,934	23,525	106,460	50.2	212,201	7,737.78	1,645.15
17	735	45	1,940	2,737	0	0	0	140,404	48,340	188,744	46.6	405,060	11,343.68	2,736.56
5	123	19	492	639	0	0	0	31,465	11,129	42,594	54.7	77,835	6,701.81	1,838.46
0	293	26	938	1,257	0	0	0	74,569	26,339	100,908	46.8	215,677	10,113.35	2,578.02
90	713	23	1,983	2,809	4	0	4	151,568	49,850	201,418	44.6	451,758	10,945.62	2,967.08
149	1,971	69	4,672	6,861	24	67	91	381,372	107,246	488,617	47.9	1,019,847	10,235.32	1,823.60
42	2,546	127	5,096	7,811	0	0	0	391,776	107,064	498,842	39.8	1,252,258	10,192.97	1,838.75
179	3,539	161	7,823	11,702	106	20	126	771,763	198,674	970,437	48.3	2,007,393	10,000.31	1,801.32
567	10,737	490	22,890	34,684	860	46	906	2,370,601	653,629	3,024,232	46.1	6,555,204	15,232.40	2,994.97
60	533	28	1,283	1,904	10	9	19	118,713	29,070	147,782	50.4	293,263	8,571.19	1,829.10
196	1,044	71	2,389	3,700	28	3	31	285,275	72,134	357,409	50.9	702,743	14,659.11	3,104.84
83	1,048	90	3,052	4,273	0	0	0	218,891	51,694	270,586	52.0	520,601	7,255.56	1,509.62
82	469	27	1,593	2,171	4	0	4	131,972	39,253	171,225	49.2	348,048	11,837.56	2,325.82
8	585	14	1,326	1,933	51	0	51	102,253	32,995	135,248	40.0	338,289	11,268.79	2,304.47
5	1,225	28	2,579	3,837	67	6	73	205,576	62,252	267,828	41.2	650,547	11,617.11	2,622.55
48	965	128	1,910	3,051	20	0	20	182,225	41,218	223,442	40.2	555,285	9,562.67	2,211.40
4,587	48,414	1,646	117,254	171,901	6,281	126	6,407	10,658,869	2,653,276	13,312,142	48.8	27,293,082	10,808.28	2,109.01
692	5,922	702	19,194	26,510	72	11	83	1,459,045	409,446	1,868,489	50.3	3,712,392	8,307.21	1,338.54
3,895	42,492	944	98,060	145,391	6,209	115	6,324	9,199,823	2,243,830	11,443,653	48.5	23,580,690	11,346.07	2,319.18
186	5,802	108	12,786	18,882	1,475	0	1,475	1,184,235	356,482	1,540,716	49.7	3,100,658	18,194.53	3,472.46
49	557	10	1,554	2,170	0	0	0	137,190	26,040	163,230	51.5	317,108	8,043.12	1,888.94
37	447	48	1,351	1,883	11	1	12	118,023	29,353	147,377	53.7	274,388	10,219.29	2,004.59
1,403	10,083	105	22,029	33,620	2,325	32	2,357	2,412,951	533,543	2,946,494	47.7	6,176,498	12,153.17	2,409.99
88	2,530	52	4,565	7,235	328	20	348	509,295	151,502	660,797	56.2	1,175,198	10,502.21	2,151.24
174	3,640	111	9,764	13,689	90	0	90	758,217	204,901	963,118	41.1	2,345,903	12,378.65	2,830.88
39	513	54	1,430	2,036	9	3	12	108,959	29,065	138,025	50.3	274,556	9,877.20	2,768.57
51	731	59	2,536	3,377	0	0	0	187,169	39,023	226,192	53.1	426,186	9,118.42	1,996.25
240	1,738	31	4,087	6,096	0	0	0	441,099	111,290	552,389	49.5	1,116,876	13,030.87	2,822.30
225	2,159	33	4,982	7,399	230	3	233	506,404	125,497	631,901	54.6	1,157,045	10,345.81	2,273.91
13	327	7	952	1,299	0	0	0	70,180	16,687	86,867	53.9	161,141	6,982.76	1,678.29
109	670	19	2,379	3,177	24	3	27	192,976	55,498	248,474	52.2	476,310	9,002.95	2,181.50
68	859	66	2,163	3,156	30	2	32	147,956	40,383	188,339	50.6	372,053	11,136.63	1,909.24
156	1,618	97	4,331	6,202	161	22	183	336,506	87,203	423,708	53.1	797,247	10,514.30	1,709.86
7	49	0	167	223	0	0	0	13,017	3,654	16,671	59.9	27,812	6,873.95	2,076.76
1,050	10,769	144	22,984	34,947	1,526	29	1,555	2,075,647	433,709	2,509,355	46.6	5,381,713	9,430.96	1,904.31

Table continues

TABLE 8

U.S. CENSUS DIVISION 4, EAST NORTH CENTRAL CONTNUED

U.S. Community Hospitals
(Nonfederal, short-term general and other special hospitals)

2012 Utilization, Personnel and Finances

CLASSIFICATION	Hospitals	Beds	Admissions	Inpatient Days	Adjusted Inpatient Days	Average Daily Census	Adjusted Average Daily Census	Average Stay (days)	Surgical Operations	NEWBORNS Bassinets	Births	OUTPATIENT VISITS Emergency	Total
Ohio	185	33,659	1,501,183	7,367,870	15,009,953	20,145	41,030	4.9	1,193,455	2,554	128,393	6,578,749	36,956,362
Nonmetropolitan	55	4,383	160,213	659,682	1,948,530	1,805	5,326	4.1	156,209	537	17,104	1,075,450	5,369,480
Metropolitan	130	29,276	1,340,970	6,708,188	13,061,423	18,340	35,704	5.0	1,037,246	2,017	111,289	5,503,299	31,586,882
Akron	8	1,796	89,834	439,372	918,461	1,201	2,510	4.9	56,931	108	7,550	417,557	2,465,021
Canton-Massillon	5	1,228	48,461	282,873	599,321	773	1,638	5.8	42,634	111	4,518	225,120	1,348,312
Cincinnati-Middletown	22	4,572	215,037	1,052,915	1,840,139	2,878	5,028	4.9	159,635	332	20,161	818,887	3,800,795
Cleveland-Elyria-Mentor	29	7,616	346,405	1,843,094	3,815,184	5,036	10,424	5.3	312,661	393	23,169	1,154,362	9,879,152
Columbus	19	5,200	250,204	1,184,836	2,237,203	3,238	6,116	4.7	191,761	407	27,122	1,073,383	5,714,680
Dayton	11	2,655	120,058	557,078	1,021,084	1,528	2,800	4.6	97,972	199	10,903	505,071	2,039,131
Lima	5	717	27,747	127,863	255,292	350	698	4.6	20,582	63	2,397	113,829	755,753
Mansfield	2	271	11,926	54,123	97,191	148	265	4.5	4,571	24	1,006	50,411	279,551
Parkersburg-Marietta-Vienna	2	177	8,768	39,073	81,128	107	222	4.5	8,623	16	302	53,206	249,200
Sandusky	1	236	8,363	41,638	76,433	114	209	5.0	12,773	15	352	59,050	288,322
Springfield	1	254	15,492	66,965	119,785	183	327	4.3	3,763	38	1,203	74,965	306,100
Toledo	12	2,429	108,151	543,285	1,104,304	1,484	3,017	5.0	80,647	164	8,600	449,807	2,730,159
Weirton-Steubenville	2	352	11,514	78,217	182,577	214	499	6.8	5,328	18	499	48,288	277,025
Wheeling	3	252	6,372	41,008	106,879	111	292	6.4	7,424	10	286	44,932	243,937
Youngstown-Warren-Boardman	8	1,521	72,638	355,848	606,442	975	1,659	4.9	31,941	119	3,221	414,431	1,209,744
Wisconsin	128	13,020	578,239	2,855,397	7,697,530	7,813	21,033	4.9	740,731	1,219	65,632	2,171,739	16,128,777
Nonmetropolitan	56	2,940	96,276	683,260	2,868,337	1,875	7,836	7.1	111,206	307	11,244	540,544	4,036,073
Metropolitan	72	10,080	481,963	2,172,137	4,829,193	5,938	13,197	4.5	629,525	912	54,388	1,631,195	12,092,704
Appleton	4	393	17,465	71,084	184,708	194	505	4.1	32,072	55	2,468	73,936	340,638
Duluth	1	25	537	3,778	46,653	10	127	7.0	3,151	0	0	15,180	21,429
Eau Claire	5	577	25,367	123,401	273,038	337	747	4.9	19,611	29	2,431	67,031	458,354
Fond du Lac	3	224	7,783	33,006	129,710	91	354	4.2	15,469	21	972	43,800	785,843
Green Bay	5	756	32,058	130,553	321,649	357	879	4.1	54,382	95	4,474	131,926	1,163,757
Janesville	4	302	15,056	66,183	169,788	181	464	4.4	16,602	29	1,962	87,269	1,443,531
La Crosse	2	409	21,533	86,156	178,810	235	488	4.0	25,298	42	2,311	43,857	395,470
Lake County-Kenosha County	3	522	23,431	94,844	233,106	259	638	4.0	22,900	60	2,983	163,329	941,876
Madison	7	1,465	70,503	363,881	846,330	994	2,312	5.2	136,739	89	7,716	178,862	1,552,523
Milwaukee-Waukesha-West Allis	24	3,970	200,566	919,372	1,792,937	2,514	4,900	4.6	223,308	312	20,196	600,431	3,757,422
Minneapolis-St. Paul-Bloomington	4	85	4,275	12,466	53,002	35	144	2.9	7,007	19	1,014	27,101	132,049
Oshkosh-Neenah	4	387	17,929	69,468	158,200	190	433	3.9	32,269	60	2,607	55,964	296,521
Racine	2	450	18,598	101,398	239,701	277	655	5.5	12,850	47	2,037	69,159	516,223
Sheboygan	2	189	8,273	28,003	78,233	77	214	3.4	13,981	28	1,223	29,484	161,491
Wausau	2	326	18,589	68,544	123,328	187	337	3.7	13,886	26	1,994	43,866	125,577

TABLE 8

U.S. CENSUS DIVISION 4, EAST NORTH CENTRAL CONTNUED

U.S. Community Hospitals
(Nonfederal, short-term general and other special hospitals)

2012 Utilization, Personnel and Finances

FULL-TIME EQUIVALENT PERSONNEL					FULL-TIME EQUIV. TRAINEES			EXPENSES						
								LABOR				TOTAL		
Physicians and Dentists	Registered Nurses	Licensed Practical Nurses	Other Salaried Personnel	Total Personnel	Medical and Dental Residents	Other Trainees	Total Trainees	Payroll (in thousands)	Employee Benefits (in thousands)	Total (in thousands)	Percent of Total	Amount (in thousands)	Adjusted per Admission	Adjusted per Inpatient Day
8,566	67,294	3,855	156,831	236,546	6,708	552	7,260	14,361,420	3,866,157	18,227,578	51.0	35,772,142	11,393.37	2,383.23
695	7,315	736	19,655	28,401	82	12	94	1,499,851	453,330	1,953,182	52.5	3,722,356	7,470.29	1,910.34
7,871	59,979	3,119	137,176	208,145	6,626	540	7,166	12,861,569	3,412,827	16,274,396	50.8	32,049,785	12,133.42	2,453.77
590	4,169	343	10,084	15,186	505	58	563	871,355	242,352	1,113,707	53.3	2,089,036	11,040.25	2,274.50
131	1,956	181	4,751	7,019	75	4	79	373,699	96,348	470,046	51.0	920,989	9,086.14	1,536.72
1,603	9,460	298	23,618	34,979	1,094	236	1,330	2,153,527	571,379	2,724,907	50.6	5,390,006	13,863.50	2,929.13
2,889	16,494	1,134	41,051	61,568	2,543	227	2,770	4,239,400	1,117,204	5,356,604	56.3	9,515,079	13,166.73	2,494.00
2,251	11,482	322	24,056	38,111	1,317	7	1,324	2,188,425	571,683	2,760,108	46.6	5,922,400	12,049.23	2,647.23
75	5,140	105	10,543	15,863	425	0	425	962,308	250,756	1,213,064	47.5	2,552,821	11,380.11	2,500.11
8	1,049	66	2,540	3,663	0	0	0	187,455	59,582	247,037	47.0	525,171	9,087.10	2,057.14
2	493	69	1,248	1,812	0	0	0	122,399	32,935	155,334	49.6	313,085	14,705.06	3,221.34
25	335	32	886	1,278	6	0	6	94,319	26,716	121,035	51.0	237,352	13,026.31	2,925.65
33	426	21	996	1,476	15	2	17	83,512	22,939	106,451	49.6	214,538	13,974.61	2,806.88
0	445	37	1,003	1,485	0	0	0	73,459	19,141	92,600	41.8	221,586	7,996.05	1,849.87
127	5,086	244	9,296	14,753	498	4	502	947,285	255,469	1,202,754	47.0	2,557,326	12,103.33	2,315.78
32	523	28	1,282	1,865	0	0	0	79,461	27,495	106,957	50.6	211,469	7,261.49	1,158.25
22	283	52	727	1,084	0	0	0	44,602	11,798	56,400	49.6	113,787	6,698.45	1,064.63
83	2,638	187	5,095	8,003	148	2	150	440,365	107,028	547,392	43.3	1,265,140	10,056.52	2,086.17
989	23,081	863	62,042	86,975	771	167	938	5,661,862	1,616,618	7,278,484	46.7	15,601,709	11,156.02	2,026.85
377	4,087	256	14,082	18,802	0	0	0	1,268,579	375,757	1,644,339	54.9	2,996,955	8,581.39	1,044.84
612	18,994	607	47,960	68,173	771	167	938	4,393,283	1,240,862	5,634,145	44.7	12,604,754	12,012.07	2,610.12
31	570	58	1,388	2,047	0	3	3	162,171	47,741	209,912	52.1	402,910	8,931.92	2,181.34
7	37	6	145	195	0	0	0	15,113	4,037	19,150	56.6	33,838	5,102.93	725.30
29	1,042	20	2,509	3,600	0	0	0	214,066	65,762	279,829	52.1	536,591	10,744.70	1,965.26
50	345	40	1,006	1,441	0	0	0	120,673	31,649	152,322	44.8	339,759	11,138.16	2,619.37
10	1,300	115	3,853	5,278	0	0	0	360,376	102,468	462,843	49.0	944,084	11,756.08	2,935.14
296	742	27	2,626	3,691	21	0	21	203,012	65,831	268,843	42.1	638,499	16,645.36	3,760.57
12	828	34	2,033	2,907	0	0	0	173,278	66,406	239,684	47.8	501,176	11,136.75	2,802.84
34	1,023	41	2,763	3,861	16	2	18	235,921	64,143	300,064	50.7	592,294	10,184.06	2,540.88
131	3,018	63	8,366	11,578	551	81	632	804,299	280,076	1,084,375	52.2	2,077,721	15,062.06	2,454.98
1	7,612	89	16,769	24,471	183	79	262	1,574,462	362,140	1,936,600	38.5	5,025,843	12,661.95	2,803.13
3	168	11	592	774	0	0	0	54,579	13,584	68,163	47.7	142,902	7,933.28	2,696.17
7	638	28	1,354	2,027	0	2	2	134,988	41,420	176,409	47.9	368,391	8,834.96	2,328.64
0	738	53	2,123	2,914	0	0	0	149,859	40,665	190,525	46.4	410,743	9,219.62	1,713.57
0	242	3	614	859	0	0	0	51,426	15,261	66,687	39.5	168,985	7,317.28	2,160.03
1	691	19	1,819	2,530	0	0	0	139,060	39,679	178,739	42.5	421,017	12,747.27	3,413.80

MSAs

TABLE 8

U.S. CENSUS DIVISION 5, EAST SOUTH CENTRAL

U.S. Community Hospitals
(Nonfederal, short-term general and other special hospitals)

2012 Utilization, Personnel and Finances

CLASSIFICATION	Hospitals	Beds	Admissions	Inpatient Days	Adjusted Inpatient Days	Average Daily Census	Adjusted Average Daily Census	Average Stay (days)	Surgical Operations	NEWBORNS Bassinets	Births	OUTPATIENT VISITS Emergency	Total
UNITED STATES	4,999	800,566	34,422,071	185,423,035	362,159,266	507,292	990,999	5.4	26,811,231	55,987	3,715,479	133,221,030	674,971,331
Nonmetropolitan	1,980	132,450	4,000,957	25,115,368	70,833,735	68,747	193,921	6.3	4,071,289	10,624	446,664	23,768,413	125,342,725
Metropolitan	3,019	668,116	30,421,114	160,307,667	291,325,531	438,545	797,078	5.3	22,739,942	45,363	3,268,815	109,452,617	549,628,606
CENSUS DIVISION 5, EAST SOUTH CENTRAL	433	62,199	2,430,269	13,150,314	26,566,788	36,229	73,246	5.4	2,133,707	4,070	209,932	9,782,661	35,577,098
Nonmetropolitan	233	20,608	611,244	3,716,402	9,360,889	10,205	25,735	6.1	573,558	1,406	54,382	3,438,170	11,162,446
Metropolitan	200	41,591	1,819,025	9,433,912	17,205,899	26,024	47,511	5.2	1,560,149	2,664	155,550	6,344,491	24,414,652
Alabama	97	14,983	650,116	3,235,410	6,383,879	8,846	17,440	5.0	633,259	1,212	54,169	2,349,349	8,136,560
Nonmetropolitan	45	3,204	109,254	517,892	1,584,079	1,420	4,331	4.7	107,301	251	9,401	654,567	1,930,598
Metropolitan	52	11,779	540,862	2,717,518	4,799,800	7,426	13,109	5.0	525,958	961	44,768	1,694,782	6,205,962
Anniston-Oxford	3	420	19,423	86,026	175,283	235	479	4.4	11,846	38	1,722	80,467	203,282
Auburn-Opelika	1	371	13,959	96,138	225,913	263	617	6.9	13,345	38	1,567	46,401	124,643
Birmingham-Hoover	14	4,346	206,264	998,352	1,668,036	2,728	4,557	4.8	224,767	268	12,098	517,540	2,523,279
Columbus	1	48	1,035	15,661	16,172	43	44	15.1	0	0	0	0	4,039
Decatur	2	175	8,204	34,470	91,425	94	249	4.2	7,070	23	507	49,915	140,335
Dothan	4	743	32,500	164,699	335,508	450	916	5.1	38,194	57	2,922	109,747	305,463
Florence-Muscle Shoals	3	574	24,061	103,532	202,334	283	554	4.3	17,956	46	1,987	90,557	221,946
Gadsden	3	593	20,133	121,088	201,354	331	550	6.0	27,517	32	1,114	61,567	143,291
Huntsville	4	1,156	57,781	282,333	555,583	771	1,517	4.9	69,419	92	6,277	198,463	948,277
Mobile	5	1,389	66,347	362,131	551,797	990	1,506	5.5	50,236	187	6,245	171,001	629,725
Montgomery	8	1,106	49,241	245,464	427,364	670	1,167	5.0	41,057	112	5,430	186,553	429,611
Tuscaloosa	4	858	41,914	207,624	349,031	568	953	5.0	24,551	68	4,899	182,571	532,071
Kentucky	106	14,180	572,294	2,908,461	6,138,913	8,191	17,277	5.1	537,974	918	53,538	2,404,826	10,570,929
Nonmetropolitan	63	5,667	206,056	1,022,448	2,531,953	2,796	6,922	5.0	192,951	438	16,647	1,061,136	4,000,014
Metropolitan	43	8,513	366,238	1,886,013	3,606,960	5,395	10,355	5.1	345,023	480	36,891	1,343,690	6,570,915
Bowling Green	3	564	23,281	123,783	213,462	338	583	5.3	18,498	19	2,343	77,339	166,943
Cincinnati-Middletown	5	908	51,435	216,759	431,029	592	1,178	4.2	30,820	38	4,511	208,259	1,117,103
Clarksville	2	164	6,798	31,720	70,969	87	195	4.7	4,154	18	616	32,485	162,615
Elizabethtown	2	308	13,397	63,719	173,655	174	474	4.8	9,961	26	1,603	55,429	333,191
Evansville	1	167	5,183	24,367	66,601	67	182	4.7	3,984	12	594	28,368	273,797
Huntington-Ashland	2	763	30,174	178,848	342,759	490	938	5.9	56,169	25	2,710	144,416	950,479
Lexington-Fayette	14	2,220	89,879	488,282	869,178	1,335	2,376	5.4	75,059	142	8,988	275,043	1,665,117
Louisville	13	3,047	128,036	674,490	1,264,199	2,082	3,951	5.3	126,985	170	13,683	458,450	1,363,290
Owensboro	1	372	18,055	84,045	175,108	230	478	4.7	19,393	30	1,843	63,901	538,380
Mississippi	98	12,882	384,078	2,505,846	5,169,379	6,842	14,120	6.5	273,139	736	37,565	1,767,684	5,088,827
Nonmetropolitan	70	7,486	173,775	1,412,688	3,199,293	3,856	8,739	8.1	135,053	427	17,603	956,958	2,659,974
Metropolitan	28	5,396	210,303	1,093,158	1,970,086	2,986	5,381	5.2	138,086	309	19,962	810,726	2,428,853
Gulfport-Biloxi	5	845	29,822	149,456	281,716	409	771	5.0	26,150	66	2,838	167,220	685,368
Hattiesburg	3	756	35,467	172,736	268,575	472	733	4.9	18,194	29	3,737	116,096	229,337
Jackson	15	3,010	108,032	599,559	1,074,735	1,637	2,935	5.5	76,809	155	9,834	330,528	916,290
Memphis	3	356	17,572	86,529	160,271	236	437	4.9	5,967	24	1,937	75,145	125,343
Pascagoula	2	429	19,410	84,878	184,789	232	505	4.4	10,966	35	1,616	121,737	472,515
Tennessee	132	20,154	823,781	4,500,597	8,874,617	12,350	24,409	5.5	689,335	1,204	64,660	3,260,802	11,780,782
Nonmetropolitan	55	4,251	122,159	763,374	2,045,564	2,133	5,743	6.2	138,253	290	10,731	765,509	2,571,860
Metropolitan	77	15,903	701,622	3,737,223	6,829,053	10,217	18,666	5.3	551,082	914	53,929	2,495,293	9,208,922
Chattanooga	6	1,532	71,134	387,048	645,009	1,058	1,763	5.4	65,689	63	7,175	276,150	899,369
Clarksville	1	247	12,339	47,259	73,737	129	202	3.8	8,712	30	288	65,030	164,552
Cleveland	2	233	10,306	42,345	96,469	116	263	4.1	8,533	22	1,052	47,624	126,570
Jackson	2	730	34,519	180,419	350,749	493	958	5.2	28,968	46	3,358	103,714	252,969
Johnson City	4	744	35,148	192,179	359,929	526	984	5.5	22,421	54	2,351	108,578	403,733
Kingsport-Bristol-Bristol	6	985	45,332	213,413	424,298	583	1,160	4.7	28,086	66	2,043	145,756	554,030
Knoxville	11	2,353	107,347	575,562	1,118,638	1,573	3,056	5.4	101,980	139	10,406	409,319	1,449,988
Memphis	15	3,620	144,754	883,371	1,572,461	2,414	4,297	6.1	89,516	186	13,262	539,066	1,202,132
Morristown	3	336	12,338	49,552	101,826	135	279	4.0	13,802	25	1,101	69,666	181,837
Nashville-Davidson--Murfreesboro	27	5,123	228,405	1,166,075	2,085,937	3,190	5,704	5.1	183,375	283	12,893	730,390	3,973,742

MSAs

TABLE 8

U.S. CENSUS DIVISION 5, EAST SOUTH CENTRAL

U.S. Community Hospitals
(Nonfederal, short-term general and other special hospitals)

2012 Utilization, Personnel and Finances

FULL-TIME EQUIVALENT PERSONNEL					FULL-TIME EQUIV. TRAINEES			EXPENSES						
								LABOR				TOTAL		
Physicians and Dentists	Registered Nurses	Licensed Practical Nurses	Other Salaried Personnel	Total Personnel	Medical and Dental Residents	Other Trainees	Total Trainees	Payroll (in thousands)	Employee Benefits (in thousands)	Total (in thousands)	Percent of Total	Amount (in thousands)	Adjusted per Admission	Adjusted per Inpatient Day
114,479	1,351,164	82,268	3,183,037	4,730,948	102,904	7,230	110,134	$296,335,931	$81,153,797	$377,489,736	49.9	$756,916,757	$11,220.70	$2,090.01
15,188	160,970	24,883	469,925	670,966	1,935	276	2,211	35,636,252	9,721,437	45,357,688	52.4	86,549,339	7,649.75	1,221.87
99,291	1,190,194	57,385	2,713,112	4,059,982	100,969	6,954	107,923	260,699,679	71,432,359	332,132,048	49.5	670,367,418	11,940.32	2,301.09
5,937	88,713	7,071	195,827	297,548	4,469	239	4,708	15,461,474	4,056,517	19,517,996	47.5	41,101,365	8,217.13	1,547.10
1,407	21,486	3,295	57,038	83,226	157	35	192	3,864,807	1,071,317	4,936,124	50.5	9,783,754	6,058.79	1,045.17
4,530	67,227	3,776	138,789	214,322	4,312	204	4,516	11,596,666	2,985,200	14,581,872	46.6	31,317,611	9,246.11	1,820.17
1,042	22,198	1,494	46,632	71,366	960	81	1,041	3,542,803	864,230	4,407,034	48.9	9,009,790	6,749.47	1,411.33
182	3,488	408	8,587	12,665	26	3	29	536,828	136,147	672,976	51.0	1,318,575	3,651.76	832.39
860	18,710	1,086	38,045	58,701	934	78	1,012	3,005,975	728,083	3,734,058	48.5	7,691,215	7,898.07	1,602.40
19	570	66	1,129	1,784	1	0	1	86,640	20,319	106,959	46.7	229,238	5,815.28	1,307.82
25	541	46	1,842	2,454	0	0	0	93,241	20,643	113,884	47.9	237,519	7,240.99	1,051.37
322	6,808	286	13,476	20,892	495	47	542	1,250,347	290,822	1,541,169	47.3	3,257,379	9,413.98	1,952.82
0	31	2	114	147	0	0	0	7,390	1,409	8,800	64.4	13,667	12,784.51	845.08
24	270	35	782	1,111	11	0	11	47,284	15,446	62,731	54.9	114,295	5,254.69	1,250.15
48	1,111	146	2,636	3,941	0	0	0	195,068	41,690	236,758	49.2	480,883	7,078.68	1,433.30
39	666	42	1,373	2,120	17	1	18	86,524	26,338	112,862	50.7	222,690	4,702.56	1,100.60
15	713	44	1,147	1,919	0	2	2	80,778	21,036	101,814	41.2	247,230	7,176.91	1,227.84
140	2,617	139	4,683	7,579	13	0	13	351,401	110,872	462,274	51.5	898,230	7,583.26	1,616.73
166	2,294	54	4,787	7,301	358	5	363	353,597	90,209	443,806	49.1	903,616	8,883.28	1,637.59
29	1,625	77	3,039	4,770	32	1	33	220,376	39,198	259,576	41.2	629,293	6,851.24	1,472.50
33	1,464	149	3,037	4,683	7	22	29	233,326	50,099	283,425	62.0	457,176	6,439.55	1,309.84
1,057	21,716	1,420	47,754	71,947	847	35	882	3,746,542	1,084,028	4,830,571	46.4	10,400,750	8,318.43	1,694.23
629	7,068	936	17,881	26,514	59	13	72	1,268,335	371,864	1,640,198	49.6	3,307,436	6,319.16	1,306.28
428	14,648	484	29,873	45,433	788	22	810	2,478,207	712,164	3,190,373	45.0	7,093,315	9,757.93	1,966.56
0	748	27	1,484	2,259	0	0	0	118,088	32,745	150,834	49.0	307,966	7,454.64	1,442.72
54	1,331	65	2,946	4,396	26	6	32	318,163	105,506	423,670	50.0	847,319	8,131.66	1,965.80
20	251	24	694	989	5	0	5	44,099	12,068	56,167	51.0	110,210	7,357.17	1,552.94
36	467	10	1,333	1,846	0	0	0	90,955	22,684	113,639	53.0	214,506	5,753.77	1,235.24
21	235	25	745	1,026	6	4	10	37,540	15,601	53,141	44.3	120,063	8,475.40	1,802.71
155	1,153	57	2,727	4,092	150	8	158	233,564	66,801	300,366	47.9	626,662	10,065.25	1,828.29
50	3,808	134	8,238	12,230	592	0	592	677,713	208,235	885,948	43.9	2,016,261	11,819.27	2,319.73
79	5,881	117	9,941	16,018	9	4	13	838,020	209,628	1,047,649	42.1	2,489,985	10,183.15	1,969.61
13	774	25	1,765	2,577	0	0	0	120,064	38,895	158,959	44.1	360,342	9,578.98	2,057.83
767	14,072	1,603	35,496	51,938	621	15	636	2,785,065	726,303	3,511,370	50.3	6,982,690	8,947.00	1,350.78
407	6,439	1,163	18,493	26,502	56	15	71	1,286,962	362,923	1,649,886	51.2	3,223,289	8,127.45	1,007.50
360	7,633	440	17,003	25,436	565	0	565	1,498,103	363,381	1,861,484	49.5	3,759,400	9,793.75	1,908.24
149	1,295	89	2,766	4,299	0	0	0	249,722	54,159	303,880	52.0	584,002	10,240.80	2,073.02
39	1,090	95	2,532	3,756	0	0	0	189,928	45,906	235,834	48.2	489,614	8,721.46	1,823.01
143	4,118	204	8,951	13,416	521	0	521	796,822	195,191	992,014	49.7	1,996,822	10,214.34	1,857.97
1	708	30	1,169	1,908	0	0	0	97,954	24,453	122,408	43.1	284,098	8,728.57	1,772.61
28	422	22	1,585	2,057	44	0	44	163,677	43,671	207,348	51.2	404,865	9,492.50	2,190.96
3,071	30,727	2,554	65,945	102,297	2,041	108	2,149	5,387,063	1,381,955	6,769,021	46.0	14,708,135	8,988.93	1,657.33
189	4,491	788	12,077	17,545	16	4	20	772,682	200,383	973,064	50.3	1,934,454	5,796.41	945.68
2,882	26,236	1,766	53,868	84,752	2,025	104	2,129	4,614,382	1,181,572	5,795,957	45.4	12,773,681	9,806.93	1,870.49
178	2,889	169	5,229	8,465	210	2	212	522,023	127,426	649,449	48.2	1,348,074	11,175.83	2,090.01
8	395	20	659	1,082	15	0	15	51,623	12,160	63,783	44.9	142,031	7,377.45	1,926.18
10	344	19	634	1,007	14	1	15	47,536	11,338	58,873	42.1	139,706	5,963.48	1,448.20
7	1,221	136	3,098	4,462	7	0	7	210,361	59,514	269,876	49.2	548,717	8,195.67	1,564.41
1	1,086	94	2,079	3,260	0	0	0	176,891	38,281	215,171	43.3	496,534	7,889.39	1,379.53
47	1,183	65	3,128	4,423	28	2	30	250,769	72,851	323,619	46.1	702,076	7,427.25	1,654.68
149	4,128	332	8,151	12,760	12	13	25	631,475	154,924	786,400	45.0	1,746,077	8,279.21	1,560.90
123	5,686	231	12,443	18,483	770	78	848	948,157	245,537	1,193,693	43.5	2,743,574	10,147.89	1,744.76
13	401	36	735	1,185	3	0	3	59,389	12,087	71,477	46.4	153,990	6,028.88	1,512.28
2,346	8,903	664	17,712	29,625	966	8	974	1,716,158	447,455	2,163,616	45.5	4,752,903	11,649.36	2,278.55

MSAs

TABLE 8

U.S. CENSUS DIVISION 6, WEST NORTH CENTRAL

U.S. Community Hospitals
(Nonfederal, short-term general and other special hospitals)

2012 Utilization, Personnel and Finances

CLASSIFICATION	Hospitals	Beds	Admissions	Inpatient Days	Adjusted Inpatient Days	Average Daily Census	Adjusted Average Daily Census	Average Stay (days)	Surgical Operations	NEWBORNS Bassinets	NEWBORNS Births	OUTPATIENT VISITS Emergency	OUTPATIENT VISITS Total
UNITED STATES	4,999	800,566	34,422,071	185,423,035	362,159,266	507,292	990,999	5.4	26,811,231	55,987	3,715,479	133,221,030	674,971,331
Nonmetropolitan	1,980	132,450	4,000,957	25,115,368	70,833,735	68,747	193,921	6.3	4,071,289	10,624	446,664	23,768,413	125,342,725
Metropolitan	3,019	668,116	30,421,114	160,307,667	291,325,531	438,545	797,078	5.3	22,739,942	45,363	3,268,815	109,452,617	549,628,606
CENSUS DIVISION 6, WEST NORTH CENTRAL	692	68,455	2,421,698	14,638,214	33,808,375	40,100	92,655	6.0	2,048,705	4,883	268,618	8,725,139	60,881,803
Nonmetropolitan	466	25,656	554,018	4,941,268	14,563,939	13,511	39,822	8.9	618,730	1,871	71,571	2,893,313	23,199,741
Metropolitan	226	42,799	1,867,680	9,696,946	19,244,436	26,589	52,833	5.2	1,429,975	3,012	197,047	5,831,826	37,682,062
Iowa	118	9,962	336,765	2,022,552	5,547,132	5,528	15,153	6.0	337,468	727	37,967	1,297,129	10,615,665
Nonmetropolitan	84	4,310	96,583	781,583	2,835,365	2,134	7,746	8.1	125,975	319	10,436	520,089	5,029,600
Metropolitan	34	5,652	240,182	1,240,969	2,711,767	3,394	7,407	5.2	211,493	408	27,531	777,040	5,586,065
Ames	2	269	10,056	64,178	144,150	176	393	6.4	9,703	17	1,030	28,839	191,685
Cedar Rapids	4	741	29,438	166,345	473,658	455	1,294	5.7	32,680	54	3,287	112,069	984,190
Davenport-Moline-Rock Island . . .	3	473	20,668	89,890	169,688	245	463	4.3	12,608	33	2,708	96,063	221,723
Des Moines	8	1,473	70,303	346,760	666,218	948	1,821	4.9	46,205	126	9,688	203,676	918,335
Dubuque	3	406	13,514	71,945	141,124	197	385	5.3	13,267	34	1,585	47,549	137,774
Iowa City	3	987	40,222	248,108	500,135	679	1,366	6.2	33,953	54	3,247	88,695	1,482,838
Omaha-Council Bluffs	3	293	13,460	54,788	117,757	150	322	4.1	13,154	22	987	58,426	245,443
Sioux City	2	395	20,010	89,233	147,816	244	404	4.5	11,664	31	2,326	60,102	334,014
Waterloo-Cedar Falls.	6	615	22,511	109,722	351,221	300	959	4.9	38,259	37	2,673	81,621	1,070,063
Kansas.	131	10,127	296,267	1,915,826	4,558,665	5,233	12,456	6.5	239,493	704	38,623	1,114,026	7,293,037
Nonmetropolitan	97	4,806	90,218	874,047	2,597,568	2,386	7,097	9.7	95,183	337	11,288	394,297	3,367,201
Metropolitan	34	5,321	206,049	1,041,779	1,961,097	2,847	5,359	5.1	144,310	367	27,335	719,729	3,925,836
Kansas City	15	2,397	98,455	499,553	959,764	1,365	2,623	5.1	76,308	181	13,209	318,259	2,038,065
Lawrence.	1	152	6,655	23,120	87,323	63	239	3.5	4,209	13	1,103	37,275	170,433
Topeka	6	864	31,776	166,276	344,672	454	942	5.2	18,351	40	3,062	100,407	747,554
Wichita	12	1,908	69,163	352,830	569,338	965	1,555	5.1	45,442	133	9,961	263,788	969,784
Minnesota.	133	14,895	583,142	3,479,304	7,840,228	9,516	21,451	6.0	469,270	1,193	64,001	1,898,093	11,430,163
Nonmetropolitan	82	5,050	103,967	1,058,885	3,190,319	2,898	8,736	10.2	124,830	375	14,765	573,626	4,225,963
Metropolitan	51	9,845	479,175	2,420,419	4,649,909	6,618	12,715	5.1	344,440	818	49,236	1,324,467	7,204,200
Duluth	10	1,264	40,015	265,268	635,498	724	1,738	6.6	40,265	105	3,234	130,470	594,193
Grand Forks	2	127	1,654	23,579	62,446	64	171	14.3	3,957	6	432	25,434	132,152
Minneapolis-St. Paul-Bloomington .	30	6,361	338,177	1,542,401	2,753,322	4,216	7,526	4.6	257,269	619	41,185	965,684	4,936,157
Rochester.	4	1,336	70,247	412,063	747,523	1,129	2,046	5.9	28,194	51	1,388	132,844	1,021,315
St. Cloud	5	757	29,082	177,108	451,120	485	1,234	6.1	14,755	37	2,997	70,035	520,383
Missouri	123	19,032	799,256	4,120,318	8,764,892	11,270	23,978	5.2	588,914	1,329	75,301	3,042,008	21,066,441
Nonmetropolitan	53	3,691	129,506	603,395	1,735,545	1,650	4,744	4.7	107,592	341	13,945	724,076	5,373,716
Metropolitan	70	15,341	669,750	3,516,923	7,029,347	9,620	19,234	5.3	481,322	988	61,356	2,317,932	15,692,725
Columbia	4	991	44,152	222,044	375,766	607	1,028	5.0	41,132	66	4,639	116,186	1,076,266
Jefferson City	3	290	15,160	59,204	139,011	163	379	3.9	11,101	24	1,383	74,947	722,312
Joplin	4	643	26,991	135,883	290,143	384	819	5.0	15,388	65	2,998	145,747	928,416
Kansas City	23	3,714	155,807	839,809	1,791,766	2,296	4,895	5.4	109,288	215	15,140	663,362	3,669,682
Springfield	5	1,459	70,023	359,410	795,081	981	2,173	5.1	64,194	83	6,662	253,214	2,456,917
St. Joseph	1	352	17,718	76,207	161,982	208	443	4.3	10,800	20	1,713	58,047	1,064,952
St. Louis	30	7,892	339,899	1,824,366	3,475,598	4,981	9,497	5.4	229,419	515	28,821	1,006,429	5,774,180
Nebraska	89	6,997	205,065	1,411,707	3,137,035	3,861	8,578	6.9	212,102	525	25,859	671,332	5,227,658
Nonmetropolitan	71	3,524	73,180	668,527	1,809,252	1,828	4,948	9.1	101,002	288	8,802	289,578	2,620,155
Metropolitan	18	3,473	131,885	743,180	1,327,783	2,033	3,630	5.6	111,100	237	17,057	381,754	2,607,503
Lincoln	5	999	39,807	241,397	375,968	660	1,029	6.1	25,322	63	4,860	107,866	420,829
Omaha-Council Bluffs	13	2,474	92,078	501,783	951,815	1,373	2,601	5.4	85,778	174	12,197	273,888	2,186,674
North Dakota	44	3,254	92,940	727,855	1,756,055	2,063	5,017	7.8	95,216	168	14,625	419,652	2,986,578
Nonmetropolitan	36	1,742	25,976	400,994	953,766	1,098	2,611	15.4	28,947	65	7,490	240,671	1,255,628
Metropolitan	8	1,512	66,964	326,861	802,289	965	2,406	4.9	66,269	103	7,135	178,981	1,730,950
Bismarck	3	531	17,949	85,160	175,290	305	692	4.7	13,133	27	1,916	42,638	599,815
Fargo	3	639	34,260	156,270	369,618	426	1,010	4.6	41,371	53	3,564	62,929	417,274
Grand Forks	2	342	14,755	85,431	257,381	234	704	5.8	11,765	23	1,655	73,414	713,861
South Dakota	54	4,188	108,263	960,652	2,204,368	2,629	6,022	8.9	106,242	237	12,242	282,899	2,262,261
Nonmetropolitan	43	2,533	34,588	553,837	1,442,124	1,517	3,940	16.0	35,201	146	4,845	150,976	1,327,478
Metropolitan	11	1,655	73,675	406,815	762,244	1,112	2,082	5.5	71,041	91	7,397	131,923	934,783
Rapid City	3	529	19,535	139,879	228,033	382	623	7.2	10,367	52	2,336	59,664	220,100
Sioux Falls	8	1,126	54,140	266,936	534,211	730	1,459	4.9	60,674	39	5,061	72,259	714,683

MSAs

TABLE 8

U.S. CENSUS DIVISION 6, WEST NORTH CENTRAL

U.S. Community Hospitals
(Nonfederal, short-term general and other special hospitals)

2012 Utilization, Personnel and Finances

FULL-TIME EQUIVALENT PERSONNEL					FULL-TIME EQUIV. TRAINEES			EXPENSES						
								LABOR				TOTAL		
Physicians and Dentists	Registered Nurses	Licensed Practical Nurses	Other Salaried Personnel	Total Personnel	Medical and Dental Residents	Other Trainees	Total Trainees	Payroll (in thousands)	Employee Benefits (in thousands)	Total (in thousands)	Percent of Total	Amount (in thousands)	Adjusted per Admission	Adjusted per Inpatient Day
114,479	1,351,164	82,268	3,183,037	4,730,948	102,904	7,230	110,134	$296,335,931	$81,153,797	$377,489,736	49.9	$756,916,757	$11,220.70	$2,090.01
15,188	160,970	24,883	469,925	670,966	1,935	276	2,211	35,636,252	9,721,437	45,357,688	52.4	86,549,339	7,649.75	1,221.87
99,291	1,190,194	57,385	2,713,112	4,059,982	100,969	6,954	107,923	260,699,679	71,432,359	332,132,048	49.5	670,367,418	11,940.32	2,301.09
10,157	105,810	9,189	265,179	390,335	3,398	373	3,771	23,077,975	6,093,337	29,171,325	51.7	56,450,154	10,479.95	1,669.71
2,915	27,159	4,873	82,432	117,379	212	58	270	6,040,315	1,579,798	7,620,121	54.1	14,089,624	8,366.45	967.43
7,242	78,651	4,316	182,747	272,956	3,186	315	3,501	17,037,659	4,513,539	21,551,204	50.9	42,360,530	11,441.28	2,201.18
1,112	14,659	1,039	38,960	55,770	718	39	757	3,035,541	835,375	3,870,920	50.2	7,709,622	9,007.47	1,389.84
441	5,227	663	15,476	21,807	28	11	39	1,076,782	285,219	1,362,005	52.3	2,602,147	7,543.40	917.75
671	9,432	376	23,484	33,963	690	28	718	1,958,758	550,156	2,508,915	49.1	5,107,475	9,995.90	1,883.45
3	334	10	903	1,250	0	0	0	67,564	19,457	87,021	49.8	174,628	8,707.88	1,211.43
55	1,279	69	3,428	4,831	0	1	1	232,952	64,911	297,864	49.3	603,612	8,111.87	1,274.36
26	701	4	1,247	1,978	11	0	11	111,788	27,738	139,527	35.7	390,419	9,543.35	2,300.80
226	2,626	30	6,537	9,419	171	5	176	573,403	137,055	710,459	51.1	1,391,361	10,227.14	2,088.45
9	551	16	1,125	1,701	0	0	0	84,073	20,246	104,319	44.4	235,087	8,681.52	1,665.82
134	2,095	27	5,165	7,421	505	17	522	460,214	175,663	635,877	52.1	1,221,200	15,582.90	2,441.74
25	401	23	883	1,332	0	5	5	73,750	22,139	95,888	43.0	223,060	7,679.27	1,894.24
60	657	23	1,548	2,288	0	0	0	130,312	31,162	161,474	50.8	317,946	9,599.23	2,150.96
133	788	174	2,648	3,743	3	0	3	224,702	51,784	276,486	50.3	550,162	7,649.64	1,566.43
1,005	14,074	1,211	31,112	47,402	3	140	143	2,680,168	666,998	3,347,167	51.4	6,513,729	9,716.88	1,428.87
370	4,392	665	13,139	18,566	3	1	4	914,239	221,339	1,135,579	55.2	2,058,739	8,058.10	792.56
635	9,682	546	17,973	28,836	0	139	139	1,765,929	445,660	2,211,588	49.6	4,454,990	10,738.41	2,271.68
213	4,986	100	8,477	13,776	0	138	138	856,119	222,487	1,078,605	46.2	2,333,568	11,262.99	2,431.40
40	306	19	791	1,156	0	0	0	69,793	15,347	85,141	50.9	167,336	6,657.21	1,916.28
283	1,393	341	3,525	5,542	0	0	0	376,842	90,749	467,591	60.2	776,165	11,405.80	2,251.89
99	2,997	86	5,180	8,362	0	1	1	463,175	117,077	580,251	49.3	1,177,921	10,288.42	2,068.93
3,646	21,988	2,296	63,238	91,168	675	92	767	6,569,952	1,798,958	8,368,909	55.5	15,069,348	12,321.86	1,922.05
774	5,015	1,319	17,344	24,452	20	5	25	1,390,215	365,890	1,756,103	53.4	3,285,934	9,832.80	1,029.97
2,872	16,973	977	45,894	66,716	655	87	742	5,179,737	1,433,069	6,612,806	56.1	11,783,414	13,257.73	2,534.12
607	1,711	201	6,208	8,727	7	1	8	609,011	165,363	774,373	61.8	1,252,572	13,840.73	1,971.01
16	188	16	532	752	0	0	0	24,176	6,557	30,733	51.1	60,110	13,723.71	962.59
1,958	11,911	447	31,148	45,464	489	70	559	3,675,153	1,008,814	4,683,969	56.2	8,327,173	13,687.54	3,024.41
258	1,900	137	4,443	6,738	143	16	159	591,263	165,638	756,900	51.3	1,476,257	11,305.99	1,974.87
33	1,263	176	3,563	5,035	16	0	16	280,134	86,696	366,831	55.0	667,301	12,139.82	1,479.21
2,662	34,048	2,703	80,165	119,578	1,801	76	1,877	6,727,805	1,777,988	8,505,800	50.0	17,024,103	9,945.86	1,942.31
694	5,308	1,183	15,720	22,905	43	24	67	1,163,472	311,653	1,475,127	58.4	2,527,142	6,762.09	1,456.11
1,968	28,740	1,520	64,445	96,673	1,758	52	1,810	5,564,333	1,466,334	7,030,673	48.5	14,496,962	10,835.16	2,062.35
49	1,821	248	4,836	6,954	360	1	361	354,543	115,660	470,203	48.2	974,535	12,863.11	2,593.46
82	572	110	1,451	2,215	9	0	9	125,058	32,055	157,113	53.5	293,824	8,014.85	2,113.68
150	1,283	73	3,200	4,706	24	0	24	270,999	59,921	330,920	53.5	618,797	10,605.83	2,132.73
525	7,017	297	15,325	23,164	196	51	247	1,425,956	334,774	1,760,733	51.9	3,389,998	11,143.10	1,891.99
283	3,087	304	9,898	13,572	25	0	25	640,332	176,074	816,406	41.6	1,961,569	12,382.94	2,467.13
143	623	153	2,296	3,215	0	0	0	219,737	54,413	274,150	61.8	443,399	11,773.44	2,737.34
736	14,337	335	27,439	42,847	1,144	0	1,144	2,527,707	693,438	3,221,148	47.3	6,814,839	10,218.77	1,960.77
481	10,563	877	23,963	35,884	42	9	51	1,875,767	518,339	2,394,108	48.1	4,972,246	11,134.40	1,585.01
270	3,732	583	10,558	15,143	18	5	23	759,351	215,875	975,228	50.9	1,916,200	9,698.45	1,059.11
211	6,831	294	13,405	20,741	24	4	28	1,116,416	302,464	1,418,880	46.4	3,056,046	12,273.87	2,301.62
20	1,657	168	3,550	5,395	0	3	3	297,949	89,786	387,735	49.1	788,892	11,407.92	2,098.30
191	5,174	126	9,855	15,346	24	1	25	818,467	212,678	1,031,145	45.5	2,267,154	12,606.85	2,381.93
672	5,044	731	14,175	20,622	133	10	143	1,050,331	239,346	1,289,675	48.4	2,666,136	10,813.64	1,518.25
195	1,706	238	4,896	7,035	99	9	108	328,503	81,911	410,413	50.9	806,025	9,906.89	845.10
477	3,338	493	9,279	13,587	34	1	35	721,828	157,435	879,262	47.3	1,860,111	11,260.23	2,318.50
235	1,177	195	3,141	4,748	2	0	2	215,980	31,764	247,744	56.7	436,809	11,686.88	2,491.92
31	1,631	262	3,584	5,508	9	1	10	275,403	71,281	346,684	35.7	970,336	11,818.23	2,625.24
211	530	36	2,554	3,331	23	0	23	230,445	54,390	284,834	62.9	452,966	9,909.13	1,759.91
579	5,434	332	13,566	19,911	26	7	33	1,138,411	256,334	1,394,746	55.9	2,494,971	10,733.23	1,131.83
171	1,779	222	5,299	7,471	1	3	4	407,753	97,913	505,666	56.6	893,437	9,231.82	619.53
408	3,655	110	8,267	12,440	25	4	29	730,658	158,421	889,080	55.5	1,601,533	11,804.19	2,101.08
57	964	44	2,106	3,171	25	4	29	172,381	21,098	193,478	62.9	307,639	9,649.30	1,349.10
351	2,691	66	6,161	9,269	0	0	0	558,277	137,323	695,602	53.8	1,293,894	12,466.10	2,422.07

MSAs

TABLE 8

U.S. CENSUS DIVISION 7, WEST SOUTH CENTRAL

U.S. Community Hospitals
(Nonfederal, short-term general and other special hospitals)

2012 Utilization, Personnel and Finances

CLASSIFICATION	Hospitals	Beds	Admissions	Inpatient Days	Adjusted Inpatient Days	Average Daily Census	Adjusted Average Daily Census	Average Stay (days)	Surgical Operations	NEWBORNS Bassinets	NEWBORNS Births	OUTPATIENT VISITS Emergency	OUTPATIENT VISITS Total
UNITED STATES	4,999	800,566	34,422,071	185,423,035	362,159,266	507,292	990,999	5.4	26,811,231	55,987	3,715,479	133,221,030	674,971,331
Nonmetropolitan	1,980	132,450	4,000,957	25,115,368	70,833,735	68,747	193,921	6.3	4,071,289	10,624	446,664	23,768,413	125,342,725
Metropolitan	3,019	668,116	30,421,114	160,307,667	291,325,531	438,545	797,078	5.3	22,739,942	45,363	3,268,815	109,452,617	549,628,606
CENSUS DIVISION 7, WEST SOUTH CENTRAL	749	97,260	3,908,065	20,396,936	37,589,018	55,733	102,742	5.2	2,755,772	7,297	516,124	16,269,062	62,161,308
Nonmetropolitan	310	16,243	517,868	2,347,590	6,210,031	6,413	16,980	4.5	413,001	1,346	60,264	3,188,742	12,710,312
Metropolitan	439	81,017	3,390,197	18,049,346	31,378,987	49,320	85,762	5.3	2,342,771	5,951	455,860	13,080,320	49,450,996
Arkansas	83	9,417	352,752	1,845,443	3,624,452	5,042	9,911	5.2	275,251	649	35,421	1,382,183	5,125,435
Nonmetropolitan	48	3,165	98,161	507,394	1,251,635	1,385	3,423	5.2	72,637	230	8,896	525,395	1,915,752
Metropolitan	35	6,252	254,591	1,338,049	2,372,817	3,657	6,488	5.3	202,614	419	26,525	856,788	3,209,683
Fayetteville-Springdale-Rogers . . .	6	922	43,158	176,484	292,707	482	800	4.1	40,725	92	6,478	174,634	520,939
Fort Smith	7	933	33,519	189,096	335,519	517	917	5.6	34,430	50	3,522	145,261	447,199
Hot Springs	3	499	17,923	99,819	175,172	272	479	5.6	16,820	24	1,604	62,036	238,440
Jonesboro	3	547	25,097	117,047	238,565	321	653	4.7	15,849	38	2,079	77,493	275,699
Little Rock-North Little Rock	14	2,876	121,509	683,968	1,183,523	1,869	3,236	5.6	87,226	167	11,314	335,089	1,512,340
Memphis	1	142	3,725	17,941	37,076	49	102	4.8	2,934	12	505	9,042	44,426
Pine Bluff	1	333	9,660	53,694	110,255	147	301	5.6	4,630	36	1,023	53,233	170,640
Louisiana	124	15,204	582,425	3,138,473	6,062,896	8,573	16,571	5.4	396,247	949	60,736	2,539,449	9,551,317
Nonmetropolitan	47	2,985	98,675	461,845	1,125,229	1,262	3,078	4.7	89,524	213	10,570	573,302	1,974,339
Metropolitan	77	12,219	483,750	2,676,628	4,937,667	7,311	13,493	5.5	306,723	736	50,166	1,966,147	7,576,978
Alexandria	6	789	32,797	188,556	320,259	514	875	5.7	17,128	55	3,021	142,421	403,205
Baton Rouge	12	2,376	80,568	527,972	1,023,307	1,443	2,797	6.6	53,523	121	9,833	290,831	1,211,612
Houma-Bayou Cane-Thibodaux . .	5	504	25,029	117,747	281,031	322	767	4.7	23,793	41	3,248	139,790	539,866
Lafayette	8	970	39,052	207,362	366,876	568	1,003	5.3	18,552	55	2,540	164,364	595,363
Lake Charles	8	755	27,310	145,636	291,482	397	796	5.3	23,953	54	3,261	123,616	417,942
Monroe	9	858	35,927	201,191	347,136	548	947	5.6	17,772	68	3,940	129,739	510,132
New Orleans-Metairie-Kenner . . .	19	3,883	158,499	864,805	1,582,534	2,362	4,326	5.5	96,120	214	17,591	681,414	2,748,362
Shreveport-Bossier City	10	2,084	84,568	423,359	725,042	1,157	1,982	5.0	55,882	128	6,732	293,972	1,150,496
Oklahoma	117	11,349	424,024	2,242,204	4,389,183	6,126	11,998	5.3	330,314	795	50,107	1,908,047	6,774,143
Nonmetropolitan	66	3,694	116,636	532,643	1,344,583	1,456	3,679	4.6	99,842	317	14,841	685,558	2,461,750
Metropolitan	51	7,655	307,388	1,709,561	3,044,600	4,670	8,319	5.6	230,472	478	35,266	1,222,489	4,312,393
Fort Smith	2	110	3,193	12,593	34,245	34	93	3.9	1,883	11	346	31,737	48,022
Lawton	2	535	15,173	122,358	246,819	335	675	8.1	10,867	32	1,638	71,447	196,869
Oklahoma City	23	4,012	155,920	919,398	1,594,053	2,511	4,356	5.9	127,294	269	19,720	701,023	2,300,115
Tulsa	24	2,998	133,102	655,212	1,169,483	1,790	3,195	4.9	90,428	166	13,562	418,282	1,767,387
Texas	425	61,290	2,548,864	13,170,816	23,512,487	35,992	64,262	5.2	1,753,960	4,904	369,860	10,439,383	40,710,413
Nonmetropolitan	149	6,399	204,396	845,708	2,488,584	2,310	6,800	4.1	150,998	586	25,957	1,404,487	6,358,471
Metropolitan	276	54,891	2,344,468	12,325,108	21,023,903	33,682	57,462	5.3	1,602,962	4,318	343,903	9,034,896	34,351,942
Abilene	5	652	23,727	120,373	217,113	329	593	5.1	19,324	46	2,748	92,341	379,840
Amarillo	5	1,039	42,556	224,780	334,178	614	913	5.3	22,301	54	4,822	113,457	404,878
Austin-Round Rock	22	2,837	136,979	659,779	1,096,749	1,801	2,993	4.8	103,803	259	24,798	656,977	1,987,500
Beaumont-Port Arthur	7	1,176	49,404	243,493	429,416	665	1,173	4.9	30,813	74	5,161	227,872	586,432
Brownsville-Harlingen	3	871	37,325	177,504	265,779	486	728	4.8	23,374	92	5,994	121,024	221,199
College Station-Bryan	4	454	23,524	95,977	183,221	262	501	4.1	19,167	70	3,382	104,496	408,069
Corpus Christi	6	1,510	59,739	329,267	508,779	899	1,390	5.5	36,587	89	6,730	239,782	559,518
Dallas-Plano-Irving	50	8,832	385,830	2,055,588	3,473,022	5,613	9,488	5.3	241,267	735	57,451	1,583,214	5,312,119
El Paso	6	1,677	80,136	380,161	610,579	1,039	1,667	4.7	49,728	164	15,664	302,289	1,263,971
Fort Worth-Arlington	28	4,747	219,562	1,150,249	1,859,702	3,142	5,080	5.2	138,575	410	33,367	1,039,152	2,778,609
Houston-Sugar Land-Baytown . . .	66	14,668	595,604	3,380,323	5,921,895	9,239	16,182	5.7	414,986	1,254	92,486	1,993,372	10,020,415
Killeen-Temple-Fort Hood	5	958	42,836	200,702	494,221	559	1,378	4.7	27,983	68	4,722	191,747	1,660,466
Laredo	2	509	25,305	120,083	200,078	328	546	4.7	21,862	63	6,028	83,341	272,955
Longview	5	640	28,946	140,107	248,649	384	679	4.8	25,440	59	3,763	143,233	310,158
Lubbock	6	1,235	58,025	266,910	488,324	727	1,333	4.6	37,156	71	5,142	174,757	731,726
McAllen-Edinburg-Mission	7	2,153	90,756	420,920	669,150	1,150	1,827	4.6	86,603	193	17,237	223,675	525,428
Midland	2	289	11,754	63,065	115,893	172	316	5.4	9,590	24	2,104	61,164	147,894
Odessa	3	592	20,681	107,374	170,000	293	464	5.2	11,323	39	3,976	77,086	331,385
San Angelo	2	413	16,923	78,782	162,356	215	444	4.7	20,571	36	1,901	77,991	192,471
San Antonio	17	5,442	233,194	1,180,637	1,923,079	3,224	5,254	5.1	148,582	317	30,007	889,964	3,901,903
Sherman-Denison	2	486	17,818	90,905	156,949	248	429	5.1	9,766	35	1,490	74,209	129,089
Texarkana TX-Texarkana AR	5	648	24,788	130,246	209,880	357	574	5.3	12,214	31	2,797	103,721	297,113
Tyler	7	1,137	50,829	284,160	490,144	776	1,339	5.6	36,029	41	3,342	148,450	985,672
Victoria	4	566	18,867	96,306	185,460	264	507	5.1	23,276	34	2,310	81,743	198,716
Waco	2	909	31,415	243,406	466,809	665	1,276	7.7	16,439	40	4,293	133,701	536,522
Wichita Falls	5	451	17,945	84,011	142,478	231	388	4.7	16,203	20	2,188	96,138	207,894

MSAs

TABLE 8

U.S. CENSUS DIVISION 7, WEST SOUTH CENTRAL

U.S. Community Hospitals
(Nonfederal, short-term general and other special hospitals)

2012 Utilization, Personnel and Finances

FULL-TIME EQUIVALENT PERSONNEL					FULL-TIME EQUIV. TRAINEES			EXPENSES						
								LABOR				TOTAL		
Physicians and Dentists	Registered Nurses	Licensed Practical Nurses	Other Salaried Personnel	Total Personnel	Medical and Dental Residents	Other Trainees	Total Trainees	Payroll (in thousands)	Employee Benefits (in thousands)	Total (in thousands)	Percent of Total	Amount (in thousands)	Adjusted per Admission	Adjusted per Inpatient Day
114,479	1,351,164	82,268	3,183,037	4,730,948	102,904	7,230	110,134	$296,335,931	$81,153,797	$377,489,736	49.9	$756,916,757	$11,220.70	$2,090.01
15,188	160,970	24,883	469,925	670,966	1,935	276	2,211	35,636,252	9,721,437	45,357,688	52.4	86,549,339	7,649.75	1,221.87
99,291	1,190,194	57,385	2,713,112	4,059,982	100,969	6,954	107,923	260,699,679	71,432,359	332,132,048	49.5	670,367,418	11,940.32	2,301.09
5,243	145,072	15,470	317,150	482,935	4,864	1,189	6,053	27,963,570	6,674,611	34,638,178	46.5	74,523,034	9,949.20	1,982.57
931	17,406	5,186	49,458	72,981	48	19	67	3,390,907	834,927	4,225,829	49.8	8,477,983	6,101.51	1,365.21
4,312	127,666	10,284	267,692	409,954	4,816	1,170	5,986	24,572,663	5,839,684	30,412,349	46.0	66,045,051	10,825.52	2,104.75
516	13,751	1,820	29,312	45,399	61	16	77	2,143,864	513,485	2,657,349	46.1	5,759,241	7,979.47	1,589.00
151	3,371	915	9,067	13,504	4	1	5	589,283	141,254	730,536	49.6	1,472,239	5,710.29	1,176.25
365	10,380	905	20,245	31,895	57	15	72	1,554,581	372,231	1,926,813	44.9	4,287,002	9,240.52	1,806.71
100	1,476	138	2,898	4,612	21	2	23	213,971	49,325	263,297	43.9	600,351	7,951.88	2,051.03
95	989	225	2,278	3,587	0	0	0	156,779	44,562	201,341	41.7	482,371	7,579.92	1,437.69
60	758	69	1,693	2,580	23	2	25	100,923	25,733	126,657	48.5	261,069	8,156.62	1,490.36
20	967	117	1,674	2,778	0	0	0	112,792	29,346	142,138	42.6	333,787	6,499.34	1,399.14
63	5,563	269	10,268	16,163	9	6	15	871,228	202,134	1,073,361	45.2	2,375,448	11,105.36	2,007.10
14	166	13	436	629	4	0	4	23,962	6,580	30,542	50.5	60,422	7,849.09	1,629.69
13	461	74	998	1,546	0	5	5	74,926	14,552	89,477	51.6	173,555	8,749.49	1,574.12
1,326	21,699	3,191	52,547	78,763	712	38	750	3,946,096	914,115	4,860,215	47.9	10,146,976	8,752.48	1,673.62
250	3,380	841	9,788	14,259	8	3	11	653,938	155,276	809,215	53.5	1,512,445	6,101.54	1,344.12
1,076	18,319	2,350	42,759	64,504	704	35	739	3,292,158	758,839	4,051,000	46.9	8,634,531	9,473.43	1,748.71
3	1,085	133	2,378	3,599	0	0	0	172,953	43,455	216,408	45.8	472,091	8,411.56	1,474.09
248	3,007	252	7,823	11,330	73	15	88	615,879	114,344	730,224	48.1	1,517,893	9,576.73	1,483.32
42	869	95	2,571	3,577	25	11	36	182,306	49,933	232,238	48.7	476,663	7,962.04	1,696.12
65	1,450	187	3,264	4,966	9	0	9	256,832	53,024	309,856	41.7	743,928	10,559.66	2,027.74
64	1,109	195	2,484	3,852	0	0	0	165,799	47,586	213,385	46.1	463,354	8,150.32	1,589.65
49	1,171	183	2,784	4,187	30	2	32	199,639	47,456	247,097	47.8	516,787	8,236.30	1,488.72
311	6,847	832	13,990	21,980	357	2	359	1,272,543	284,763	1,557,306	46.5	3,345,863	11,348.64	2,114.24
294	2,781	473	7,465	11,013	210	5	215	426,207	118,278	544,486	49.6	1,097,952	7,219.24	1,514.33
761	14,449	1,941	35,683	52,834	307	94	401	2,731,685	661,066	3,392,748	45.5	7,462,798	8,543.69	1,700.27
347	3,890	960	10,724	15,921	36	4	40	748,498	182,052	930,548	49.9	1,864,039	6,293.41	1,386.33
414	10,559	981	24,959	36,913	271	90	361	1,983,188	479,014	2,462,200	44.0	5,598,759	9,698.21	1,838.91
3	70	52	346	471	0	0	0	15,390	3,234	18,625	56.9	32,748	3,219.09	956.28
87	382	165	1,319	1,953	12	6	18	107,293	19,669	126,961	48.1	263,984	8,698.85	1,069.54
258	5,795	446	13,090	19,589	101	83	184	1,103,866	277,350	1,381,214	43.5	3,173,615	11,053.27	1,990.91
66	4,312	318	10,204	14,900	158	1	159	756,638	178,761	935,400	43.9	2,128,413	8,525.31	1,819.96
2,640	95,173	8,518	199,608	305,939	3,784	1,041	4,825	19,141,924	4,585,945	23,727,866	46.4	51,154,020	10,801.59	2,175.61
183	6,765	2,470	19,879	29,297	0	11	11	1,399,189	356,346	1,755,530	48.4	3,629,261	6,176.42	1,458.36
2,457	88,408	6,048	179,729	276,642	3,784	1,030	4,814	17,742,736	4,229,599	21,972,336	46.2	47,524,759	11,456.76	2,260.51
2	836	183	1,814	2,835	0	25	25	145,885	31,218	177,102	46.5	380,673	8,881.77	1,753.34
44	1,382	125	2,897	4,448	0	2	2	196,197	41,365	237,563	41.2	577,033	8,719.67	1,726.72
295	5,935	256	10,299	16,785	243	75	318	1,092,301	231,784	1,324,085	51.5	2,570,127	10,765.65	2,343.40
1	1,569	160	2,508	4,238	0	0	0	251,351	58,485	309,837	43.3	716,232	7,883.94	1,667.92
1	756	90	1,246	2,093	0	0	0	167,840	29,253	197,093	36.0	547,007	9,768.86	2,058.13
39	754	106	1,638	2,537	0	0	0	145,240	39,161	184,401	47.1	391,507	8,628.05	2,136.80
45	2,176	154	3,899	6,274	150	5	155	366,112	84,088	450,199	48.3	932,725	9,920.92	1,833.26
322	16,327	510	29,919	47,078	1,192	4	1,196	3,325,653	781,833	4,107,485	46.2	8,899,961	13,194.33	2,562.60
13	2,379	96	4,623	7,111	0	0	0	421,435	91,633	513,067	39.2	1,308,684	10,005.38	2,143.35
25	8,606	571	16,054	25,256	252	0	252	1,609,178	418,160	2,027,340	47.1	4,308,837	11,607.05	2,316.95
972	25,104	1,283	54,749	82,108	1,056	894	1,950	5,972,414	1,490,118	7,462,533	48.2	15,483,341	14,115.27	2,614.59
517	1,771	215	5,364	7,867	463	0	463	394,984	87,939	482,924	50.7	952,382	8,971.19	1,927.04
0	619	40	1,310	1,969	0	0	0	89,248	20,927	110,174	30.6	360,367	8,484.61	1,801.13
0	1,038	40	1,930	3,008	0	0	0	155,642	36,827	192,469	45.0	427,861	7,956.79	1,720.74
0	2,157	184	3,816	6,157	0	0	0	330,429	90,835	421,264	50.9	827,456	7,202.29	1,694.48
0	2,606	179	5,120	7,905	0	0	0	410,061	86,328	496,389	45.1	1,099,467	7,449.21	1,643.08
1	489	24	1,106	1,620	0	0	0	92,667	23,305	115,972	44.0	263,692	11,230.49	2,275.31
0	707	83	1,419	2,209	0	0	0	124,907	38,482	163,389	42.5	384,114	11,497.31	2,259.49
0	583	113	1,362	2,058	0	0	0	104,263	26,056	130,319	48.3	269,890	7,728.81	1,662.34
56	7,220	669	15,794	23,739	382	17	399	1,341,562	280,744	1,622,307	39.6	4,100,717	10,615.81	2,132.37
0	548	56	1,126	1,730	0	0	0	93,185	23,109	116,294	44.4	261,720	8,550.14	1,667.55
0	858	149	1,575	2,582	0	0	0	120,427	25,984	146,411	41.7	351,311	8,237.46	1,673.87
60	1,849	380	4,924	7,213	46	7	53	364,279	100,230	464,508	43.3	1,073,925	11,386.22	2,191.04
18	655	116	1,388	2,177	0	1	1	116,279	27,358	143,636	53.6	267,748	7,089.84	1,443.70
46	892	164	2,226	3,328	0	0	0	181,171	39,465	220,636	48.5	454,715	7,558.68	974.09
0	592	102	1,623	2,317	0	0	0	130,026	24,913	154,939	49.5	313,268	9,720.98	2,198.71

MSAs

MSAs

CLASSIFICATION	Hospitals	Beds	Admissions	Inpatient Days	Adjusted Inpatient Days	Average Daily Census	Adjusted Average Daily Census	Average Stay (days)	Surgical Operations	NEWBORNS Bassinets	Births	OUTPATIENT VISITS Emergency	Total
UNITED STATES	4,999	800,566	34,422,071	185,423,035	362,159,266	507,292	990,999	5.4	26,811,231	55,987	3,715,479	133,221,030	674,971,331
Nonmetropolitan	1,980	132,450	4,000,957	25,115,368	70,833,735	68,747	193,921	6.3	4,071,289	10,624	446,664	23,768,413	125,342,725
Metropolitan	3,019	668,116	30,421,114	160,307,667	291,325,531	438,545	797,078	5.3	22,739,942	45,363	3,268,815	109,452,617	549,628,606
CENSUS DIVISION 8, MOUNTAIN . . .	388	47,501	2,060,596	10,231,226	20,427,488	27,970	55,846	5.0	1,597,100	4,074	269,841	7,821,770	40,258,247
Nonmetropolitan	195	9,314	236,397	1,683,119	5,138,082	4,600	14,047	7.1	275,621	906	43,838	1,518,940	8,441,499
Metropolitan	193	38,187	1,824,199	8,548,107	15,289,406	23,370	41,799	4.7	1,321,479	3,168	226,003	6,302,830	31,816,748
Arizona	72	13,527	674,808	2,977,605	5,180,526	8,144	14,165	4.4	462,159	994	73,033	2,309,621	8,737,017
Nonmetropolitan	14	550	24,036	95,900	319,488	263	874	4.0	23,866	62	4,258	133,812	594,289
Metropolitan	58	12,977	650,772	2,881,705	4,861,038	7,881	13,291	4.4	438,293	932	68,775	2,175,809	8,142,728
Flagstaff	3	365	17,701	72,663	168,733	199	461	4.1	14,498	44	1,919	80,343	911,527
Lake Havasu City-Kingman	4	523	26,361	114,102	224,279	313	614	4.3	16,300	33	2,619	128,932	586,914
Phoenix-Mesa-Scottsdale	36	8,672	453,587	1,994,511	3,260,854	5,454	8,916	4.4	300,046	673	47,780	1,369,235	4,763,615
Prescott	3	316	15,812	53,276	110,854	145	303	3.4	9,286	11	1,446	93,444	200,403
Tucson	10	2,691	120,832	570,030	942,578	1,559	2,576	4.7	87,991	152	11,646	434,132	1,503,782
Yuma	2	410	16,479	77,123	153,740	211	421	4.7	10,172	19	3,365	69,723	176,487
Colorado	82	10,244	444,430	2,253,793	4,611,457	6,165	12,609	5.1	366,912	929	58,253	1,818,858	8,958,787
Nonmetropolitan	38	1,541	37,687	256,213	931,872	704	2,550	6.8	46,978	158	7,668	270,059	1,705,163
Metropolitan	44	8,703	406,743	1,997,580	3,679,585	5,461	10,059	4.9	319,934	771	50,585	1,548,799	7,253,624
Boulder	4	628	34,020	133,806	260,661	365	713	3.9	26,095	94	6,939	119,181	700,473
Colorado Springs	5	962	64,210	293,194	596,055	802	1,630	4.6	39,360	86	4,652	217,244	632,649
Denver-Aurora	24	5,190	228,922	1,174,861	2,018,666	3,211	5,518	5.1	184,889	434	28,507	851,087	3,726,585
Fort Collins-Loveland	4	551	29,026	117,819	245,955	323	673	4.1	22,714	53	4,171	116,345	914,900
Grand Junction	3	502	14,583	102,251	218,302	280	596	7.0	11,800	32	2,176	69,419	494,004
Greeley	2	298	15,375	66,596	119,552	182	327	4.3	13,781	38	2,007	53,827	514,114
Pueblo	2	572	20,607	109,053	220,394	298	602	5.3	21,295	34	2,133	121,696	270,899
Idaho	40	3,305	123,794	611,785	1,449,171	1,668	3,961	4.9	122,228	286	20,117	543,272	4,350,570
Nonmetropolitan	26	1,038	30,492	178,873	547,185	488	1,496	5.9	37,422	119	6,506	178,847	1,377,951
Metropolitan	14	2,267	93,302	432,912	901,986	1,180	2,465	4.6	84,806	167	13,611	364,425	2,972,619
Boise City-Nampa	8	1,309	55,744	231,370	487,066	630	1,331	4.2	48,826	107	7,823	208,512	2,140,180
Coeur d'Alene	1	254	11,305	60,250	128,884	165	352	5.3	10,958	18	1,635	47,415	328,662
Idaho Falls	1	309	11,923	64,044	98,783	175	270	5.4	11,348	10	1,628	41,653	177,537
Lewiston	1	119	4,950	23,081	47,698	63	130	4.7	2,462	12	755	29,361	117,201
Logan	1	65	439	12,934	39,786	35	109	29.5	888	5	214	1,047	5,447
Pocatello	2	211	8,941	41,233	99,769	112	273	4.6	10,324	15	1,556	36,437	203,592
Montana	48	3,710	93,423	809,199	2,089,390	2,211	5,709	8.7	76,415	212	10,191	366,756	3,585,038
Nonmetropolitan	42	2,274	40,452	484,683	1,344,764	1,325	3,674	12.0	37,112	133	4,544	212,202	1,456,963
Metropolitan	6	1,436	52,971	324,516	744,626	886	2,035	6.1	39,303	79	5,647	154,554	2,128,075
Billings	3	647	26,626	155,281	394,888	424	1,079	5.8	20,969	34	2,759	72,537	1,469,200
Great Falls	1	463	12,698	106,171	229,136	290	626	8.4	7,817	24	1,438	35,949	351,241
Missoula	2	326	13,647	63,064	120,602	172	330	4.6	10,517	21	1,450	46,068	307,634
Nevada	38	5,504	260,781	1,361,402	2,182,360	3,723	5,968	5.2	151,878	288	26,384	865,371	2,910,827
Nonmetropolitan	11	365	10,146	65,011	194,629	177	533	6.4	14,485	26	961	78,394	451,096
Metropolitan	27	5,139	250,635	1,296,391	1,987,731	3,546	5,435	5.2	137,393	262	25,423	786,977	2,459,731
Carson City	1	190	10,161	43,448	76,312	119	209	4.3	5,928	12	893	32,246	221,434
Las Vegas-Paradise	19	3,757	188,866	999,553	1,494,645	2,735	4,087	5.3	93,578	179	19,586	580,786	1,637,016
Reno-Sparks	7	1,192	51,608	253,390	416,774	692	1,139	4.9	37,887	71	4,944	173,945	601,281

MSAs

| FULL-TIME EQUIVALENT PERSONNEL | | | | | FULL-TIME EQUIV. TRAINEES | | | EXPENSES | | | | | | |
| | | | | | | | | LABOR | | | | TOTAL | | |
Physicians and Dentists	Registered Nurses	Licensed Practical Nurses	Other Salaried Personnel	Total Personnel	Medical and Dental Residents	Other Trainees	Total Trainees	Payroll (in thousands)	Employee Benefits (in thousands)	Total (in thousands)	Percent of Total	Amount (in thousands)	Adjusted per Admission	Adjusted per Inpatient Day
114,479	1,351,164	82,268	3,183,037	4,730,948	102,904	7,230	110,134	$296,335,931	$81,153,797	$377,489,736	49.9	$756,916,757	$11,220.70	$2,090.01
15,188	160,970	24,883	469,925	670,966	1,935	276	2,211	35,636,252	9,721,437	45,357,688	52.4	86,549,339	7,649.75	1,221.87
99,291	1,190,194	57,385	2,713,112	4,059,982	100,969	6,954	107,923	260,699,679	71,432,359	332,132,048	49.5	670,367,418	11,940.32	2,301.09
5,816	80,111	3,695	180,536	270,158	2,502	408	2,910	16,668,357	4,231,698	20,900,046	48.2	43,346,402	10,915.95	2,121.96
1,302	10,826	1,287	34,631	48,046	33	9	42	2,658,544	656,008	3,314,550	52.4	6,331,150	9,046.39	1,232.20
4,514	69,285	2,408	145,905	222,112	2,469	399	2,868	14,009,813	3,575,690	17,585,496	47.5	37,015,251	11,315.95	2,420.97
1,503	24,064	670	47,435	73,672	1,148	123	1,271	4,630,731	1,119,133	5,749,864	47.5	12,112,684	10,238.45	2,338.12
74	870	85	2,858	3,887	2	4	6	215,740	52,696	268,436	51.7	519,715	6,733.63	1,626.71
1,429	23,194	585	44,577	69,785	1,146	119	1,265	4,414,991	1,066,437	5,481,428	47.3	11,592,969	10,483.06	2,384.88
116	779	5	1,886	2,786	1	9	10	198,309	48,616	246,925	52.6	469,581	10,777.62	2,782.98
72	964	62	2,309	3,407	16	0	16	192,307	47,715	240,023	52.1	460,313	8,945.76	2,052.41
1,115	15,787	363	28,985	46,250	1,053	90	1,143	3,006,099	760,721	3,766,818	47.2	7,981,847	10,715.85	2,447.78
49	612	2	1,539	2,202	0	7	7	155,982	38,190	194,172	55.7	348,403	10,468.53	3,142.90
69	4,489	139	8,539	13,236	76	1	77	732,428	132,425	864,855	43.3	1,995,593	9,991.95	2,117.16
8	563	14	1,319	1,904	0	12	12	129,865	38,770	168,635	50.0	337,232	10,223.80	2,193.52
1,195	18,907	573	41,819	62,494	412	185	597	4,189,313	1,019,513	5,208,825	47.6	10,941,849	12,605.06	2,372.75
273	2,052	209	6,898	9,432	2	0	2	576,832	148,338	725,170	52.1	1,391,925	11,762.29	1,493.69
922	16,855	364	34,921	53,062	410	185	595	3,612,480	871,175	4,483,655	46.9	9,549,924	12,738.09	2,595.38
88	1,292	30	3,077	4,487	2	2	4	297,296	67,170	364,467	48.6	749,245	11,332.80	2,874.40
76	1,636	29	3,864	5,605	0	18	18	385,411	100,080	485,491	45.3	1,070,676	8,211.21	1,796.27
636	10,810	234	21,040	32,720	301	165	466	2,252,337	536,603	2,788,940	47.2	5,905,200	14,799.89	2,925.30
20	1,200	33	2,099	3,352	22	0	22	241,743	67,959	309,703	47.1	657,339	11,371.67	2,672.60
59	563	15	1,502	2,139	24	0	24	156,157	36,059	192,215	47.6	404,175	14,909.80	1,851.45
4	543	10	1,369	1,926	33	0	33	124,646	27,619	152,265	43.2	352,596	12,890.10	2,949.31
39	811	13	1,970	2,833	28	0	28	154,890	35,684	190,574	46.4	410,692	9,792.61	1,863.45
790	5,858	543	17,219	24,410	19	6	25	1,260,075	320,364	1,580,437	50.5	3,127,968	11,112.02	2,158.45
170	1,448	258	4,941	6,817	3	1	4	329,231	84,220	413,448	50.3	822,208	9,107.10	1,502.61
620	4,410	285	12,278	17,593	16	5	21	930,844	236,145	1,166,989	50.6	2,305,760	12,058.66	2,556.32
484	2,806	152	8,826	12,268	12	5	17	601,702	155,822	757,525	50.3	1,504,677	12,733.91	3,089.27
70	428	11	1,377	1,886	0	0	0	127,190	30,361	157,551	54.3	290,285	12,003.69	2,252.30
2	542	41	610	1,195	0	0	0	65,936	19,090	85,026	49.3	172,559	9,383.32	1,746.85
15	208	14	532	769	4	0	4	53,938	14,811	68,749	50.5	136,007	13,296.17	2,851.41
4	51	9	165	229	0	0	0	6,235	1,793	8,028	54.6	14,701	10,889.32	369.49
45	375	58	768	1,246	0	0	0	75,843	14,267	90,110	48.1	187,532	9,923.91	1,879.66
883	4,215	625	13,865	19,588	0	2	2	1,130,765	259,358	1,390,123	52.2	2,660,996	11,414.70	1,273.58
368	2,115	281	7,411	10,175	0	0	0	510,685	122,166	632,852	53.8	1,175,553	10,192.07	874.17
515	2,100	344	6,454	9,413	0	2	2	620,080	137,192	757,271	51.0	1,485,443	12,612.01	1,994.88
344	968	185	3,448	4,945	0	0	0	364,201	76,195	440,395	54.7	805,789	12,562.38	2,040.55
58	545	72	1,477	2,152	0	0	0	136,281	27,555	163,836	50.1	327,075	11,934.88	1,427.43
113	587	87	1,529	2,316	0	2	2	119,598	33,442	153,040	43.4	352,579	13,440.80	2,923.49
148	7,857	358	15,308	23,671	71	2	73	1,578,249	439,967	2,018,214	48.1	4,199,883	9,860.01	1,924.47
30	394	36	1,201	1,661	0	0	0	98,203	23,652	121,854	51.2	238,022	8,131.40	1,222.95
118	7,463	322	14,107	22,010	71	2	73	1,480,046	416,315	1,896,360	47.9	3,961,860	9,987.57	1,993.16
1	315	6	754	1,076	0	0	0	72,129	17,691	89,821	48.0	187,242	10,491.49	2,453.63
116	5,346	287	10,255	16,004	71	2	73	1,118,169	330,863	1,449,031	51.4	2,820,580	9,707.06	1,887.12
1	1,802	29	3,098	4,930	0	0	0	289,748	67,761	357,508	37.5	954,039	10,809.17	2,289.10

Table continues

TABLE 8

U.S. CENSUS DIVISION 8, MOUNTAIN
CONTINUED

U.S. Community Hospitals
(Nonfederal, short-term general and other special hospitals)

2012 Utilization, Personnel and Finances

CLASSIFICATION	Hospitals	Beds	Admissions	Inpatient Days	Adjusted Inpatient Days	Average Daily Census	Adjusted Average Daily Census	Average Stay (days)	Surgical Operations	NEWBORNS Bassinets	NEWBORNS Births	OUTPATIENT VISITS Emergency	OUTPATIENT VISITS Total
New Mexico.	37	4,076	177,744	850,391	1,854,778	2,325	5,071	4.8	139,556	520	23,924	793,582	4,155,560
Nonmetropolitan	23	1,403	52,299	205,860	532,146	562	1,455	3.9	54,698	174	8,681	388,307	1,275,196
Metropolitan	14	2,673	125,445	644,531	1,322,632	1,763	3,616	5.1	84,858	346	15,243	405,275	2,880,364
Albuquerque	9	1,767	81,869	458,694	961,809	1,255	2,629	5.6	55,979	254	10,625	233,114	2,283,609
Farmington	1	232	10,834	45,145	88,452	123	242	4.2	5,735	22	1,292	48,052	161,885
Las Cruces.	3	406	19,621	87,980	164,828	241	451	4.5	14,788	46	2,118	70,013	271,472
Santa Fe	1	268	13,121	52,712	107,543	144	294	4.0	8,356	24	1,208	54,096	163,398
Utah	47	5,212	241,436	992,015	2,120,824	2,711	5,797	4.1	237,972	679	51,575	894,661	6,353,873
Nonmetropolitan	19	634	16,282	103,989	470,594	283	1,286	6.4	31,500	108	7,062	103,287	654,929
Metropolitan	28	4,578	225,154	888,026	1,650,230	2,428	4,511	3.9	206,472	571	44,513	791,374	5,698,944
Logan	2	150	8,163	22,969	55,035	63	151	2.8	9,306	34	2,670	31,369	331,086
Ogden-Clearfield	4	796	37,715	136,593	243,915	373	667	3.6	26,415	103	7,791	139,924	515,340
Provo-Orem	6	729	38,067	143,628	261,514	393	714	3.8	32,144	133	11,014	125,269	679,835
Salt Lake City	15	2,642	125,742	532,612	991,036	1,456	2,709	4.2	126,739	285	20,762	452,055	3,716,341
St. George	1	261	15,467	52,224	98,730	143	270	3.4	11,868	16	2,276	42,757	456,342
Wyoming	24	1,923	44,180	375,036	938,982	1,023	2,566	8.5	39,980	166	6,364	229,649	1,206,575
Nonmetropolitan	22	1,509	25,003	292,590	797,404	798	2,179	11.7	29,560	126	4,158	154,032	925,912
Metropolitan	2	414	19,177	82,446	141,578	225	387	4.3	10,420	40	2,206	75,617	280,663
Casper	1	192	8,826	34,114	53,733	93	147	3.9	5,131	24	1,061	36,094	81,728
Cheyenne.	1	222	10,351	48,332	87,845	132	240	4.7	5,289	16	1,145	39,523	198,935

MSAs

TABLE 8

U.S. CENSUS DIVISION 8, MOUNTAIN
CONTINUED

U.S. Community Hospitals
(Nonfederal, short-term general and other special hospitals)

2012 Utilization, Personnel and Finances

FULL-TIME EQUIVALENT PERSONNEL					FULL-TIME EQUIV. TRAINEES			EXPENSES						
								LABOR				TOTAL		
Physicians and Dentists	Registered Nurses	Licensed Practical Nurses	Other Salaried Personnel	Total Personnel	Medical and Dental Residents	Other Trainees	Total Trainees	Payroll (in thousands)	Employee Benefits (in thousands)	Total (in thousands)	Percent of Total	Amount (in thousands)	Adjusted per Admission	Adjusted per Inpatient Day
781	7,452	403	16,197	24,833	71	31	102	1,597,569	360,593	1,958,162	48.9	4,003,332	10,304.93	2,158.39
157	1,929	178	5,115	7,379	24	1	25	446,664	100,619	547,285	51.9	1,054,119	7,777.92	1,980.88
624	5,523	225	11,082	17,454	47	30	77	1,150,904	259,974	1,410,877	47.8	2,949,213	11,658.81	2,229.81
468	4,154	186	7,490	12,298	18	26	44	835,040	180,468	1,015,507	47.2	2,150,014	12,777.93	2,235.39
69	458	3	1,081	1,611	0	0	0	116,423	34,734	151,157	61.4	246,073	11,592.47	2,782.00
8	556	25	1,228	1,817	25	0	25	107,126	22,501	129,626	43.7	296,837	8,087.55	1,800.89
79	355	11	1,283	1,728	4	4	8	92,316	22,270	114,587	44.7	256,289	9,573.73	2,383.13
270	9,672	385	22,536	32,863	780	57	837	1,776,407	569,120	2,345,523	45.8	5,117,474	10,531.04	2,412.96
53	654	126	2,137	2,970	1	3	4	139,923	38,933	178,854	48.5	368,411	5,960.58	782.86
217	9,018	259	20,399	29,893	779	54	833	1,636,484	530,187	2,166,669	45.6	4,749,062	11,197.08	2,877.82
0	253	13	625	891	0	0	0	43,661	17,136	60,796	46.6	130,363	6,610.04	2,368.73
19	1,243	70	2,482	3,814	24	0	24	220,597	65,479	286,075	44.8	638,392	9,486.61	2,617.27
25	1,420	40	3,108	4,593	48	4	52	233,222	77,214	310,434	48.3	642,916	8,951.51	2,458.44
166	5,647	135	12,817	18,765	707	50	757	1,045,539	334,595	1,380,134	45.8	3,012,568	12,762.09	3,039.82
7	455	1	1,367	1,830	0	0	0	93,466	35,764	129,230	39.8	324,824	11,108.88	3,290.02
246	2,086	138	6,157	8,627	1	2	3	505,249	143,650	648,898	54.9	1,182,217	11,278.54	1,259.04
177	1,364	114	4,070	5,725	1	0	1	341,266	85,385	426,651	56.0	761,197	10,556.79	954.59
69	722	24	2,087	2,902	0	2	2	163,983	58,265	222,247	52.8	421,020	12,869.31	2,973.76
0	310	6	701	1,017	0	2	2	64,548	32,223	96,771	51.0	189,678	13,643.93	3,530.01
69	412	18	1,386	1,885	0	0	0	99,435	26,042	125,476	54.2	231,342	12,296.91	2,633.52

MSAs

TABLE 8

U.S. CENSUS DIVISION 9, PACIFIC

U.S. Community Hospitals
(Nonfederal, short-term general and other special hospitals)

2012 Utilization, Personnel and Finances

CLASSIFICATION	Hospitals	Beds	Admissions	Inpatient Days	Adjusted Inpatient Days	Average Daily Census	Adjusted Average Daily Census	Average Stay (days)	Surgical Operations	NEWBORNS Bassinets	NEWBORNS Births	OUTPATIENT VISITS Emergency	OUTPATIENT VISITS Total
UNITED STATES	4,999	800,566	34,422,071	185,423,035	362,159,266	507,292	990,999	5.4	26,811,231	55,987	3,715,479	133,221,030	674,971,331
Nonmetropolitan	1,980	132,450	4,000,957	25,115,368	70,833,735	68,747	193,921	6.3	4,071,289	10,624	446,664	23,768,413	125,342,725
Metropolitan	3,019	668,116	30,421,114	160,307,667	291,325,531	438,545	797,078	5.3	22,739,942	45,363	3,268,815	109,452,617	549,628,606
CENSUS DIVISION 9, PACIFIC	541	94,194	4,403,646	22,168,393	38,294,550	60,609	104,681	5.0	3,004,231	7,064	621,481	16,342,076	78,483,065
Nonmetropolitan	120	5,530	188,207	1,076,449	3,126,350	2,942	8,545	5.7	217,491	567	32,320	1,319,590	7,196,356
Metropolitan	421	88,664	4,215,439	21,091,944	35,168,200	57,667	96,136	5.0	2,786,740	6,497	589,161	15,022,486	71,286,709
Alaska	23	1,549	56,131	341,987	772,996	934	2,117	6.1	56,505	163	8,522	290,711	1,452,226
Nonmetropolitan	17	564	12,986	111,045	346,632	303	950	8.6	20,432	57	2,857	94,853	447,346
Metropolitan	6	985	43,145	230,942	426,364	631	1,167	5.4	36,073	106	5,665	195,858	1,004,880
Anchorage	5	768	37,761	183,951	309,648	503	848	4.9	31,110	90	4,554	160,607	619,419
Fairbanks	1	217	5,384	46,991	116,716	128	319	8.7	4,963	16	1,111	35,251	385,461
California	349	71,004	3,304,230	16,919,921	27,674,218	46,264	75,658	5.1	2,117,543	5,087	482,313	11,859,123	52,224,855
Nonmetropolitan	31	1,379	51,485	276,697	748,152	757	2,045	5.4	63,517	127	9,150	425,762	2,247,354
Metropolitan	318	69,625	3,252,745	16,643,224	26,926,066	45,507	73,613	5.1	2,054,026	4,960	473,163	11,433,361	49,977,501
Bakersfield	10	1,527	71,204	353,355	601,804	967	1,645	5.0	36,779	95	12,227	254,648	666,601
Chico	4	529	30,063	135,993	264,227	372	724	4.5	16,517	43	3,512	130,127	779,170
El Centro	2	272	12,868	46,177	104,339	126	285	3.6	9,456	32	3,462	87,344	299,602
Fresno	8	1,770	84,901	435,437	692,190	1,189	1,893	5.1	45,601	101	14,154	302,257	1,293,336
Hanford-Corcoran	3	268	13,431	50,610	115,940	139	317	3.8	9,813	30	2,905	48,940	362,763
Los Angeles-Long Beach-Glendale	89	20,601	987,053	4,948,766	7,693,481	13,532	21,034	5.0	550,074	1,380	131,144	2,691,022	12,160,801
Madera	2	446	17,688	101,479	156,947	278	429	5.7	16,706	10	1,703	121,249	377,076
Merced	2	232	12,422	48,358	89,066	132	243	3.9	6,870	24	3,546	86,934	253,347
Modesto.	4	1,386	52,901	325,114	507,385	889	1,386	6.1	33,121	109	8,264	225,914	468,243
Napa.	2	290	13,481	61,102	101,954	167	279	4.5	12,641	12	1,087	36,735	298,884
Oakland-Fremont-Hayward	19	4,385	203,443	1,022,249	1,723,117	2,795	4,708	5.0	113,423	352	29,224	815,501	4,234,191
Oxnard-Thousand Oaks-Ventura. .	6	1,099	61,376	290,444	564,307	796	1,544	4.7	33,419	93	9,914	251,660	1,091,992
Redding.	3	489	21,088	121,734	211,850	333	579	5.8	10,945	14	2,040	88,927	213,784
Riverside-San Bernardino-Ontario.	34	6,916	344,614	1,658,184	2,716,562	4,534	7,429	4.8	217,824	507	50,544	1,271,606	4,045,943
Sacramento--Arden-Arcade--Rose-ville	17	4,036	194,397	977,975	1,548,527	2,673	4,233	5.0	147,525	276	23,076	750,853	2,824,866
Salinas	4	676	32,881	146,829	207,586	401	568	4.5	18,343	81	6,532	146,766	545,914
San Diego-Carlsbad-San Marcos .	21	5,558	286,339	1,473,689	2,236,897	4,029	6,113	5.1	198,505	359	42,483	876,318	2,868,993
San Francisco-San Mateo-Redwood City	19	5,484	168,746	1,330,084	2,101,376	3,636	5,744	7.9	129,483	220	19,658	671,700	4,818,866
San Jose-Sunnyvale-Santa Clara .	11	3,060	154,560	777,539	1,305,438	2,126	3,568	5.0	119,964	327	30,430	725,931	4,984,071
San Luis Obispo-Paso Robles . . .	4	465	18,141	70,346	106,469	192	292	3.9	11,727	38	2,655	88,749	257,481
Santa Ana-Anaheim-Irvine	24	5,586	256,030	1,225,419	2,000,211	3,351	5,470	4.8	178,070	368	39,136	748,098	3,307,667
Santa Barbara-Santa Maria.	5	859	33,547	203,323	327,732	555	896	6.1	25,053	52	5,479	138,085	435,760
Santa Cruz-Watsonville	3	410	19,342	89,124	167,183	244	458	4.6	15,728	55	4,255	66,946	278,835
Santa Rosa-Petaluma	7	693	33,641	148,070	289,187	404	790	4.4	28,095	50	5,058	151,914	477,794
Stockton	7	1,130	55,857	241,561	440,972	662	1,205	4.3	32,973	218	7,922	291,420	1,220,323
Vallejo-Fairfield	4	571	26,806	121,331	230,954	332	632	4.5	16,109	45	3,895	124,288	405,761
Visalia-Porterville	3	675	34,473	189,038	328,776	516	898	5.5	15,658	53	7,031	208,810	855,935
Yuba City.	1	212	11,452	49,894	91,589	137	251	4.4	3,604	16	1,827	30,619	149,502
Hawaii	24	2,803	109,270	745,956	1,451,702	2,038	3,970	6.8	75,387	197	11,085	399,437	2,034,660
Nonmetropolitan	12	930	29,007	236,453	535,013	646	1,463	8.2	19,800	71	4,552	120,654	333,749
Metropolitan	12	1,873	80,263	509,503	916,689	1,392	2,507	6.3	55,587	126	6,533	278,783	1,700,911
Honolulu	12	1,873	80,263	509,503	916,689	1,392	2,507	6.3	55,587	126	6,533	278,783	1,700,911

TABLE 8

U.S. Community Hospitals
(Nonfederal, short-term general and other special hospitals)

2012 Utilization, Personnel and Finances

FULL-TIME EQUIVALENT PERSONNEL					FULL-TIME EQUIV. TRAINEES			EXPENSES						
								LABOR				TOTAL		
Physicians and Dentists	Registered Nurses	Licensed Practical Nurses	Other Salaried Personnel	Total Personnel	Medical and Dental Residents	Other Trainees	Total Trainees	Payroll (in thousands)	Employee Benefits (in thousands)	Total (in thousands)	Percent of Total	Amount (in thousands)	Adjusted per Admission	Adjusted per Inpatient Day
114,479	1,351,164	82,268	3,183,037	4,730,948	102,904	7,230	110,134	$296,335,931	$81,153,797	$377,489,736	49.9	$756,916,757	$11,220.70	$2,090.01
15,188	160,970	24,883	469,925	670,966	1,935	276	2,211	35,636,252	9,721,437	45,357,688	52.4	86,549,339	7,649.75	1,221.87
99,291	1,190,194	57,385	2,713,112	4,059,982	100,969	6,954	107,923	260,699,679	71,432,359	332,132,048	49.5	670,367,418	11,940.32	2,301.09
12,488	180,384	9,254	399,039	601,165	11,578	767	12,345	44,626,157	14,558,895	59,185,051	52.1	113,537,965	14,826.48	2,964.86
893	8,934	859	26,310	36,996	41	17	58	2,452,195	810,228	3,262,425	54.9	5,940,305	11,314.50	1,900.08
11,595	171,450	8,395	372,729	564,169	11,537	750	12,287	42,173,962	13,748,667	55,922,626	52.0	107,597,660	15,084.98	3,059.52
164	2,660	167	6,900	9,891	57	6	63	707,994	217,448	925,441	52.4	1,765,709	14,410.66	2,284.24
88	822	92	2,636	3,638	6	5	11	275,199	91,502	366,700	57.3	639,706	14,801.16	1,845.49
76	1,838	75	4,264	6,253	51	1	52	432,795	125,946	558,741	49.6	1,126,003	14,197.85	2,640.94
70	1,608	72	3,424	5,174	51	1	52	347,979	102,334	450,313	49.2	914,384	13,867.97	2,952.98
6	230	3	840	1,079	0	0	0	84,816	23,612	108,428	51.2	211,618	15,824.30	1,813.11
7,656	134,124	7,388	285,877	435,045	8,488	660	9,148	32,507,582	10,987,256	43,494,833	52.4	83,074,054	15,228.71	3,001.86
81	2,505	252	6,559	9,397	7	6	13	622,398	235,416	857,814	53.3	1,610,470	12,161.28	2,152.60
7,575	131,619	7,136	279,318	425,648	8,481	654	9,135	31,885,185	10,751,840	42,637,019	52.3	81,463,585	15,305.03	3,025.45
133	2,628	175	5,341	8,277	163	2	165	562,991	189,925	752,917	55.3	1,362,248	11,767.35	2,263.61
63	1,055	105	2,812	4,035	21	1	22	296,216	87,734	383,951	52.0	738,144	12,872.20	2,793.60
0	382	21	1,109	1,512	0	0	0	82,266	25,718	107,984	49.1	220,057	7,564.69	2,109.06
62	2,992	194	6,147	9,395	15	3	18	567,679	139,640	707,319	47.3	1,494,996	10,713.36	2,159.81
40	435	45	1,201	1,721	7	3	10	134,445	36,779	171,224	54.6	313,375	9,634.90	2,702.91
2,925	39,984	2,467	83,686	129,062	4,147	180	4,327	8,861,505	2,725,468	11,586,972	49.0	23,646,308	15,305.45	3,073.55
1	644	54	1,986	2,685	0	4	4	198,724	83,801	282,525	56.8	497,738	17,701.74	3,171.37
1	380	27	916	1,324	24	0	24	104,461	36,800	141,261	49.6	284,594	12,040.21	3,195.32
11	2,494	81	3,434	6,020	3	0	3	437,368	172,922	610,290	53.0	1,151,764	14,502.56	2,270.00
18	599	24	1,317	1,958	4	1	5	150,510	66,703	217,212	51.5	421,540	18,799.44	4,134.61
268	7,641	532	19,651	28,092	200	20	220	2,502,925	1,052,075	3,555,000	58.6	6,068,334	17,579.13	3,521.72
126	1,911	130	4,472	6,639	65	4	69	574,212	163,250	737,462	54.2	1,359,413	11,277.32	2,409.00
8	887	24	1,347	2,266	25	0	25	176,455	63,084	239,539	47.3	506,530	15,845.39	2,390.98
1,023	12,571	858	25,294	39,746	1,119	57	1,176	2,421,887	715,942	3,137,829	49.7	6,310,604	11,132.62	2,323.01
258	8,740	288	16,560	25,846	780	29	809	2,375,484	812,394	3,187,877	54.4	5,855,406	18,751.28	3,781.27
64	1,224	71	2,822	4,181	39	3	42	388,624	212,455	601,078	61.5	977,286	21,041.34	4,707.86
973	12,382	364	20,835	34,554	696	278	974	2,395,625	706,737	3,102,362	49.5	6,266,004	14,327.83	2,801.20
199	7,717	496	20,574	28,986	270	19	289	2,836,550	1,017,335	3,853,884	57.8	6,669,571	23,197.30	3,173.91
899	7,211	311	16,185	24,606	440	20	460	2,593,575	1,003,687	3,597,262	56.8	6,334,239	24,328.59	4,852.19
6	785	23	1,080	1,894	6	0	6	140,732	40,386	181,118	51.4	352,049	12,777.61	3,306.58
117	10,283	375	21,779	32,554	154	9	163	2,078,870	741,185	2,820,055	49.8	5,659,043	13,229.57	2,829.22
21	1,431	75	2,776	4,303	61	1	62	334,765	113,998	448,762	50.8	883,337	17,167.84	2,695.30
50	821	45	1,792	2,708	28	2	30	213,998	59,292	273,290	56.4	484,862	13,105.09	2,900.19
16	1,201	82	3,271	4,570	35	2	37	303,160	130,766	433,926	50.4	860,400	13,667.56	2,975.24
166	2,240	108	5,661	8,175	116	5	121	504,241	170,857	675,098	58.8	1,148,493	11,162.01	2,604.46
70	1,358	54	3,189	4,671	34	5	39	291,915	85,283	377,197	52.3	721,582	14,286.20	3,124.35
22	1,195	85	3,040	4,342	11	5	16	261,045	71,540	332,584	52.6	631,727	10,490.66	1,921.45
35	428	22	1,041	1,526	18	1	19	94,958	26,083	121,041	49.6	243,942	11,604.14	2,663.44
478	4,297	278	11,408	16,461	111	6	117	1,174,360	333,675	1,508,037	52.8	2,855,850	13,777.21	1,967.24
148	1,120	117	2,977	4,362	16	0	16	279,391	107,102	386,494	56.1	688,924	11,066.69	1,287.68
330	3,177	161	8,431	12,099	95	6	101	894,969	226,573	1,121,543	51.8	2,166,926	14,940.61	2,363.86
330	3,177	161	8,431	12,099	95	6	101	894,969	226,573	1,121,543	51.8	2,166,926	14,940.61	2,363.86

Table continues

MSAs

TABLE 8

U.S. CENSUS DIVISION 9, PACIFIC
CONTINUED

U.S. Community Hospitals
(Nonfederal, short-term general and other special hospitals)

2012 Utilization, Personnel and Finances

MSAs

CLASSIFICATION	Hospitals	Beds	Admissions	Inpatient Days	Adjusted Inpatient Days	Average Daily Census	Adjusted Average Daily Census	Average Stay (days)	Surgical Operations	NEWBORNS		OUTPATIENT VISITS	
										Bassinets	Births	Emergency	Total
Oregon.................	58	6,706	336,677	1,429,092	2,930,633	3,907	8,003	4.2	322,898	639	43,472	1,402,280	9,804,779
Nonmetropolitan	28	1,302	55,216	222,561	708,874	609	1,934	4.0	59,471	166	7,972	369,254	2,474,123
Metropolitan.................	30	5,404	281,461	1,206,531	2,221,759	3,298	6,069	4.3	263,427	473	35,500	1,033,026	7,330,656
Bend...................	2	308	16,585	64,848	107,505	178	294	3.9	17,848	33	1,900	53,275	235,103
Corvallis................	1	165	9,355	40,281	76,469	110	209	4.3	10,771	20	1,073	23,553	220,619
Eugene-Springfield	5	631	34,005	143,671	243,937	393	667	4.2	23,261	50	3,485	130,597	398,081
Medford.................	3	467	22,423	98,184	168,071	269	459	4.4	20,754	40	2,379	78,837	713,694
Portland-Vancouver-Beaverton...	15	3,331	174,057	760,336	1,412,968	2,077	3,859	4.4	173,265	298	21,730	607,336	5,127,029
Salem..................	4	502	25,036	99,211	212,809	271	581	4.0	17,528	32	4,933	139,428	636,130
Washington.................	87	12,132	597,338	2,731,437	5,465,001	7,466	14,933	4.6	431,898	978	76,089	2,390,525	12,966,545
Nonmetropolitan	32	1,355	39,513	229,693	787,679	627	2,153	5.8	54,271	146	7,789	309,067	1,693,784
Metropolitan.................	55	10,777	557,825	2,501,744	4,677,322	6,839	12,780	4.5	377,627	832	68,300	2,081,458	11,272,761
Bellingham	1	253	15,303	59,480	109,185	163	298	3.9	7,072	24	1,978	19,182	93,659
Bremerton-Silverdale	1	262	13,809	56,263	103,280	154	282	4.1	10,434	24	1,938	51,139	249,694
Kennewick-Richland-Pasco	4	438	22,651	86,451	178,467	237	487	3.8	15,762	37	4,660	163,558	711,983
Lewiston	1	35	1,320	5,286	19,047	14	52	4.0	2,615	0	0	24,492	126,552
Longview	1	202	9,690	41,728	76,599	114	210	4.3	3,836	27	708	63,356	309,349
Mount Vernon-Anacortes	3	205	11,729	42,123	124,989	115	341	3.6	15,137	27	1,504	53,753	703,431
Olympia.................	2	479	26,344	110,208	157,859	302	431	4.2	12,025	46	2,681	82,472	324,322
Portland-Vancouver-Beaverton...	2	644	24,398	91,737	157,107	251	430	3.8	11,971	60	3,210	73,977	359,374
Seattle-Bellevue-Everett	21	4,773	259,042	1,245,166	2,374,822	3,403	6,489	4.8	180,099	364	31,584	866,031	6,068,502
Spokane	6	1,435	60,131	315,319	518,409	862	1,417	5.2	45,215	65	5,718	225,136	659,649
Tacoma.................	6	1,291	77,472	312,254	576,148	853	1,574	4.0	48,579	77	9,054	284,095	781,842
Wenatchee................	3	232	10,958	42,409	79,033	116	216	3.9	7,244	25	1,380	33,272	229,860
Yakima	4	528	24,978	93,320	202,377	255	553	3.7	17,638	56	3,885	140,995	654,544

TABLE 8

U.S. CENSUS DIVISION 9, PACIFIC CONTINUED

U.S. Community Hospitals
(Nonfederal, short-term general and other special hospitals)

2012 Utilization, Personnel and Finances

FULL-TIME EQUIVALENT PERSONNEL					FULL-TIME EQUIV. TRAINEES			EXPENSES						
								LABOR				TOTAL		
Physicians and Dentists	Registered Nurses	Licensed Practical Nurses	Other Salaried Personnel	Total Personnel	Medical and Dental Residents	Other Trainees	Total Trainees	Payroll (in thousands)	Employee Benefits (in thousands)	Total (in thousands)	Percent of Total	Amount (in thousands)	Adjusted per Admission	Adjusted per Inpatient Day
1,483	14,209	218	31,248	47,158	1,197	22	1,219	3,489,513	1,177,175	4,666,688	51.3	9,102,610	13,171.93	3,106.02
363	2,331	92	7,334	10,120	1	3	4	687,896	216,261	904,157	56.1	1,610,757	9,857.27	2,272.28
1,120	11,878	126	23,914	37,038	1,196	19	1,215	2,801,618	960,914	3,762,531	50.2	7,491,853	14,198.45	3,372.04
54	664	2	1,667	2,387	0	0	0	189,125	61,949	251,073	52.1	481,491	17,171.57	4,478.78
99	323	13	955	1,390	69	2	71	131,720	42,778	174,498	53.4	326,995	18,412.92	4,276.18
85	1,081	18	2,635	3,819	0	0	0	273,518	87,970	361,488	46.5	777,576	13,608.03	3,187.61
37	747	11	1,750	2,545	0	2	2	185,376	77,452	262,828	46.8	561,053	14,389.67	3,338.19
739	7,867	74	14,201	22,881	1,127	15	1,142	1,729,983	610,353	2,340,336	50.0	4,682,489	14,198.39	3,313.94
106	1,196	8	2,706	4,016	0	0	0	291,896	80,412	372,308	56.2	662,248	11,840.03	3,111.94
2,707	25,094	1,203	63,606	92,610	1,725	73	1,798	6,746,708	1,843,342	8,590,052	51.3	16,739,743	14,164.48	3,063.08
213	2,156	306	6,804	9,479	11	3	14	587,312	159,948	747,260	53.7	1,390,449	11,239.49	1,765.25
2,494	22,938	897	56,802	83,131	1,714	70	1,784	6,159,395	1,683,394	7,842,792	51.1	15,349,294	14,506.47	3,281.64
64	735	39	1,816	2,654	33	2	35	159,421	51,855	211,276	53.0	398,414	14,182.97	3,648.98
43	529	26	1,243	1,841	20	2	22	142,732	38,174	180,906	54.6	331,532	13,078.68	3,210.03
59	1,023	54	2,396	3,532	12	1	13	229,108	58,932	288,041	52.2	551,610	11,671.07	3,090.82
12	92	13	287	404	1	2	3	21,396	4,848	26,244	45.7	57,460	12,081.52	3,016.73
34	403	21	987	1,445	17	1	18	103,321	28,381	131,702	49.6	265,427	14,921.71	3,465.15
81	308	13	1,477	1,879	8	0	8	152,313	35,909	188,222	51.3	367,202	10,344.59	2,937.87
6	857	39	1,658	2,560	6	0	6	170,425	49,632	220,057	46.8	470,215	12,298.34	2,978.70
134	1,285	40	2,941	4,400	64	4	68	213,452	58,702	272,154	57.6	472,493	11,329.67	3,007.46
1,554	11,631	362	30,185	43,732	1,409	52	1,461	3,423,641	905,482	4,329,124	52.2	8,297,280	16,583.78	3,493.85
76	2,110	33	4,485	6,704	36	3	39	536,866	159,414	696,282	48.4	1,437,304	14,236.93	2,772.53
347	2,490	157	5,889	8,883	87	2	89	710,710	199,018	909,728	46.5	1,955,316	13,647.39	3,393.77
38	414	31	1,116	1,599	7	1	8	105,181	25,608	130,788	56.0	233,349	12,132.09	2,952.55
46	1,061	69	2,322	3,498	14	0	14	190,829	67,439	258,268	50.5	511,695	9,198.34	2,528.42

MSAs

Statistics for Health Care Systems and their Hospitals

The following tables describing health care systems refers to information in section B of the 2014 *AHA Guide*. Table 1 shows the number of health care systems by type of control. Table 2 provides a breakdown of the number of systems that own, lease, sponsor or contract manage hospitals within each control category. Table 3 gives the number of hospitals and beds in each control category as well as total hospitals and beds. Finally, Table 4 shows the percentage of hospitals and beds in each control category.

For more information on health care systems, please write to the Section for Health Care Systems, 155 N. Wacker Drive, Chicago, Illinois 60606 or call 312/422–3000.

Table 1. Health Care Systems, by Type of Organizaton Control

Type of Control	Code	Number of Systems
Catholic (Roman) church–related	CC	36
Other church–related	CO	10
Subtotal, church–related		46
Other not–for–profit	NP	305
Subtotal, not–for–profit		351
Investor Owned	IO	82
Federal Government	FG	5
Total		438

Table 2. Health Care Systems, by Type of Ownership and Control

Type of Ownership	Catholic Church–Related (CC)	Other Church–Related (CO)	Total Church–Related (CC + CO)	Other Not–for–Profit (NP)	Total Not–for–Profit (CC, CO, + NP)	Investor–Owned (IO)	Federal Government (FG)	All Systems
Systems that only own, lease or sponsor	28	6	34	270	304	74	5	383
Systems that only contract–manage	0	0	0	1	1	2	0	3
Systems that manage, own, lease, or sponsor	8	3	11	27	38	6	0	44
Total	36	9	45	298	343	82	5	430

Table 3. Hospitals and Beds in Health Care Systems, by Type of Ownership and Control

Type of Ownership	Catholic Church–Related (CC) H	Catholic Church–Related (CC) B	Other Church–Related (CO) H	Other Church–Related (CO) B	Total Church–Related (CC + CO) H	Total Church–Related (CC + CO) B	Other Not–for–Profit (NP) H	Other Not–for–Profit (NP) B	Total Not–for–Profit (CC, CO, + NP) H	Total Not–for–Profit (CC, CO, + NP) B	Investor–Owned (IO) H	Investor–Owned (IO) B	Federal Government (FG) H	Federal Government (FG) B	All Systems H	All Systems B
Owned, leased or sponsored	558	104,621	87	18,958	645	123,579	1,427	310,671	2,072	434,250	1,303	152,872	209	38,972	3,584	626,094
Contract–managed	41	1,709	6	662	47	2,371	80	6,043	127	8,414	113	6,959	0	0	240	15,373
Total	599	106,330	93	19,620	692	125,950	1,507	316,714	2,199	442,664	1,416	159,831	209	38,972	3,824	641,467

H = hospitals; **B** = beds.

Table 4. Hospitals and Beds in Health Care Systems, by Type of Ownership and Control as a Percentage of All Systems

Type of Ownership	Catholic Church–Related (CC) H	Catholic Church–Related (CC) B	Other Church–Related (CO) H	Other Church–Related (CO) B	Total Church–Related (CC + CO) H	Total Church–Related (CC + CO) B	Other Not–for–Profit (NP) H	Other Not–for–Profit (NP) B	Total Not–for–Profit (CC, CO, + NP) H	Total Not–for–Profit (CC, CO, + NP) B	Investor–Owned (IO) H	Investor–Owned (IO) B	Federal Government (FG) H	Federal Government (FG) B	All Systems H	All Systems B
Owned, leased or sponsored	15.6	16.7	2.4	3.0	18.0	19.7	39.8	49.6	57.8	69.4	36.4	24.4	5.8	6.2	100.0	100.0
Contract–managed	17.1	11.1	2.5	4.3	19.6	15.4	33.3	39.3	52.9	54.7	47.1	45.3	0.0	0.0	100.0	100.0
Total	15.7	16.6	2.4	3.1	18.1	19.6	39.4	49.4	57.5	69.0	37.0	24.9	5.5	6.1	100.0	100.0

H = hospitals; **B** = beds.
*Please note that figures may not always equal the provided subtotal or total percentages due to rounding.

This glossary explains specific terms as they are used in the tables and text of AHA Hospital Statistics

Ablation of Barrett's esophagus:
Premalignant condition that can lead to adenocarcinoma of the esophagus. The non surgical ablation of the premalignant tissue in Barrett's esophagus by the application of thermal energy or light through an endoscope passed from the mouth into the esophagus.

Acute long term care: Providers specialized acute hospital care to medically complex patients who are critically ill, have multisystem complications and/or failure, and require hospitalization averaging 25 days, in a facility offering specialized treatment programs and therapeutic intervention on a 24 hour/7day a week basis.

Adjusted average daily census: An estimate of the average number of patients (both inpatients and outpatients) receiving care each day during the reporting period, which is usually 12 months. The figure is derived by dividing the number of inpatient day equivalents (also called adjusted inpatient days) by the number of days in the reporting period.

Adjusted inpatient days: An aggregate figure reflecting the number of days of inpatient care, plus an estimate of the volume of outpatient services, expressed in units equivalent to an inpatient day in terms of level of effort. The figure is derived by first multiplying the number of outpatient visits by the ratio of outpatient revenue per outpatient visit to inpatient revenue per inpatient day. The product (which represents the number of patient days attributable to outpatient services) is then added to the number of *inpatient days*. Originally, the purpose of this calculation was to summarize overall productivity and calculate a unit cost that would include both inpatient and outpatient activities.

Formula 1:

$$\frac{\text{total expenses}}{\text{inpatient days} + \text{outpatient visits} \left(\frac{\frac{\text{outpatient revenue}}{\text{per outpatient visit}}}{\frac{\text{inpatient revenue}}{\text{per inpatient day}}} \right)}$$

However, the value of this calculation has changed over the years as the outpatient share of total revenue has grown and third-party payers have exerted a greater influence on pricing.

Admissions: The number of patients, excluding newborns, accepted for inpatient service during the reporting period; the number includes patients who visit the emergency room and are later admitted for inpatient service.

Adult Cardiac Surgery: Includes minimally invasive procedures that include surgery done with only a small incision or no incision at all, such as through a laparoscope or an endoscope and more invasive major surgical procedures that include open chest and open heart surgery.

Adult Cardiology Services: An organized clinical service offering diagnostic and interventional procedures to manage the full range of adult heart conditions.

Adult day care program: Program providing supervision, medical and psychological care, and social activities for older adults who live at home or in another family setting, but cannot be alone or prefer to be with others during the day. May include intake assessment, health monitoring, occupational therapy, personal care, noon meal, and transportation services.

Adult Diagnostic/invasive catheterization: (also called coronary angiography or coronary arteriography) is used to assist in diagnosing complex heart conditions. Cardiac angiography involves the insertion of a tiny catheter into the artery in the groin then carefully threading the catheter up into the aorta where the coronary arteries originate. Once the catheter is in place, a dye is injected which allows the cardiologist to see the size, shape, and distribution of the coronary arteries. These images are used to diagnose heart disease and to determine, among other things, whether or not surgery is indicated.

Adult Interventional cardiac catheterization: Non surgical procedure that utilizes the same basic principles as diagnostic catheterization and then uses advanced techniques to improve the heart's function. It can be a less-invasive alternative to heart surgery.

Airborne infection isolation room: A single-occupancy room for patient care where environmental factors are controlled in an effort to minimize the transmission of those infectious agents, usually spread person to person by droplet nuclei associated with coughing and inhalation. Such rooms typically have specific ventilation requirements for controlled ventilation, air pressure and filtration.

Alcoholism-drug abuse or dependency inpatient care: Provides diagnosis and therapeutic services to patients with alcoholism or other drug dependencies. Includes care for inpatient/residential treatment for patients whose course of treatment involves more intensive care than provided in an outpatient setting or where patient requires supervised withdrawal.

Alcoholism-drug abuse or dependency outpatient services: Organized hospital services that provide medical care and/or rehabilitative treatment services to outpatients for whom the primary diagnosis is alcoholism or other chemical dependency.

Alzheimer Center: Facility that offers care to persons with Alzheimer's disease and their families through an integrated program of clinical services, research, and education.

Ambulance services: Provision of ambulance services to the ill and injured who require medical attention on a scheduled or unscheduled basis.

Ambulatory Surgery Center: Facility that provides care to patients requiring surgery who are admitted and discharged on the same day. Ambulatory surgery centers are distinct from same day surgical units within the hospital outpatient departments for purposes of Medicare payments.

Arthritis treatment center: Specifically equipped and staffed center for the diagnosis and treatment of arthritis and other joint disorders.

Assisted living: A special combination of housing, supportive services, personalized assistance and health care designed to respond to the individual needs of those who need help in activities of daily living and instrumental activities of daily living. Supportive services are available, 24 hours a day, to meet scheduled and unscheduled needs, in a way that promotes maximum independence and dignity for each resident and encourages the involvement of a resident's family, neighbor and friends.

Assistive Technology Center: A program providing access to specialized hardware and software with adaptations allowing individuals greater independence with mobility, dexterity, or increased communication options.

Auxiliary: A volunteer community organization formed to assist the hospital in carrying out its purpose and to serve as a link between the institution and the community.

Average daily census: The average number of people served on an inpatient basis on a single day during the reporting period; the figure is calculated by dividing the number of inpatient days by the number of days in the reporting period.

Bariatric/weight control services: Bariatrics is the medical practice of weight reduction.

Beds: Number of beds regularly maintained (set up and staffed for use) for inpatients as of the close of the reporting period. Excludes newborn bassinets.

Bed-size category: Hospitals are categorized by the number of beds set up and staffed for use at the end of the reporting period. The eight categories in Hospital Statistics are: 6 to 24 beds; 25 to 49; 50 to 99; 100 to 199; 200 to 299; 300 to 399; 400 to 499; and 500 or more.

Birthing room-LDR room-LDRP room: A single-room type of maternity care with a more homelike setting for families than the traditional three-room unit (labor/delivery/recovery) with a separate postpartum area. A birthing room combines labor and delivery in one room. An LDR room accommodates three stages in the birthing process—labor, delivery, and recovery. An LDRP room accommodates all four stages of the birth process—labor, delivery, recovery, and postpartum.

Births: Total number of infants born in the hospital during the reporting period. Births do not include infants transferred from other institutions, and are excluded from admission and discharge figures.

Blood Donor Center: A facility that performs, or is responsible for the collection, processing, testing or distribution of blood and components.

Bone marrow transplant: See definition for Transplant service on page 214.

Breast cancer screening/mammograms: Mammography screening – The use of breast x-ray to detect unsuspected breast cancer in asymptomatic women. Diagnostic mammography – The x-ray imaging of breast tissue in symptomatic women who are considered to have a substantial likelihood of having breast cancer already.

Burn care: Provides care to severely burned patients. Severely burned patients are those with any of the following: (1) second-degree burns of more than 25% total body surface area for adults or 20% total body surface area for children: (2) third-degree burns of more than 10% total body surface area; (3) any severe burns of the hands, face, eyes, ears, or feet; or (4) all inhalation injuries, electrical burns, complicated burn injuries involving fractures and other major traumas, and all other poor risk factors.

Cardiac electrophysiology: Evaluation and management of patients with complex rhythm or conduction abnormalities, including diagnostic testing, treatment of arrhythmias by catheter ablation or drug therapy, and pacemaker/defibrillator implantation and follow-up.

Cardiac intensive care: Provides patient care of a more specialized nature than the usual medical and surgical care, on the basis of physicians' orders and approved nursing care plans. The unit is staffed with specially trained nursing personnel and contains monitoring and specialized support or treatment equipment for patients who, because of heart seizure, open-heart surgery, or other life-threatening conditions, require intensified, comprehensive observation and care. May include myocardial infarction, pulmonary care, and heart transplant units.

Cardiac Rehabilitation: A medically supervised program to help heart patients recover quickly and improve their overall physical and mental functioning. The goal is to reduce risk of another cardiac event or to keep an already present heart condition from getting worse. Cardiac rehabilitation programs include: counseling to patients, an exercise program, helping patients modify risk factors such as smoking and high blood pressure, providing vocational guidance to enable the patient to return to work, supplying information on physical limitations and lending emotional support.

Case management: A system of assessment, treatment planning, referral and follow-up that ensures the provision of comprehensive and continuous services and the coordination of payment and reimbursement for care.

Chaplaincy/pastoral care services: A service ministering religious activities and providing pastoral counseling to patients, their families, and staff of a health care organization.

Chemotherapy: An organized program for the treatment of cancer by the use of drugs or chemicals.

Children's wellness program: A program that encourages improved health status and a healthful lifestyle of children through health education, exercise, nutrition and health promotion.

Chiropractic services: An organized clinical service including spinal manipulation or adjustment and related diagnostic and therapeutic services.

Closed physician-hospital organization (Closed PHO): A joint venture between the hospital and physicians who have been selected on the basis of cost-effectiveness and/or high quality. The PHO can act as a unified agent in managed care contracting, own a managed care plan, own and operate ambulatory care centers or ancillary services projects, or provide administrative services to physician members.

Community health education: Education that provides health information to individuals and populations, as well as support for personal, family and community health decisions with the objective of improving health status.

Community hospitals: All nonfederal, short-term general, and special hospitals whose facilities and services are available to the public. (Special hospitals include obstetrics and gynecology; eye, ear, nose, and throat; rehabilitation; orthopedic; and other individually described specialty services.) Short-term general and special childrens hospitals are also considered to be community hospitals.

A hospital may include a nursing-home-type unit and still be classified as short-term, provided that the majority of its patients are admitted to units where the average length of stay is less than 30 days. Therefore, statistics for community hospitals often include some data about such nursing-home-type units. An example is furnished by Montana, where in 1995 63.6 percent of all hospitals classified as community hospitals include nursing-home-type units. Expense, revenue, utilization, and personnel data for these hospitals include data about their nursing-home-type units. Thus, total admissions to Montana community hospitals in 1995 were 96,154; total inpatient days, 997,759; total expenses, $791,806,393; and total payroll expenses, $352,583,331. If nursing-home-type unit data were excluded, these same items would be 94,034; 457,340; 752,567,865; and $328,911841, respectively.

Note that before 1972, hospital units of institutions such as prison and college infirmaries were included in the category of community hospitals. Including these units made this category equivalent to the short-term general and other special hospitals category. Although these hospital units are few in number and small in size, this change in definition should be taken into consideration when comparing data.

Community outreach: A program that systematically interacts with the community to identify those in need of services, alerting persons and their families to the availability of services, locating needed services, and enabling persons to enter the service delivery system.

Complementary and alternative medicine services: Organized hospital services or formal arrangements to providers that provide care or treatment not based solely on traditional western allopathic medical teachings as instructed in most U.S. medical schools. Includes any of the following: acupuncture, chiropractic, homeopathy, osteopathy, diet and lifestyle changes, herbal medicine, message therapy, etc.

Computer assisted orthopedic surgery (CAOS): Orthopedic surgery using computer technology, enabling three-dimensional graphic models to visualize a patient's anatomy.

Control: The type of organization responsible for establishing policy concerning the overall operation of hospitals. The three major categories are government (including federal, state, and local); nongovernment (nonprofit); and investor-owned (for-profit).

Crisis prevention: Services provided in order to promote physical and mental well being and the early identification of disease and ill health prior to the onset and recognition of symptoms so as to permit early treatment.

CT scanner: Computed tomographic scanner for head or whole body scans.

Deduction from revenue: The difference between revenue at full established rates (gross) and the payment actually received from payers (net).

Dental Services: An organized dental service or dentists on staff, not necessarily involving special facilities, providing dental or oral services to inpatients or outpatients.

Diagnostic radioisotope facility: The use of radioactive isotopes (Radiopharmaceuticals) as tracers or indicators to detect an abnormal condition or disease.

Electrodiagnostic Services: Diagnostic testing services for nerve and muscle function including services such as nerve conduction studies and needle electromyography.

Electron beam computed tomography (EBCT): A high tech computed tomography scan used to detect coronary artery disease by measuring coronary calcifications. This imaging procedure uses electron beams which are magnetically steered to produce a visual of the coronary artery and the images are produced faster than conventional CT scans.

Emergency department: Hospital facilities for the provision of unscheduled outpatient services to patients whose conditions require immediate care.

Emergency room visits: The number of visits to the emergency unit. When emergency outpatients are admitted to the inpatient areas of the hospital, they are counted as emergency room visits and subsequently, as inpatient admissions.

Emergency services: Health services that are provided after the onset of a medical condition that manifests itself by symptoms of sufficient severity, including severe pain, that the absence of immediate medical attention could reasonably be expected by a prudent layperson, who possesses an average knowledge of health and medicine, to result in placing the patient's health in serious jeopardy.

Enabling services: A program that is designed to help the patient access health care services by offering any of the following: transportation services and/or referrals to local social services agencies.

End of Life: Services offered to patients suffering from chronic, severe, and life-threatening diseases including comprehensive services that give patients and caregivers the resources and the confidence to manage symptoms, avoid emergency room admissions and frequent hospitalization, and remain in familiar and comfortable settings.

Endoscopic retrograde cholangiopancreatography (ERCP):
A procedure in which a catheter is introduced through an endoscope into the bile ducts and pancreatic ducts. Injection of contrast materials permits detailed x-ray of these structures. The procedure is used diagnostically as well as therapeutically to relieve obstruction or remove stones.

Endoscopic ultrasound:
Specially designed endoscope that incorporates an ultrasound transductor used to obtain detailed images of organs in the chest and abdomen. The endoscope can be passed through the mouth or the anus. When combined with needle biopsy the procedure can assist in diagnosis and staging of cancer.

Enrollment (insurance) assistance services:
A program that provides enrollment assistance for patients who are potentially eligible for public health insurance programs such as Medicaid, State Children's Health Insurance, or local/state indigent care programs. The specific services offered could include explanation of benefits, assist applicants in completing the application and locating all relevant documents, conduct eligibility interviews, and/or forward applications and documentation to state/local social service or health agency.

Equity model:
An arrangement that allows established practitioners to become shareholders in a professional corporation in exchange for tangible and intangible assets of their existing practices.

Esophageal impedance study:
A test in which a catheter is placed through the nose into the esophagus to measure whether gas or liquids are passing from the stomach into the esophagus and causing symptoms.

Expenses:
Includes all expenses for the reporting period including payroll, non-payroll, and all nonoperating expenses. *Payroll expenses* include all salaries and wages. *Non-payroll expenses* are all professional fees and those salary expenditures excluded from payroll. *Labor related expenses* are defined as payroll expenses plus employee benefits.

Non-labor related expenses are all other non-payroll expenses. *Bad debt* has been reclassified from a "reduction in revenue" to an expense in accordance with the revised AICPA Audit Guide. However, for purposes of historical consistency, the expense total that appears throughout *AHA Hospital Statistics does not include "bad debt" as an expense item.* Note: Financial data may not add due to rounding.

Extracorporeal shock wave lithotripter (ESWL):
A medical device used for treating stones in the kidney or urethra. The device disintegrates kidney stones noninvasively through the transmission of acoustic shock waves directed at the stones.

Fertility Clinic:
A specialized program set in an infertility center that provides counseling and education as well as advanced reproductive techniques such as: injectable therapy, reproductive surgeries, treatment for endometriosis, male factor infertility, tubal reversals, in vitro fertilization (IVF), donor eggs, and other such services to help patients achieve successful pregnancies.

Fitness center:
Provides exercise, testing, or evaluation programs and fitness activities to the community and hospital employees.

Foundation:
A corporation, organized as a hospital affiliate or subsidiary, that purchases both tangible and intangible assets of one or more medical group practices. Physicians remain in a separate corporate entity but sign a professional services agreement with the foundation.

Freestanding outpatient care center:
A facility owned and operated by the hospital, that is physically separate from the hospital and provides various medical treatments and diagnostic services on an outpatient basis only. Laboratory and radiology services are usually available.

Full-field digital mammography (FFDM):
Combines the x-ray generators and tubes used in analog screen-film mammography (SFM) with a detector plate that converts the x-rays into a digital signal.

Full time equivalent employees (FTE):
Full time personnel on payroll plus one half of the part time personnel on payroll. For purposes of *AHA Hospital Statistics*, full time and part time medical and dental residents/interns and other trainees are excluded from the calculation.

General medical-surgical care: Provides acute care to patients in medical and surgical units on the basis of physicians' orders and approved nursing care plans.

Genetic testing/counseling: A service equipped with adequate laboratory facilities and directed by a qualified physician to advise parents and prospective parents on potential problems in cases of genetic defects. A genetic test is the analysis of human DNA, RNA, chromosomes, proteins, and certain metabolites in order to detect heritable disease-related genotypes, mutations, phenotypes, or karyotypes for clinical purposes. Genetic tests can have diverse purposes, including the diagnosis of genetic diseases in newborns, children, and adults; the identification of future health risks; the prediction of drug responses; and the assessment of risks to future children.

Geriatric services: The branch of medicine dealing with the physiology of aging and the diagnosis and treatment of disease affecting the aged. Services could include: Adult day care; Alzheimer's diagnostic-assessment services; Comprehensive geriatric assessment; Emergency response system; Geriatric acute care unit; and/or Geriatric clinics.

Government, nonfederal, state, local: Controlled by an agency of state, county, or city government.

Gross inpatient revenue: Revenue from services rendered to inpatients at full established rates (also known as "charges").

Gross outpatient revenue: Revenue from services rendered to outpatients at full established rates.

Group practice without walls: In this organization, the hospital sponsors the formation of a physician group or provides capital to physicians to establish one. The group shares administrative expenses, although the physicians remain independent practitioners.

Group Purchasing Organization: An organization whose primary function is to negotiate contracts for the purpose of purchasing for members of the group or has a central supply site for its members.

Health fair: Community health education events that focus on the prevention of disease and promotion of health through such activities as audiovisual exhibits and free diagnostic services.

Health maintenance organization (HMO): A health care organization that acts as both insurer and provider of comprehensive but specified medical services in return for prospective per capita (capitation) payments.

Health Research: Organized hospital research program in any of the following areas: basic research, clinical research, community health research, and/or research on innovative health care delivery.

Health screening: A preliminary procedure such as a test or examination to detect the most characteristic sign or signs of a disorder that may require further investigation.

Heart transplant: See definition for Transplant services on page 214.

Hemodialysis: Provision of equipment and personnel for the treatment of renal insufficiency on an inpatient or outpatient basis.

HIV-AIDS services: (could include). *HIV-AIDS unit* – Special unit or team designated and equipped specifically for diagnosis, treatment, continuing care planning, and counseling services for HIV-AIDS patients and their families. *General inpatient care for HIV-AIDS* – Inpatient diagnosis and treatment for human immunodeficiency virus and acquired immunodeficiency syndrome patients, but dedicated unit is not available. *Specialized outpatient program for HIV-AIDS* – Special outpatient program providing diagnostic, treatment, continuing care planning, and counseling for HIV-AIDS patients and their families.

Home health services: Service providing nursing, therapy, and health-related homemaker or social services in the patient's home.

Hospice: A program providing palliative care, chiefly medical relief of pain and supportive services, addressing the emotional, social, financial, and legal needs of terminally ill patients and their families. Care can be provided in a variety of settings, both inpatient and at home.

Hospital unit: The hospital operation, excluding activity pertaining to nursing-home-type unit (as described below), for the following items: Admissions, Beds, FTEs (full-time, part-time, and total), Inpatient Days, Length of Stay, Net Revenue, and Total Expense.

Hospital unit of institutions: A hospital unit that is not open to the public and is contained within a nonhospital unit. An example is an infirmary that is contained within a college.

Hospitals in a network: Hospitals participating in a group that may include other hospitals, physicians, other providers, insurers, and/or community agencies that work together to coordinate and deliver a broad spectrum of services to the community.

Hospitals in a system: Hospitals belonging to a corporate body that owns and/or manages health provider facilities or health-related subsidiaries; the system may also own non-health-related facilities.

Image-guided radiation therapy (IGRT): Automated system for image-guided radiation therapy that enables clinicians to obtain high-resolution x-ray images to pinpoint tumor sites, adjust patient positioning when necessary, and complete a treatment, all within the standard treatment time slot, allowing for more effective cancer treatments.

Immunization program: Program that plans, coordinates and conducts immunization services in the community.

Indemnity fee for service: The traditional type of health insurance, in which the insured is reimbursed for covered expenses without regard to choice of provider. Payment up to a stated limit may be made either to the individual incurring and claiming the expense, or directly to providers.

Independent practice association (IPA): An IPA is a legal entity that holds managed care contracts and contracts with physicians, usually in solo practice, to provide care either on a fee-for-services or capitated basis. The purpose of an IPA is to assist solo physicians in obtaining managed care contracts.

Indigent care clinic: Health care services for uninsured and underinsured persons where care is free of charge or charged on a sliding scale. This would include "free clinics" staffed by volunteer practitioners, but could also be staffed by employees with sponsoring health care organizations subsidizing the cost of service.

Inpatient days: The number of adult and pediatric days of care, excluding newborn days of care, rendered during the entire reporting period.

Inpatient palliative care unit: An inpatient palliative care ward is a physically discreet, inpatient nursing unit where the focus is palliative care. The patient care focus is on symptom relief for complex patients who may be continuing to undergo primary treatment. Care is delivered by palliative medicine specialists.

Inpatient surgeries: Surgical services provided to patients who remain in the hospital overnight.

Insurance product: In tables 3 through 6, insurance product refers to a hospital-owned insurance product.

Integrated salary model: In this arrangement, physicians are salaried by the hospital or other entity of a health system to provide medical services for primary care and specialty care.

Intensity-Modulated Radiation Therapy (IMRT): A type of three-dimensional radiation therapy, which improves the targeting of treatment delivery in a way that is likely to decrease damage to normal tissues and allows varying intensities.

Intermediate nursing care: Provides health-related services (skilled nursing care and social services) to residents with a variety of physical conditions or functional disabilities. These residents do not require the care provided by a hospital or skilled nursing facility, but do need supervision and support services.

Intraoperative magnetic resonance imaging. An integrated surgery system which provides an MRI system in an operating room. The system allows for immediate evaluation of the degree to tumor resection while the patient is undergoing a surgical resection. Intraoperative MRI exists when a MRI (low-field or high-field) is placed in the operating theater and is used during surgical resection without moving the patient from the operating room to the diagnostic imaging suite.

Investor-owned, for-profit: Investor-owned, for-profit hospitals are those controlled on a for-profit basis by an individual, partnership, or profit-making corporation.

Kidney transplant: See definition for Transplant sevices on page 214.

Labor-related expenses: Payroll expenses plus employee benefits. *Non-labor-related expenses refers* to all other nonpayroll expenses, such as interest depreciation, supplies, purchased services, professional fees, and others.

Length of stay (LOS): LOS refers to the average number of days a patient stays at the facility. Short-term hospitals are those where the average LOS is less than 30 days. Long-term hospitals are those where the average LOS is 30 days or more. The figure is derived by dividing the number of inpatient days by the number of admissions.

Note that this publication carries two LOS variables: *total facility length of stay and hospital unit length of stay. Total facility* includes admissions and inpatient days from nursing-home-type units under control of the hospital. In *hospital unit length of stay,* nursing home utilization is subtracted.

Licensed practical nurse (LPN): A nurse who has graduated from an approved school of practical (vocational) nursing and works under the supervision of registered nurses and/or physicians.

Linguistic/Translation services: Services provided by the hospital designed to make health care more accessible to non-English speaking patients and their physicians.

Liver transplant: See definition for Transplant on page 214.

Long-term: Hospitals are classified either short-term or long-term according to the average length of stay (LOS). A long-term hospital is one in which the average LOS is 30 days or more.

Lung transplant: See definition for Transplant services on page 214.

Magnetic resonance imaging (MRI): The use of a uniform magnetic field and radio frequencies to study tissue and structure of the body. This procedure enables the visualization of biochemical activity of the cell in vivo without the use of ionizing radiation, radio-isotopic substances, or high-frequency sound.

Magnetoencephalography: a noninvasive neurophysiological measurement tool used to study magnetic fields generated by neuronal activity of the brain. The primary uses of MEG include assisting surgeons in localizing the source of epilepsy, sensory mapping, and the study of brain function. When it is combined with structural imaging, it is known as magnetic source imaging (MSI).

Managed care: A term covering a broad spectrum of arrangements for health care delivery and financing, including managed indemnity plans (MIP), health maintenance organizations (HMO), preferred provider organizations (PPO), point-of-service plans (POS), and direct contracting arrangements between employers and providers.

Managed care contract: A contract between the hospital and a managed care organization.

Management services organization (MSO): A corporation owned by the hospital or a physician/hospital joint venture that provides management services to one or more medical group practices. As part of a full-service management agreement, the MSO purchases the tangible assets of the practices and leases them back, employs all non-physician staff, and provides all supplies/administrative systems for a fee.

Meals on wheels: A hospital sponsored program which delivers meals to people, usually the elderly, who are unable to prepare their own meals. Low cost, nutritional meals are delivered to individuals' homes on a regular basis.

Medical surgical intensive care: Provides patient care of a more intensive nature than the usual medical and surgical care, on the basis of physicians' orders and approved nursing care plans. These units are staffed with specially trained nursing personnel and contain monitoring and specialized support equipment for patients who, because of shock, trauma, or other life-threatening conditions, require intensified, comprehensive observation and care. Includes mixed intensive care units.

Mobile health services: Vans and other vehicles used to deliver primary care services.

Multi-slice spiral computed tomography (<64 slice CT): A specialized computed tomography procedure that provides three-dimensional processing and allows narrower and multiple slices with increased spatial resolution and faster scanning times as compared to a regular computed tomography scan.

Multi-slice spiral computed tomography (64+ slice CT): Involves the acquisition of volumetric tomographic x-ray absorption data expressed in Hounsfield units using multiple rows of detectors. 64+ systems reconstruct the equivalent of 64 or greater slices to cover the imaged volume.

Neonatal intensive care: A unit that must be separate from the newborn nursery providing intensive care to all sick infants including those with the very lowest birth weights (less than 1500 grams). NICU has potential for providing mechanical ventilation, neonatal surgery, and special care for the sickest infants born in the hospital or transferred from another institution. A full-time neonatologist serves as director of the NICU.

Neonatal intermediate care: A unit that must be separate from the normal newborn nursery and that provides intermediate and/or recovery care and some specialized services, including immediate resuscitation, intravenous therapy, and capacity for prolonged oxygen therapy and monitoring.

Net patient revenue: The estimated net realizable amounts from patients, third-party payers, and others for services rendered. The number includes estimated retroactive adjustments called for by agreements with third-party payers; retroactive adjustments are accrued on an estimated basis in the period the related services are rendered and then adjusted later as final settlements are determined.

Net total revenue: Net patient revenue plus all other revenue, including contributions, endowment revenue, governmental grants, and all other payments not made on behalf of individual patients.

Neurological services: Services provided by the hospital dealing with the operative and nonoperative management of disorders of the central, peripheral, and autonomic nervous system.

Nongovernment, nonprofit: Hospitals that are nongovernment, nonprofit are controlled by not-for-profit organizations, including religious organizations (Catholic hospitals, for example), fraternal societies, and others.

Nursing-home-type unit/facility: A unit/facility that primarily offers the following type of services to a majority of all admissions:

- *Skilled nursing*: The provision of medical and nursing care services, health-related services, and social services under the supervision of a registered nurse on a 24-hour basis.

- *Intermediate care*: The provision, on a regular basis, of health-related care and services to individuals who do not require the degree of care or treatment that a skilled nursing unit is designed to provide.

- *Personal care*: The provision of general supervision and direct personal care services for residents who require

assistance in activities of daily living but who do not need nursing services or inpatient care. Medical and nursing services are available as needed.

- *Sheltered/residential care*: The provision of general supervision and protective services for residents who do not need nursing services or continuous personal care services in the conduct of daily life. Medical and nursing services are available as needed.

Nutrition programs: Those services within a health care facility which are designed to provide inexpensive, nutritionally sound meals to patients.

Obstetrics: Levels should be designated: (1) unit provides services for uncomplicated maternity and newborn cases; (2) unit provides services for uncomplicated cases, the majority of complicated problems, and special neonatal services; and (3) unit provides services for all serious illnesses and abnormalities and is supervised by a full-time maternal/fetal specialist.

Occupational health services: Includes services designed to protect the safety of employees from hazards in the work environment.

Oncology services: Inpatient and outpatient services for patients with cancer, including comprehensive care, support and guidance in addition to patient education and prevention, chemotherapy, counseling and other treatment methods.

Open physician hospital organization (Open PHO): A joint venture between the hospital and all members of the medical staff who wish to participate. The open PHO can act as a unified agent in managed care contracting, own a managed care plan, own and operate ambulatory care centers or ancillary services projects, or provide administrative services to physician members.

Optical colonoscopy: An examination of the interior of the colon using a long, flexible, lighted tube with a small built-in camera.

Orthopedic services: Services provided for the prevention or correction of injuries or disorders of the skeletal system and associated muscles, joints and ligaments.

Osteopathic hospitals: Osteopathic medicine is a medical practice based on a theory that diseases are due chiefly to a loss of structural integrity, which can be restored by manipulation of the neuro-muscular and skeletal systems, supplemented by therapeutic measures (such as medicine or surgery).

Other Intensive Care: A specially staffed, specialty equipped, separate section of a hospital dedicated to the observation, care, and treatment of patients with life threatening illnesses, injuries, or complications from which recovery is possible. It provides special expertise and facilities for the support of vital function and utilizes the skill of medical nursing and other staff experienced in the management of these problems.

Other long-term care: Provision of long-term care other than skilled nursing care or intermediate care for those who do not require daily medical or nursing services, but may require some assistance in the activities of daily living. This can include residential care, elderly care, or sheltered care facilities for developmentally disabled.

Other special care: Provides care to patients requiring care more intensive than that provided in the acute area, yet not sufficiently intensive to require admission to an intensive care unit. Patients admitted to this area are usually transferred here from an intensive care unit once their condition has improved. These units are sometimes referred to as definitive observation, step-down, or progressive care units.

Other transplant: See definition for Transplant services on page 214.

Outpatient care: Treatment provided to patients who do not remain in the hospital for overnight care. Hospitals may deliver outpatient care on site or through a facility owned and operated by the hospital, but physically separate from the hospital. In addition to treating minor illnesses or injuries, a free-standing center will stabilize seriously ill or injured patients before transporting them to a hospital. Laboratory and radiology services are usually available.

Outpatient care center (Freestanding): A facility owned and operated by the hospital, but physically separate from the hospital, that provides various medical treatments on an outpatient basis only. In addition to treating minor illnesses or injuries, the center will stabilize seriously ill or injured patients before transporting them to a hospital. Laboratory and radiology services are usually available.

Outpatient care center-services (Hospital-based): Organized hospital health care services offered by appointment on an ambulatory basis. Services may include outpatient surgery, examination, diagnosis, and treatment of a variety of medical conditions on a nonemergency basis, and laboratory and other diagnostic testing as ordered by staff or outside physician referral.

Outpatient surgery: Scheduled surgical services provided to patients who do not remain in the hospital overnight. The surgery may be performed in operating suites also used for inpatient surgery, specially designated surgical suites for outpatient surgery, or procedure rooms within an outpatient care facility.

Outpatient visit: A visit by a patient who is not lodged in the hospital while receiving medical, dental, or other services. Each visit an outpatient makes to a discrete unit constitutes one visit regardless of the number of diagnostic and/or therapeutic treatments that the patient receives. Total outpatient visits should include all clinic visits, referred visits, observation services, outpatient surgeries, and emergency room visits.

Pain Management Program: A recognized clinical service or program providing specialized medical care, drugs or therapies for the management of acute or chronic pain or other distressing symptom, administered by specially trained physicians and other clinicians, to patients suffering from acute illness of diverse causes.

Palliative Care Inpatient Unit: An inpatient palliative care ward is a physically discreet, inpatient nursing unit where the focus is palliative care. The patient care focus is on symptom relief for complex patients who may be continuing to undergo primary treatment. Care is delivered by palliative medicine specialists.

Palliative care program: An organized program providing specialized medical care, drugs or therapies for the management of acute or chronic pain and/or the control of symptoms administered by specially trained physicians and other clinicians; and supportive care services, such as counseling on advanced directives, spiritual care, and social services, to patients with advanced disease and their families.

Patient Controlled Analgesia (PCA). Patient-controlled Analgesia (PCA) is intravenously administered pain medicine under the patient's control. The patient has a button on the end of a cord than can be pushed at will, whenever more pain medicine is desired. This button will only deliver more pain medicine at pre-determined intervals, as programmed by the doctor's order.

Patient education center: Written goals and objectives for the patient and/or family related to therapeutic regimens, medical procedures, and self care.

Patient representative services: Organized hospital services providing personnel through whom patients and staff can seek solutions to institutional problems affecting the delivery of high-quality care and services.

Payroll expenses: Includes all salaries and wages. All professional fees and salary expenditures excluded from payroll, such as employee benefits, are defined as nonpayroll expenses and are included in total expenses.

Pediatric Cardiac Surgery: Includes minimally invasive procedures that include surgery done with only a small incision or no incision at all, such as through a laparoscope or an endoscope and more invasive major surgical procedures that include open chest and open heart surgery.

Pediatric Cardiology Services: An organized clinical service offering diagnostic and interventional procedures to manage the full range of pediatric heart conditions.

Pediatric Diagnostic/invasive catheterization: (also called coronary angiography or coronary arteriography) is used to assist in diagnosing complex heart conditions. Cardiac angiography involves the insertion of a tiny catheter into the artery in the groin then carefully threading the catheter up into the aorta where the coronary arteries originate. Once the catheter is in place, a dye is injected which allows the cardiologist to see the size, shape, and distribution of the coronary arteries. These images are used to diagnose heart disease and to determine, among other things, whether or not surgery is indicated.

Pediatric intensive care: Provides care to pediatric patients that is of a more intensive nature than that usually provided to pediatric patients. The unit is staffed with specially trained personnel and contains monitoring and specialized support equipment for treatment of patients who, because of shock, trauma, or other life-threatening conditions, require intensified, comprehensive observation and care.

Pediatric Interventional cardiac catheterization: Non surgical procedure that utilizes the same basic principles as diagnostic

catheterization and then uses advanced techniques to improve the heart's function. It can be a less-invasive alternative to heart surgery.

Pediatric medical-surgical care: Provides acute care to pediatric patients on the basis of physicians' orders and approved nursing care plans.

Personnel: Number of persons on the hospital payroll at the end of the reporting period. Personnel are recorded in *Hospital Statistics* as full-time equivalents (FTEs), which are calculated by adding the number of full-time personnel to one-half the number of part-time personnel, excluding medical and dental residents, interns, and other trainees. *Per 100 adjusted census* indicates the ratio of personnel to adjusted average daily census, calculated on a per-100 basis.

Physical rehabilitation inpatient care: Provides care encompassing a comprehensive array of restoration services for the disabled and all support services necessary to help patients attain their maximum functional capacity.

Physical rehabilitation outpatient services: Outpatient program providing medical, health-related, therapy, social, and/or vocational services to help disabled persons attain or retain their maximum functional capacity.

Population: Population refers to the residential population of the United States. This includes both civilian and military personnel. Note that population is being used to calculate the values *for community health indicators per 1000 population.*

Positron emission tomography/CT (PET/CT): Provides metabolic functional information for the monitoring of chemotherapy, radiotherapy and surgical planning.

Positron emission tomography scanner (PET): A nuclear medicine imaging technology which uses radioactive (positron emitting) isotopes created in a cyclotron or generator and computers to produce composite pictures of the brain and heart at work. PET scanning produces sectional images depicting metabolic activity or blood flow rather than anatomy.

Preferred provider organization (PPO): A pre-set arrangement in which purchasers and providers agree to furnish specified health services to a group of employees/patients.

Primary care department: A unit or clinic within the hospital that provides primary care services (e.g. general pediatric care, general internal medicine, family practice, gynecology) through hospital-salaried medical and/or nursing staff, focusing on evaluating and diagnosing medical problems and providing medical treatment on an outpatient basis.

Prosthetic and Orthotic Services: Services providing comprehensive prosthetic and orthotic evaluation, fitting, and training.

Proton beam therapy: A form of radiation therapy which administers proton beams. While producing the same biologic effects as x-ray beams, the energy distribution of protons differs from conventional x-ray beams in that they can be more precisely focused in tissue volumes in a three-dimensional pattern resulting in less surrounding tissue damage than conventional radiation therapy permitting administration of higher doses.

Psychiatric child-adolescent services: Provides care to emotionally disturbed children and adolescents, including those admitted for diagnosis and those admitted for treatment.

Psychiatric consultation-liaison services: Provides organized psychiatric consultation/liaison services to nonpsychiatric hospital staff and/or departments on psychological aspects of medical care that may be generic or specific to individual patients.

Psychiatric education services: Provides psychiatric educational services to community agencies and workers such as schools, police, courts, public health nurses, welfare agencies, clergy, and so forth. The purpose is to expand the mental health knowledge and competence of personnel not working in the mental health field and to promote good mental health through improved understanding, attitudes, and behavioral patterns.

Psychiatric emergency services: Services of facilities available on a 24-hour basis to provide immediate unscheduled out-patient care, diagnosis, evaluation, crisis intervention, and assistance to persons suffering acute emotional or mental distress.

Psychiatric geriatric services: Provides care to emotionally disturbed elderly patients, including those admitted for diagnosis and those admitted for treatment.

Psychiatric inpatient care: Provides acute or long-term care to emotionally disturbed patients, including patients admitted for diagnosis and those admitted for treatment of psychiatric problems, on the basis of physicians'

orders and approved nursing care plans. Long-term care may include intensive supervision to the chronically mentally ill, mentally disordered, or other mentally incompetent persons.

Psychiatric outpatient services: Provides medical care, including diagnosis and treatment, of psychiatric outpatients.

Psychiatric partial hospitalization program: Organized hospital services of intensive day/evening outpatient services of three hours of more duration, distinguished from other outpatient visits of one hour.

Radiology, diagnostic: The branch of radiology that deals with the utilization of all modalities of radiant energy in medical diagnoses and therapeutic procedures using radiologic guidance. This includes, but is not restricted to, imaging techniques and methodologies utilizing radiation emitted by x-ray tubes, radionnuclides, and ultrasonographic devices and the radiofrequency electromagnetic radiation emitted by atoms.

Radiology, therapeutic: The branch of medicine concerned with radioactive substances and using various techniques of visualization, with the diagnosis and treatment of disease using any of the various sources of radiant energy. Services could include: megavoltage radiation therapy; radioactive implants; stereotactic radiosurgery; therapeutic radioisotope facility; X-ray radiation therapy.

Registered nurse (RN): A nurse who has graduated from an approved school of nursing and who is currently registered by the state. RNs are responsible for the nature and quality of all nursing care that patients receive. In these tables, the number of RNs does not include those registered nurses more appropriately reported in other occupational categories, such as facility administrators, which are listed under *all other personnel* (Tables 1 and 2).

Rehabilitation services: A wide array of restoration services for disabled and recuperating patients, including all support services necessary to help them attain their maximum functional capacity.

Retirement housing: A facility which provides social activities to senior citizens, usually retired persons, who do not require health care but some short-term skilled nursing care may be provided. A retirement center may furnish housing and may also have acute hospital and long-term care facilities, or it may arrange for acute and long term care through affiliated institutions.

Robot-assisted walking therapy:
A form of physical therapy that uses a robotic device to assist patients who are relearning how to walk.

Robotic surgery: The use of mechanical guidance devices to remotely manipulate surgical instrumentation.

Rural: A rural hospital is located outside a Metropolitan Statistical Area (MSA), as designated by the U.S. Office of Management and Budget (OMB) effective June 6, 2003. An urban area is a geographically defined, integrated social and economic unit with a large population nucleus. Micropolitan areas, which are new to the OMB June 6, 2003 definitions, continue to be classified as rural for purposes of this publication.

Rural Health Clinic: A clinic located in a rural, medically under-served area in the United States that has a separate reimbursement structure from the standard medical office under the Medicare and Medicaid programs.

Satellite Emergency Department:
A facility owned and operated by the hospital but physically separate from the hospital for the provision of unscheduled outpatient services to patients whose conditions require immediate care. A freestanding ED is not physically connected to a hospital, but has all necessary emergency staffing and equipment on-site.

Shaped beam radiation system:
A precise, non-invasive treatment that involves targeting beams of radiation that mirrors the exact size and shape of a tumor at a specific area of a tumor to shrink or destroy cancerous cells. This procedure delivers a therapeutic dose of radiation that conforms precisely to the shape of the tumor, thus minimizing the risk to nearby tissues.

Simulated rehabilitation environment:
Rehabilitation focused on retraining functional skills in a contextually appropriate environment (simulated home and community settings) or in a traditional setting (gymnasium) using motor learning principles.

Single photon emission computerized tomography (SPECT): A nuclear medicine imaging technology that combines existing technology of gamma camera imaging with computed tomographic imaging technology to provide a more precise and clear image.

Skilled nursing care: Provides non-acute medical and skilled nursing care services, therapy, and social services under the supervision of a licensed registered nurse on a 24-hour basis.

Sleep Center: Specially equipped and staffed center for the diagnosis and treatment of sleep disorders.

Social work services (could include)**:**
Organized services that are properly directed and sufficiently staffed by qualified individuals who provide assistance and counseling to patients and their families in dealing with social, emotional, and environmental problems associated with illness or disability, often in the context of financial or discharge planning coordination.

Sports medicine: Provision of diagnostic screening and assessment and clinical and rehabilitation services for the prevention and treatment of sports-related injuries.

Stereotactic radiosurgery: Stereotactic radiosurgery (SRS) is a radiotherapy modality that delivers a high dosage of radiation to a discrete treatment area in as few as one treatment session. Includes gamma knife, cyberknife, etc.

Support groups: A hospital sponsored program that allows a group of individuals with the same or similar problems who meet periodically to share experiences, problems, and solutions in order to support each other.

Surgical operations: Those surgical operations, whether major or minor, performed in the operating room(s). A surgical operation involving more than one surgical procedure is still considered only one surgical operation.

Swing bed services: A hospital bed that can be used to provide either acute or long-term care depending on community or patient needs. To be eligible a hospital must have a Medicare provider agreement in place, have fewer than 100 beds, be located in a rural area, do not have a 24 hour nursing service waiver in effect, have not been terminated from the program in the prior two years, and meet various service conditions.

Teen outreach services: A program focusing on the teenager which encourages an improved health status and a healthful lifestyle including physical, emotional, mental, social, spiritual and economic health through education, exercise, nutrition and health promotion.

Tissue transplant: See definition for Transplant sevices on page 214.

Tobacco treatment/cessation program:
Organized hospital services with the purpose of ending tobacco-use habits of patients addicted to tobacco/nicotine.

Transplant services. The branch of medicine that transfers an organ or tissue from one person to another or from one body part to another to replace a diseased structure or to restore function or to change appearance. Services could include: bone marrow transplant program; heart, lung, kidney, intestine, or tissue transplant. The other transplant services include transplant services other than bone marrow, heart, kidney, liver, lung, tissue and heart/lung or other multi-transplant surgeries.

Transportation to health facilities:
A long-term care support service designed to assist the mobility of the elderly. Some programs offer improved financial access by offering reduced rates and barrier-free buses or vans with ramps and lifts to assist the elderly or handicapped; others offer subsidies for public transport systems or operate mini-bus services exclusively for use by senior citizens.

Trauma center (certified): A facility to provide emergency and specialized intensive care to critically ill and injured patients. **Level 1:** A regional resource trauma center, which is capable of providing total care for every aspect of injury and plays a leadership role in trauma research and education. **Level 2:** A community trauma center, which is capable of providing trauma care to all but the most severely injured patients who require highly specialized care. **Level 3:** A rural trauma hospital, which is capable of providing care to a large number of injury victims and can resuscitate and stabilize more severely injured patients so that they can be transported to Level 1 or 2 facilities.

Ultrasound: The use of acoustic waves above the range of 20,000 cycles per second to visualize internal body structures.

Urban: An urban hospital is located inside a Metropolitan Statistical Area (MSA), designated by the U.S. Office of Management and Budget effective June 6, 2003. An urban areas is a geographically defined, integrated social and economic unit with a large population base. Micropolitan areas, which are new to the OMB June 6, 2003 definitions, are not considered to be urban for purposes of this publication.

Urgent care center: A facility that provides care and treatment for problems that are not life-threatening but require attention over the short term.

Virtual colonoscopy: Noninvasive screening procedure used to visualize, analyze and detect cancerous or potentially cancerous polyps in the colon.

Volunteer services department:
An organized hospital department responsible for coordinating the services of volunteers working within the institution.

Women's health center/services:
An area set aside for coordinated education and treatment services specifically for and promoted to women as provided by this special unit. Services may or may not include obstetrics but include a range of services other than OB.

Wound Management Services:
Services for patients with chronic wounds and nonhealing wounds often resulting from diabetes, poor circulation, improper seating and immunocompromising conditions. The goals are to progress chronic wounds through stages of healing, reduce and eliminate infections, increase physical function to minimize complications from current wounds and prevent future chronic wounds. Wound management services are provided on an inpatient or outpatient basis, depending on the intensity of service needed.

2012 AHA Annual Survey
Health Forum, L.L.C.

A. REPORTING PERIOD (please refer to the instructions and definitions at the end of this questionnaire)

Report data for a full 12-month period, preferably your last completed fiscal year (366 days). (Be consistent in using the same reporting period for responses throughout various sections of this survey.)

1. Reporting Period used (beginning and ending date) ...... __ __ / __ __ / __ __ __ __ to __ __ / __ __ / __ __ __ __
   Month   Day   Year   Month   Day   Year

2. a. Were you in operation 12 full months
      at the end of your reporting period .... YES ☐ NO ☐

   b. Number of days open
      during reporting period .... _____

3. Indicate the beginning of your current fiscal year .... __ __ / __ __ / __ __ __ __
   Month   Day   Year

B. ORGANIZATIONAL STRUCTURE

1. CONTROL

Indicate the type of organization that is responsible for establishing policy for overall operation of your hospital. CHECK ONLY ONE:

Government, nonfederal
☐ 12 State
☐ 13 County
☐ 14 City
☐ 15 City-County
☐ 16 Hospital district or authority

Nongovernment, not-for profit (NFP)
☐ 21 Church-operated
☐ 23 Other not-for-profit (including NFP Corporation)

Investor-owned, for-profit
☐ 31 Individual
☐ 32 Partnership
☐ 33 Corporation

Government, federal
☐ 41 Air Force
☐ 42 Army
☐ 43 Navy
☐ 44 Public Health Service

☐ 45 Veterans' Affairs
☐ 46 Federal other than 41-45 or 47-48
☐ 47 PHS Indian Service
☐ 48 Department of Justice

2. SERVICE

Indicate the ONE category that BEST describes your hospital or the type of service it provides to the MAJORITY of patients:

☐ 10 General medical and surgical
☐ 11 Hospital unit of an institution (prison hospital, college infirmary)
☐ 12 Hospital unit within an institution for the mentally retarded
☐ 13 Surgical
☐ 22 Psychiatric
☐ 33 Tuberculosis and other respiratory diseases
☐ 41 Cancer
☐ 42 Heart
☐ 44 Obstetrics and gynecology
☐ 45 Eye, ear, nose, and throat

☐ 46 Rehabilitation
☐ 47 Orthopedic
☐ 48 Chronic disease
☐ 62 Institution for the mentally retarded
☐ 80 Acute long-term care hospital
☐ 82 Alcoholism and other chemical dependency
☐ 49 Other-specify treatment area: _____
_____

3. OTHER

a. Does your hospital restrict admissions primarily to children? .... YES ☐ NO ☐

B. ORGANIZATIONAL STRUCTURE (continued)

b. Does the hospital itself operate subsidiary corporations? .... YES ☐   NO ☐

c. Is the hospital contract managed? If yes, please provide the name, city, and state of the organization .. YES ☐   NO ☐

     Name: _____ City: _____ State: _____

d. Is the hospital a participant in a network? ....YES ☐   NO ☐
     If yes, please provide the name, city and state and telephone number of the network. If the hospital participates in more than one network, please provide the name, city, and state and telephone number of the network on page 15, under supplemental information.

     Name: _____ City: _____ State: _____ Telephone_____

e. Is your hospital owned in whole or in part by physicians or a physician group?... YES ☐ NO ☐

f. If you checked 80 Acute long-term care hospital (LTCH) in the Section B2 (Service), please indicate if you are a freestanding LTCH or a LTCH arranged within a general acute care hospital.
    ☐ Free standing LTCH   ☐ LTCH arranged in a general acute care hospital

     If you are arranged in a general acute care hospital, what is your host hospital's name?
     Name_____ City_____ State_____

4. NATIONAL PROVIDER IDENTIFIER (NPI)

a. Does your hospital have its National Provider Identifier (NPI) from the National Plan and Provider Enumeration System?
     YES ☐   NO ☐

    If yes, please report the ten digit NPI _ _ _ _ _ _ _ _ _ _

b. Does your hospital also have a Subpart NPI? YES ☐   NO ☐

If yes, please report the Subpart NPI and provide the relevant taxonomy code to indicate the type of service provided. If you have multiple Subpart NPIs please report them all (in the supplemental section on page 15 at the end of this questionnaire, or on a separate sheet).

Subpart NPI 1 _ _ _ _ _ _ _ _ _ _   Taxonomy Code _ _

Subpart NPI 2 _ _ _ _ _ _ _ _ _ _   Taxonomy Code _ _

Subpart NPI 3 _ _ _ _ _ _ _ _ _ _   Taxonomy Code _ _

Taxonomy Codes
Ambulatory Health Care Facility   01
Medicare Defined Swing Bed Unit   02
Psychiatric Unit   03
Rehabilitation Unit   04
Rehabilitation, Substance Use Disorder Unit   05
Laboratory   06
Nursing and Custodial Care Facility   07
Residential Treatment Facility   08
Respite Care Facility   09
Other 10

C. FACILITIES AND SERVICES

For each service or facility listed below, please check all the categories that describe how each item is provided **as of the last day of the reporting period**. Check all categories that apply for an item. Leave all categories blank for a facility or service that is not provided. Column 3 refers to the networks that were identified in section B, question 3d. If you check column (1) C1-19, please include the number of staffed beds.
The sum of the beds reported in 1-19 should equal Section D(1b), beds set up and staffed on page 9.

	(1) Owned or provided by my hospital or its subsidiary	(2) Provided by my Health System (in my local community)	(3) Provided by my network (in my local community)	(4) Provided through a formal contractual arrangement or joint venture with another provider that is not in my system or network (in my local community)
1. General medical-surgical care ....(#Beds_____)	☐	☐	☐	☐
2. Pediatric medical-surgical care ....(#Beds_____)	☐	☐	☐	☐
3. Obstetrics [Level of unit (1-3): (___)]..........(#Beds_____)	☐	☐	☐	☐
4. Medical-surgical intensive care ....(#Beds_____)	☐	☐	☐	☐
5. Cardiac intensive care ....(#Beds_____)	☐	☐	☐	☐
6. Neonatal intensive care ....(#Beds_____)	☐	☐	☐	☐
7. Neonatal intermediate care ....(#Beds_____)	☐	☐	☐	☐
8. Pediatric intensive care ....(#Beds_____)	☐	☐	☐	☐
9. Burn care..(#Beds_____)	☐	☐	☐	☐
10. Other special care _____........(#Beds_____)	☐	☐	☐	☐
11. Other intensive care_____..........(#Beds_____)	☐	☐	☐	☐
12. Physical rehabilitation ....(#Beds_____)	☐	☐	☐	☐
13. Alcoholism-drug abuse or dependency care ....(#Beds_____)	☐	☐	☐	☐
14. Psychiatric care ....(#Beds_____)	☐	☐	☐	☐
15. Skilled nursing care ....(#Beds_____)	☐	☐	☐	☐
16. Intermediate nursing care ....(#Beds_____)	☐	☐	☐	☐
17. Acute long-term care................................(#Beds_____)	☐	☐	☐	☐
18. Other long-term care................................(#Beds_____)	☐	☐	☐	☐
19. Other care (specify):_____..........(#Beds_____)	☐	☐	☐	☐
20. Adult day care program................................	☐	☐	☐	☐
21. Airborne infection isolation room (# rooms _____)	☐	☐	☐	☐
22. Alcoholism-drug abuse or dependency outpatient services	☐	☐	☐	☐
23. Alzheimer Center................................	☐	☐	☐	☐
24. Ambulance services................................	☐	☐	☐	☐
25. Ambulatory surgery center................................	☐	☐	☐	☐
26. Arthritis treatment center................................	☐	☐	☐	☐
27. Assisted living	☐	☐	☐	☐
28. Auxiliary	☐	☐	☐	☐
29. Bariatric/weight control services	☐	☐	☐	☐
30. Birthing room/LDR room/LDRP room	☐	☐	☐	☐
31. Blood Donor Center	☐	☐	☐	☐
32. Breast cancer screening/mammograms	☐	☐	☐	☐

C. FACILITIES AND SERVICES (continued)

	(1) Owned or provided by my hospital or its subsidiary	(2) Provided by my Health System (in my local community)	(3) Provided by my network (in my local community)	(4) Provided through a formal contractual arrangement or joint venture with another provider that is not in my system or network (in my local community)
33. Cardiology and cardiac surgery services				
a. Adult cardiology services	☐	☐	☐	☐
b. Pediatric cardiology services	☐	☐	☐	☐
c. Adult diagnostic catheterization	☐	☐	☐	☐
d. Pediatric diagnostic catheterization	☐	☐	☐	☐
e. Adult interventional cardiac catheterization	☐	☐	☐	☐
f. Pediatric interventional cardiac catheterization	☐	☐	☐	☐
g. Adult cardiac surgery	☐	☐	☐	☐
h. Pediatric cardiac surgery	☐	☐	☐	☐
i. Adult cardiac electrophysiology	☐	☐	☐	☐
j. Pediatric cardiac electrophysiology	☐	☐	☐	☐
k. Cardiac rehabilitation	☐	☐	☐	☐
34. Case management	☐	☐	☐	☐
35. Chaplaincy/pastoral care services	☐	☐	☐	☐
36. Chemotherapy	☐	☐	☐	☐
37. Children's wellness program	☐	☐	☐	☐
38. Chiropractic services	☐	☐	☐	☐
39. Community outreach	☐	☐	☐	☐
40. Complementary and alternative medicine services	☐	☐	☐	☐
41. Computer assisted orthopedic surgery (CAOS)	☐	☐	☐	☐
42. Crisis prevention	☐	☐	☐	☐
43. Dental services	☐	☐	☐	☐
44. Emergency services				
a. Emergency department	☐	☐	☐	☐
b. Pediatric emergency department	☐	☐	☐	☐
c. Satellite emergency department	☐	☐	☐	☐
d. If you checked column 1 (44c), is the department open 24 hours a day, 7 days a week?	Yes ☐	No ☐		
e. Trauma center (certified) [Level of unit (1-3) ____]	☐	☐	☐	☐
45. Enabling services	☐	☐	☐	☐
46. Endoscopic services				
a. Optical colonoscopy	☐	☐	☐	☐
b. Endoscopic ultrasound	☐	☐	☐	☐
c. Ablation of Barrett's esophagus	☐	☐	☐	☐
d. Esophageal impedance study	☐	☐	☐	☐
e. Endoscopic retrograde cholangiopancreatography (ERCP)	☐	☐	☐	☐
47. Enrollment (insurance) assistance services	☐	☐	☐	☐
48. Extracorporeal shock wave lithotripter (ESWL)	☐	☐	☐	☐
49. Fertility clinic	☐	☐	☐	☐
50. Fitness center	☐	☐	☐	☐
51. Freestanding outpatient care center	☐	☐	☐	☐
52. Geriatric services	☐	☐	☐	☐
53. Health fair	☐	☐	☐	☐

C. FACILITIES AND SERVICES (continued)

	(1) Owned or provided by my hospital or its subsidiary	(2) Provided by my Health System (in my local community)	(3) Provided by my network (in my local community)	(4) Provided through a formal contractual arrangement or joint venture with another provider that is not in my system or network (in my local community)
54. Community health education	☐	☐	☐	☐
55. Genetic testing/counseling	☐	☐	☐	☐
56. Health screenings	☐	☐	☐	☐
57. Health research	☐	☐	☐	☐
58. Hemodialysis	☐	☐	☐	☐
59. HIV/AIDS services	☐	☐	☐	☐
60. Home health services	☐	☐	☐	☐
61. Hospice program	☐	☐	☐	☐
62. Hospital-based outpatient care center services	☐	☐	☐	☐
63. Immunization program	☐	☐	☐	☐
64. Indigent care clinic	☐	☐	☐	☐
65. Linguistic/translation services	☐	☐	☐	☐
66. Meal on wheels	☐	☐	☐	☐
67. Mobile health services	☐	☐	☐	☐
68. Neurological services	☐	☐	☐	☐
69. Nutrition program	☐	☐	☐	☐
70. Occupational health services	☐	☐	☐	☐
71. Oncology services	☐	☐	☐	☐
72. Orthopedic services	☐	☐	☐	☐
73. Outpatient surgery	☐	☐	☐	☐
74. Pain management program	☐	☐	☐	☐
75. Palliative care program	☐	☐	☐	☐
76. Palliative care inpatient unit	☐	☐	☐	☐
77. Patient controlled analgesia (PCA)	☐	☐	☐	☐
78. Patient education center	☐	☐	☐	☐
79. Patient representative services	☐	☐	☐	☐
80. Physical rehabilitation services				
a. Assistive technology center	☐	☐	☐	☐
b. Electrodiagnostic services	☐	☐	☐	☐
c. Physical rehabilitation outpatient services	☐	☐	☐	☐
d. Prosthetic and orthotic services	☐	☐	☐	☐
e. Robot-assisted walking therapy	☐	☐	☐	☐
f. Simulated rehabilitation environment	☐	☐	☐	☐
81. Primary care department	☐	☐	☐	☐
82. Psychiatric services				
a. Psychiatric child-adolescent services	☐	☐	☐	☐
b. Psychiatric consultation-liaison services	☐	☐	☐	☐
c. Psychiatric education services	☐	☐	☐	☐
d. Psychiatric emergency services	☐	☐	☐	☐
e. Psychiatric geriatric services	☐	☐	☐	☐
f. Psychiatric outpatient services	☐	☐	☐	☐
g. Psychiatric partial hospitalization services	☐	☐	☐	☐
h. Psychiatric residential treatment	☐	☐	☐	☐

C. FACILITIES AND SERVICES (continued)

	(1) Owned or provided by my hospital or its subsidiary	(2) Provided by my Health System (in my local community)	(3) Provided by my network (in my local community)	(4) Provided through a formal contractual arrangement or joint venture with another provider that is not in my system or network (in my local community)
83. Radiology, diagnostic				
a. CT Scanner	☐	☐	☐	☐
b. Diagnostic radioisotope facility	☐	☐	☐	☐
c. Electron beam computed tomography (EBCT)	☐	☐	☐	☐
d. Full-field digital mammography (FFDM)	☐	☐	☐	☐
e. Magnetic resonance imaging (MRI)	☐	☐	☐	☐
f. Intraoperative magnetic resonance imaging	☐	☐	☐	☐
g. Magnetoencephalography (MEG)	☐	☐	☐	☐
h. Multi-slice spiral computed tomography (<64+ slice CT)	☐	☐	☐	☐
i. Multi-slice spiral computed tomography (64+ slice CT)	☐	☐	☐	☐
j. Positron emission tomography (PET)	☐	☐	☐	☐
k. Positron emission tomography/CT (PET/CT)	☐	☐	☐	☐
l. Single photon emission computerized tomography (SPECT)	☐	☐	☐	☐
m. Ultrasound	☐	☐	☐	☐
84. Radiology, therapeutic				
a. Image-guided radiation therapy (IGRT)	☐	☐	☐	☐
b. Intensity-modulated radiation therapy (IMRT)	☐	☐	☐	☐
c. Proton beam therapy	☐	☐	☐	☐
d. Shaped beam radiation system	☐	☐	☐	☐
e. Stereotactic radiosurgery	☐	☐	☐	☐
85. Retirement housing	☐	☐	☐	☐
86. Robotic surgery	☐	☐	☐	☐
87. Rural health clinic	☐	☐	☐	☐
88. Sleep center	☐	☐	☐	☐
89. Social work services	☐	☐	☐	☐
90. Sports medicine	☐	☐	☐	☐
91. Support groups	☐	☐	☐	☐
92. Swing bed services	☐	☐	☐	☐
93. Teen outreach services	☐	☐	☐	☐
94. Tobacco treatment/cessation program	☐	☐	☐	☐
95. Transplant services				
a. Bone marrow	☐	☐	☐	☐
b. Heart	☐	☐	☐	☐
c. Kidney	☐	☐	☐	☐
d. Liver	☐	☐	☐	☐
e. Lung	☐	☐	☐	☐
f. Tissue	☐	☐	☐	☐
g. Other	☐	☐	☐	☐

C. FACILITIES AND SERVICES (continued)

	(1) Owned or provided by my hospital or its subsidiary	(2) Provided by my Health System (in my local community)	(3) Provided by my network (in my local community)	(4) Provided through a formal contractual arrangement or joint venture with another provider that is not in my system or network (in my local community)
96. Transportation to health services	☐	☐	☐	☐
97. Urgent care center..	☐	☐	☐	☐
98. Virtual colonoscopy	☐	☐	☐	☐
99. Volunteer services department	☐	☐	☐	☐
100. Women's health center/services	☐	☐	☐	☐
101. Wound management services...................................	☐	☐	☐	☐

102a. In which of the following physician arrangements does your hospital or system/network participate? Column 3 refers to the networks that were identified in section B, question 3d. For hospital level physician arrangements that are reported in column 1, please report the number of physicians involved.

	(1) My Hospital		(2) My Health System	(3) My Health Network
a. Independent Practice Association (IPA)	☐	(# of physicians _____)	☐	☐
b. Group practice without walls	☐	(# of physicians _____)	☐	☐
c. Open Physician-Hospital Organization (PHO)	☐	(# of physicians _____)	☐	☐
d. Closed Physician-Hospital Organization (PHO)..........	☐	(# of physicians _____)	☐	☐
e. Management Service Organization (MSO)	☐	(# of physicians _____)	☐	☐
f. Integrated Salary Model	☐	(# of physicians _____)	☐	☐
g. Equity Model	☐	(# of physicians _____)	☐	☐
h. Foundation..	☐	(# of physicians _____)	☐	☐
i. Other, please specify _____	☐	(# of physicians _____)	☐	☐

102b. Looking across all the relationships identified in question 102a, what is the total number of physicians (count each physician only once) that are engaged in an arrangement with your hospital that allows for joint contracting with payers or shared responsibility for financial risk or clinical performance between the hospital and physician (arrangement may be at the hospital, system or network level)? # of physicians _____

103a. Does your hospital participate in any joint venture arrangements with physicians or physician groups? YES ☐   NO ☐

103b. If your hospital participates in any joint ventures with physicians or physician groups, please indicate which types of services are involved in those joint ventures (Check all that apply)

- a. ☐ Limited service hospital
- b. ☐ Ambulatory surgical centers
- c. ☐ Imaging centers
- d. ☐ Other _____

103c. If you selected 'a. Limited Service Hospital', please tell us what type(s) of services are provided. (Check all that apply.)

- a. ☐ Cardiac
- b. ☐ Orthopedic
- c. ☐ Surgical
- d. ☐ Other _____

103d. Does your hospital participate in joint venture arrangements with organizations other than physician groups? YES ☐   NO ☐

C. FACILITIES AND SERVICES (continued)

104a. Has your hospital or health care system established an accountable care organization (ACO)? YES ☐ NO ☐

104b. If yes, please indicate the patient population that participates in the ACO. (Check all that apply):

    a. ☐ Medicaid

    b. ☐ Medicare

    c. ☐ Privately insured

    d. ☐ Other, please specify_____

105. Does your hospital have an established medical home program? YES ☐ NO ☐

106. Does your hospital participate in a bundled payment program involving inpatient, physician, and/or post acute care services where the hospital receives a single payment from a payer for a package of services and then distributes payments to participating providers of care (such as a single fee for hospital and physician services for a specific procedure, e.g. hip replacement, CABG)? YES ☐ NO ☐

107. Does your hospital, health system or health network have an equity interest in any of the following insurance products? (Check all that apply) Contractual relationships with HMOs and PPOs should not be reported here but in Question 108. Column 3 refers to the networks that were identified in section B, question 3d.

	(1) My Hospital	(2) My Health System	(3) My Health Network	(4) Joint Venture with Insurer
1. Health Maintenance Organization	☐	☐	☐	☐
2. Preferred Provider Organization.	☐	☐	☐	☐
3. Indemnity Fee for Service Plan	☐	☐	☐	☐

108. Does your hospital have a formal written contract that specifies the obligations of each party with:

    a. Health maintenance organization (HMO) ....YES ☐ NO ☐ b. If YES, how many contracts? _____

    c. Preferred provider organization (PPO) ....YES ☐ NO ☐ d. If YES, how many contracts? _____

109. What percentage of the hospital's net patient revenue is paid on a capitated basis? If the hospital does not participate in capitated arrangements, please enter "0") _____ %

110. What percentage of the hospital's net patient revenue is paid on a shared risk basis? _____ %

111. Does your hospital contract directly with employers or a coalition of employers to provide care on a capitated, predetermined, or shared risk basis? ....YES ☐ NO ☐

112. If your hospital has arrangements to care for a specific group of enrollees in exchange for a capitated payment, how many lives are covered? _____

D. TOTAL FACILITY BEDS, UTILIZATION, FINANCES, AND STAFFING

Please report beds, utilization, financial, and staffing data for the 12-month period that is consistent with the period reported on page 1. Report financial data for reporting period only. Include within your operations all activities that are wholly owned by the hospital, including subsidiary corporations regardless of where the activity is physically located. Please do not include within your operations distinct and separate divisions that may be owned by your hospital's parent corporation. If final figures are not available, please estimate. Round to the nearest dollar. Report all personnel who were on the payroll and whose payroll expenses are reported in D3f. (Please refer to specific definitions on pages 21-23.)

	(1) Total Facility	(2) Nursing Home Unit/Facility
Fill out column (2) if hospital owns and operates a nursing home type unit/facility. Column (1) should be the combined total of hospital plus nursing home unit/facility.		

1. BEDS AND UTILIZATION

	(1) Total Facility	(2) Nursing Home Unit/Facility
a. Total licensed beds..	_____	_____
b. Beds set up and staffed for use at the end of the reporting period	_____	_____
c. Bassinets set up and staffed for use at the end of the reporting period	_____	
d. Births (exclude fetal deaths)	_____	
e. Admissions (exclude newborns, include neonatal & swing admissions)	_____	_____
f. Inpatient days (exclude newborns, include neonatal & swing days)	_____	_____
g. Emergency department visits..	_____	
h. Total outpatient visits (include emergency department visits & outpatient surgeries)....	_____	
i. Inpatient surgical operations	_____	
j. Number of operating rooms	_____	
k. Outpatient surgical operations..	_____	

2. MEDICARE/MEDICAID UTILIZATION (exclude newborns, include neonatal & swing days and deaths)

	(1) Total Facility	(2) Nursing Home Unit/Facility
a1. Total Medicare (Title XVIII) inpatient discharges (including Medicare Managed Care)	_____	_____
a2. How many Medicare inpatient discharges were Medicare Managed Care	_____	_____
b1. Total Medicare (Title XVIII) inpatient days (including Medicare Managed Care)	_____	_____
b2. How many Medicare inpatient days were Medicare Managed Care	_____	_____
c1. Total Medicaid (Title XIX) inpatient discharges (including Medicaid Managed Care)	_____	_____
c2. How many Medicaid inpatient discharges were Medicaid Managed Care	_____	_____
d1. Total Medicaid (Title XIX) inpatient days (including Medicaid Managed Care)	_____	_____
d2. How many Medicaid inpatient days were Medicaid Managed Care	_____	_____

3. FINANCIAL

	(1) Total Facility	(2) Nursing Home Unit/Facility
*a. Net patient revenue (treat bad debt as a deduction from revenue)...................	_____.00	_____.00
*b. Tax appropriations	_____.00	
*c. Other operating revenue	_____.00	
*d. Nonoperating revenue	_____.00	
*e. TOTAL REVENUE (add 3a thru 3d)	_____.00	_____.00
f. Payroll expenses (only)	_____.00	_____.00
g. Employee benefits	_____.00	_____.00
h. Depreciation expense (for reporting period only)	_____.00	
i. Interest expense	_____.00	
j. Supply expense..	_____.00	
k. TOTAL EXPENSES (Payroll plus all non-payroll expenses. Exclude bad debt)	_____.00	_____.00

*4. REVENUE BY TYPE

	(1) Total Facility
a. Total gross inpatient revenue..	_____.00
b. Total gross outpatient revenue	_____.00
c. Total gross patient revenue	_____.00

D. TOTAL FACILITY BEDS, UTILIZATION, FINANCES, AND STAFFING (continued)

*5. UNCOMPENSATED CARE & PROVIDER TAXES

a. Bad debt **(Revenue forgone at full established rates. Include in gross revenue)** .... _____ .00

b. Financial Assistance (includes Charity Care) (Revenue forgone at full-established rates. Include in gross revenue.)........ _____ .00

c. Is your bad debt reported here (5a) reported on the basis of full charges? YES ☐ NO ☐

d. Does your state have a provider Medicaid tax/assessment program? YES ☐ NO ☐

e. If yes, please report the total gross amount paid into the program.. _____ .00

f. Due to differing accounting standards please indicate whether the provider tax/assessment amount is included in:

    1. Total expense YES ☐ NO ☐

    2. Deductions from net patient revenue YES ☐ NO ☐

*6. REVENUE BY PAYOR (report total facility gross and net figures)

		(1) Gross	(2) Net
*a. GOVERNMENT (1) Medicare:			
a) Fee for service patient revenue		.00	.00
b) Managed care revenue		.00	.00
c) Total (a + b)		**.00**	**.00**
(2) Medicaid:			
a) Fee for service patient revenue		.00	.00
b) Managed care revenue		.00	.00
c) Medicaid Disproportionate Share Hospital Payments (DSH)			.00
d) Medicaid supplemental payments: not including Medicaid Disproportionate Share Hospital Payments (DSH)			.00
e) Total (a + b + c + d)		**.00**	**.00**
(3) Other government:		.00	.00
*b. NONGOVERNMENT (1) Self-pay		.00	.00
(2) Third-party payors:			
a) Managed care (includes HMO and PPO)		.00	.00
b) Other third-party payors		.00	.00
c) Total third-party payors (a + b)		**.00**	**.00**
(3) All Other nongovernment:		.00	.00
*c. **TOTAL**		**.00**	**.00**

(Total gross should equal 4c on page 9. Total net should equal 3a on page 9.)

Are the financial data on pages 9 and 10 from your audited financial statement? .... YES ☐ NO ☐

7. FIXED ASSETS

a. Property, plant and equipment at <u>cost</u> .... _____ .00

b. Accumulated <u>depreciation</u> .... _____ .00

c. Net property, plant and equipment (a-b) .... _____ .00

d. Total gross square feet of your physical plant used for or in support of your healthcare activities .... _____

8. TOTAL CAPITAL EXPENSES

Include all expenses used to acquire assets, including buildings, remodeling projects, equipment, or property. _____ .00

D. TOTAL FACILITY BEDS, UTILIZATION, FINANCES, AND STAFFING (continued)

9. INFORMATION TECHNOLOGY

*a. IT operating expense..._____.00

*b. IT capital expense..._____.00

*c. Number of employed IT staff (in FTEs) ...._____

*d. Number of outsourced IT staff (in FTEs).._____

e. Does your hospital have an electronic health record (see definition)?

☐ Yes, fully implemented   ☐ Yes, partially implemented   ☐ No

10. STAFFING

Report full-time (35 hours or more) and part-time (less than 35 hours) personnel who were on the hospital/facility **payroll at the end of your reporting period.** Include members of religious orders for whom dollar equivalents were reported. Exclude private-duty nurses, volunteers, and all personnel whose salary is financed entirely by outside research grants. Exclude physicians and dentists who are paid on a fee basis. FTE is the total number of hours worked by all employees over the full (12 month) reporting period divided by the normal number of hours worked by a full-time employee for that same time period. For example, if your hospital considers a normal workweek for a full-time employee to be 40 hours, a total of 2,080 would be worked over a full year (52 weeks). If the total number of hours worked by all employees on the payroll is 208,000, then the number of Full-Time Equivalents (FTE) is 100 (employees). The FTE calculation for a specific occupational category such as registered nurses is exactly the same. The calculation for each occupational category should be based on the number of hours worked by staff employed in that specific category.

For each occupational category, please report the number of staff vacancies as of the last day of your reporting period. A vacancy is defined as a budgeted staff position which is unfilled as of the last day of the reporting period and for which the hospital is actively seeking either a full-time or part-time permanent replacement. Personnel who work in more than one area should be included only in the category of their primary responsibility and should be counted only once.

	(1) Full-Time (35 hr/wk or more) On Payroll	(2) Part-Time (Less than 35hr/wk) On Payroll	(3) FTE	(4) Vacancies
a. Physicians..	_____	_____	_____	_____
b. Dentists...	_____	_____	_____	_____
c. Medical and dental residents/interns.............	_____	_____	_____	_____
d. Other trainees......................................	_____	_____	_____	_____
e. Registered nurses..................................	_____	_____	_____	_____
f. Licensed practical (vocational) nurses............	_____	_____	_____	_____
g. Nursing assistive personnel.......................	_____	_____	_____	_____
h. Radiology technicians..............................	_____	_____	_____	_____
i. Laboratory technicians.............................	_____	_____	_____	_____
j. Pharmacists, licensed..............................	_____	_____	_____	_____
k. Pharmacy technicians..............................	_____	_____	_____	_____
l. Respiratory therapists.............................	_____	_____	_____	_____
m. All other personnel.................................	_____	_____	_____	_____
n. Total facility personnel (add 10a through 10m).....	_____	_____	_____	_____

(Total facility personnel should include hospital plus nursing home type unit/facility personnel reported in 10o and 10p.)

o. Nursing home type unit/facility registered nurses............	_____	_____	_____	_____
p. Total nursing home type unit/facility personnel................	_____	_____	_____	_____

11. PRIVILEGED PHYSICIANS

Report the total number of physicians with privileges at your hospital by type of relationship with the hospital. <u>The sum of the physicians reported in 11a-11f should equal the total number of privileged physicians (11g) in the hospital.</u>

	(1) Total Employed	(2) Total Individual Contract	(3) Total Group Contract	(4) Not Employed or Under Contract	(5) Total Privileged
a. Primary care (general practitioner, general internal medicine, family practice, general pediatrics, obstetrics/gynecology, geriatrics)	_____	_____	_____	_____	_____
b. Emergency medicine	_____	_____	_____	_____	_____
c. Hospitalist	_____	_____	_____	_____	_____
d. Intensivist	_____	_____	_____	_____	_____
e. Radiologist/pathologist/anesthesiologist	_____	_____	_____	_____	_____
f. Other specialist	_____	_____	_____	_____	_____
g. Total (add 11a-11f)	_____	_____	_____	_____	_____

12. HOSPITALISTS

a. Do hospitalists provide care for patients in your hospital? .... YES ☐   NO ☐ **(if yes, please report in D.11c.)**

b. If yes, please report the total number of full-time equivalents (FTE) hospitalists......................FTE _____

13. INTENSIVISTS

a. Do intensivists provide care for patients in your hospital? (If no, please skip to 14.) YES ☐   NO ☐ **(if yes, please report in D.11d.)**

b. If yes, please report the total number of FTE intensivists and assign them to the following areas. Please indicate whether the intensive care area is closed to intensivists. (Meaning that only intensivists are authorized to care for ICU patients.)

		FTE	Closed to Intensivists
1.	Medical-surgical intensive care	_____	☐
2.	Cardiac intensive care	_____	☐
3.	Neonatal intensive care	_____	☐
4.	Pediatric intensive care	_____	☐
5.	Other intensive care	_____	☐
6.	**Total**	_____	

14. ADVANCED PRACTICE REGISTERED NURSES

a. Do advanced practice nurses provide care for patients in your hospital? .... YES ☐   NO ☐ (if no, please skip to 15.)

b. If yes, please report the number of full time, part time and FTE advanced practice nurses employed or contracted to provide care for patients in your hospital.

_____ Full-time   _____ Part-time   _____ FTE

c. If yes, please indicate the type of service the nurses provide (Please check all that apply).

☐ Primary care   ☐ Anesthesia services (Certified registered nurse anesthetist)   ☐ Emergency department care

☐ Other specialty care   ☐ Patient education   ☐ Case management   ☐ Other

15. FOREIGN EDUCATED NURSES

a. Did your facility hire more foreign-educated nurses (including contract or agency nurses) to help fill RN vacancies in 2012 vs. 2011?

More ☐   Less ☐   Same ☐   Did not hire foreign nurses ☐

b. If yes, from which countries/continents are you recruiting foreign-educated nurses?

Africa ☐   South Korea ☐   Canada ☐   Philippines ☐   China ☐   India ☐   Other ☐

E. SUPPLEMENTAL INFORMATION

1. CARE COORDINATION

Please indicate activities that your organization is engaged in to coordinate care across settings and extent to which they are used.

		Not used at all	Used minimally	Used moderately	Used Widely	Used hospital-wide
a.	Use of predictive analytic tools to identify individual patients at high risk for poor outcomes or extraordinary resource use.	☐	☐	☐	☐	☐
b.	Telephonic outreach to discharge patients within 72 hours of discharge.	☐	☐	☐	☐	☐

2. DIVERSITY, LANGUAGE AND LEADERSHIP

		YES	NO
a.	Does your hospital gather information on a patient's race/ethnicity at any point during their stay?	☐	☐
b.	Does your hospital gather information on a patient's primary language at any point during their stay?	☐	☐
c.	Does your hospital or health system currently have or plan to develop, execute, or evaluate a diversity strategy or plan?	☐	☐
d.	Does your hospital educate all clinical staff during orientation about how to address the unique cultural and linguistic factors affecting the care of diverse patients and communities?	☐	☐
e.	Does your hospital require all employees to attend diversity training?	☐	☐
f.	Does the hospital's strategic plan include goals for improving quality of care of culturally and linguistically-diverse patient population?	☐	☐

3. OTHER

a. Does your hospital provide services through one or more satellite facilities?   YES ☐   NO ☐

b. Does the hospital participate in a group purchasing arrangement?   YES ☐   NO ☐

If yes, please provide the name, city, and state of the group purchasing organization. If the hospital participates in more than one group purchasing organization, please provide the name, city, state and telephone number of the group purchasing organization(s) on page 13 (3e), under supplemental information

Name: _____   City: _____   State: _____

c. Does the hospital purchase medical/surgical supplies directly through a distributor?   YES ☐   NO ☐
If yes, please provide the name of the distributor.

Name: _____

d. If your hospital hired RNs during the reporting period, how many were new graduates from nursing schools? _____

e. Use this space to describe your community benefit activities as well as any partners you are currently working with on such activities. Also use this space or additional sheets if more space is required for comments or to elaborate on any information supplied on this survey. Refer to the response by page, section and item name.

_____

_____

_____

_____

_____

_____

_____

_____

_____

As declared previously, hospital specific revenue data are treated as confidential. AHA's policy is not to release these data without written permission from your institution. The AHA will however, share these data with your respective state hospital association and if requested with your appropriate metropolitan/regional association.

On occasion, the AHA is asked to provide these data to external organizations, both public and private, for their use in analyzing crucial health care policy or research issues. The AHA is requesting your permission to allow us to release your confidential data to those requests that we consider legitimate and worthwhile. In every instance of disclosure, the receiving organization will be prohibited from releasing hospital specific information.

Please indicate below whether or not you agree to these types of disclosure:

[   ] I hereby grant AHA permission to release my hospital's revenue data to external users that the AHA determines have a legitimate and worthwhile need to gain access to these data subject to the user's agreement with the AHA not to release hospital specific information.

_____
Chief Executive Officer   Date

[   ] I do not grant AHA permission to release my confidential data.

_____
Chief Executive Officer   Date

Does your hospital or health system have an Internet or Homepage address?   Yes ☐ No ☐

If yes, please provide the address: http:// _____

Thank you for your cooperation in completing this survey. If there are any questions about your responses to this survey, who should be contacted?

_____   (___) _____
Name (please print)   Title   (Area Code) Telephone Number

____ / ____ / ____   _____   (___) _____
Date of Completion   Chief Executive Officer   Hospital's Main Fax Number

Contact Email address: _____

NOTE: PLEASE PHOTOCOPY THE INFORMATION FOR YOUR HOSPITAL FILE BEFORE RETURNING THE ORIGINAL FORM TO THE AMERICAN HOSPITAL ASSOCIATION. ALSO, PLEASE FORWARD A PHOTOCOPY OF THE COMPLETED QUESTIONNAIRE TO YOUR STATE HOSPITAL ASSOCIATION.

THANK YOU

INSTRUCTIONS AND DEFINITIONS FOR THE 2012 ANNUAL SURVEY OF HOSPITALS.
For purposes of this survey, a hospital is defined as the organization or corporate entity licensed or registered as a hospital by a state to provide diagnostic and therapeutic patient services for a variety of medical conditions, both surgical and nonsurgical.

1. Reporting period used (beginning and ending date): Record the beginning and ending dates of the reporting period in an eight-digit number: for example, January 1, 2009 should be shown as 01/01/2009. Number of days should equal the time span between the two dates that the hospital was open. If you are reporting for less than 366 days, utilization and finances should be presented for days reported only.
2. Were you in operation 12 full months at the end of your reporting period? If you are reporting for less than 366 days, utilization and finances should be presented for days reported only.
3. Number of days open during reporting period: Number of days should equal the time span between the two dates that the hospital was open.

SECTION B
ORGANIZATIONAL STRUCTURE
Instructions and Definitions

1. **CONTROL**
   Check the box to the left of the type of organization that is responsible for establishing policy for overall operation of the hospital.
   Government, nonfederal.
   State. Controlled by an agency of state government.
   County. Controlled by an agency of county government.
   City. Controlled by an agency of municipal government.
   City-County. Controlled jointly by agencies of municipal and county governments.
   Hospital district or authority. Controlled by a political subdivision of a state, county, or city created solely for the purpose of establishing and maintaining medical care or health-related care institutions.
   Nongovernment, not for profit. Controlled by not-for-profit organizations, including religious organizations (Catholic hospitals, for example), community hospitals, cooperative hospitals, hospitals operated by fraternal societies, and so forth.
   Investor owned, for profit. Controlled on a for profit basis by an individual, partnership, or a profit making corporation.
   Government, federal. Controlled by an agency or department of the federal government.

2. **SERVICE**
   Indicate the ONE category that best describes the type of service that your hospital provides to the majority of patients.
   General medical and surgical. Provides diagnostic and therapeutic services to patients for a variety of medical conditions, both surgical and nonsurgical.
   Hospital unit of an institution. Provides diagnostic and therapeutic services to patients in an institution.
   Hospital unit within an institution for the mentally retarded. Provides diagnostic and therapeutic services to patients in an institution for the mentally retarded.
   Surgical. An acute care specialty hospital where 2/3 or more of its inpatient claims are for surgical/diagnosis related groups.
   Psychiatric. Provides diagnostic and therapeutic services to patients with mental or emotional disorders.
   Tuberculosis and other respiratory diseases. Provides medical care and rehabilitative services to patients for whom the primary diagnosis is tuberculosis or other respiratory diseases.
   Cancer. Provides medical care to patients for whom the primary diagnosis is cancer.
   Heart. Provides diagnosis and treatment of heart disease.
   Obstetrics and gynecology. Provides medical and surgical treatment to pregnant women and to mothers following delivery. Also provides diagnostic and therapeutic services to women with diseases or disorders of the reproductive organs.
   Eye, ear, nose, and throat. Provides diagnosis and treatment of diseases and injuries of the eyes, ears, nose, and throat.
   Rehabilitation. Provides a comprehensive array of restoration services for the disabled and all support services necessary to help them attain their maximum functional capacity.
   Orthopedic. Provides corrective treatment of deformities, diseases, and ailments of the locomotive apparatus, especially affecting the limbs, bones, muscles, and joints.
   Chronic disease. Provides medical and skilled nursing services to patients with long-term illnesses who are not in an acute phase, but who require an intensity of services not available in nursing homes.
   Institution for the mentally retarded. Provides health-related care on a regular basis to patients with psychiatric or developmental impairment who cannot be treated in a skilled nursing unit.
   Acute long term care hospital. Provides high acuity interdisciplinary services to medically complex patients that require more intensive recuperation and care than can be provided in a typical nursing facility.
   Alcoholism and other chemical dependency. Provides diagnostic and therapeutic services to patients with alcoholism or other drug dependencies.

3. **OTHER**
   a. **Children admissions.** A hospital whose primary focus is the health and treatment of children and adolescents.
   b. **Subsidiary.** A company that is wholly controlled by another or one that is more than 50% owned by another organization.
   c. **Contract managed.** General day-to-day management of an entire organization by another organization under a formal contract. Managing organization reports directly to the board of trustees or owners of the managed organization; managed organization retains total legal responsibility and ownership of the facility's assets and liabilities.
   d. **Network.** A group of hospitals, physicians, other providers, insurers and/or community agencies that voluntarily work together to coordinate and deliver health services

4. **National Provider Identifier (NPI)** is a unique identification number for covered health care providers. Covered health care providers and all health plans and health care clearinghouses must use the NPIs in the administrative and financial transactions adopted under HIPAA. The NPI is a 10-position, intelligence-free numeric identifier (10-digit number).

Owned/provided by the hospital or its subsidiary. All patient revenues, expenses and utilization related to the provision of the service are reflected in the hospital's statistics reported elsewhere in this survey.

Provided by my Health System (in my local community). Another health care provider in the same system as your hospital provides the service and patient revenue, expenses, and utilization related to the provision of the service are recorded at the point where the service was provided and would not be reflected in your hospital's statistics reported elsewhere in this survey. (A system is a corporate body that owns, leases, religiously sponsors and/or manages health provider)

Provided by my network (in my local community). Another health care provider in the same network as your hospital provides the service and patient revenue, expenses and utilization related to the provision of the service are recorded at the point where the service was provided and would not be reflected in your hospital's statistics reported elsewhere in this survey. (A network is a group of hospitals, physicians, other providers, insurers and/or community agencies that voluntarily work together to coordinate and deliver health services. When reporting a service for a network, please indicate the name of the network in Section B, question d.)

Provided through a formal contractual arrangement or joint venture with another provider that is not in my system or network. All patient revenues and utilization related to the provision of the service are recorded at the site where the service was provided and would not be reflected in your hospital statistics reported elsewhere in this survey. (A joint venture is a contractual arrangement between two or more parties forming an unincorporated business. The participants in the arrangement remain independent and separate outside of the venture's purpose.)

1. **General medical-surgical care.** Provides acute care to patients in medical and surgical units on the basis of physicians' orders and approved nursing care plans.
2. **Pediatric medical-surgical care.** Provides acute care to pediatric patients on the basis of physicians' orders and approved nursing care plans.
3. **Obstetrics.** Level should be designated: (1) unit provides services for uncomplicated maternity and newborn cases; (2) unit provides services for uncomplicated cases, the majority of complicated problems, and special neonatal services; and (3) unit provides services for all serious illnesses and abnormalities and is supervised by a full-time maternal/fetal specialist.
4. **Medical surgical intensive care.** Provides patient care of a more intensive nature than the usual medical and surgical care, on the basis of physicians' orders and approved nursing care plans. These units are staffed with specially trained nursing personnel and contain monitoring and specialized support equipment for patients who because of shock, trauma or other life-threatening conditions require intensified comprehensive observation and care. Includes mixed intensive care units.
5. **Cardiac intensive care.** Provides patient care of a more specialized nature than the usual medical and surgical care, on the basis of physicians' orders and approved nursing care plans. The unit is staffed with specially trained nursing personnel and contains monitoring and specialized support or treatment equipment for patients who, because of heart seizure, open-heart surgery, or other life-threatening conditions, require intensified, comprehensive observation and care. May include myocardial infarction, pulmonary care, and heart transplant units.
6. **Neonatal intensive care.** A unit that must be separate from the newborn nursery providing intensive care to all sick infants including those with the very lowest birth weights (less than 1500 grams). NICU has potential for providing mechanical ventilation, neonatal surgery, and special care for the sickest infants born in the hospital or transferred from another institution. A full-time neonatologist serves as director of the NICU.
7. **Neonatal intermediate care.** A unit that must be separate from the normal newborn nursery and that provides intermediate and/or recovery care and some specialized services, including immediate resuscitation, intravenous therapy, and capacity for prolonged oxygen therapy and monitoring.
8. **Pediatric intensive care.** Provides care to pediatric patients that is of a more intensive nature than that usually provided to pediatric patients. The unit is staffed with specially trained personnel and contains monitoring and specialized support equipment for treatment of patients who, because of shock, trauma, or other life-threatening conditions, require intensified, comprehensive observation and care.
9. **Burn care.** Provides care to severely burned patients. Severely burned patients are those with any of the following: (1) second-degree burns of more than 25% total body surface area for adults or 20% total body surface area for children: (2) third-degree burns of more than 10% total body surface area; (3) any severe burns of the hands, face, eyes, ears, or feet; or (4) all inhalation injuries, electrical burns, complicated burn injuries involving fractures and other major traumas, and all other poor risk factors.
10. **Other special care.** Provides care to patients requiring care more intensive than that provided in the acute area, yet not sufficiently intensive to require admission to an intensive care unit. Patients admitted to this area are usually transferred here from an intensive care unit once their condition has improved. These units are sometimes referred to as definitive observation, step-down or progressive care units.
11. **Other intensive care.** A specially staffed, specialty equipped, separate section of a hospital dedicated to the observation, care, and treatment of patients with life threatening illnesses, injuries, or complications from which recovery is possible. It provides special expertise and facilities for the support of vital function and utilizes the skill of medical nursing and other staff experienced in the management of these problems.
12. **Physical rehabilitation.** Provides care encompassing a comprehensive array of restoration services for the disabled and all support services necessary to help patients attain their maximum functional capacity.
13. **Alcoholism-drug abuse or dependency care.** Provides diagnosis and therapeutic services to patients with alcoholism or other drug dependencies. Includes care for inpatient/residential treatment for patients whose course of treatment involves more intensive care than provided in an outpatient setting or where patient requires supervised withdrawal.
14. **Psychiatric care.** Provides acute or long-term care to emotionally disturbed patients, including patients admitted for diagnosis and those admitted for treatment of psychiatric problems, on the basis of physicians' orders and approved nursing care plans. Long-term care may include intensive supervision to the chronically mentally ill, mentally disordered, or other mentally incompetent persons.
15. **Skilled nursing care.** Provides non-acute medical and skilled nursing care services, therapy, and social services under the supervision of a licensed registered nurse on a 24-hour basis.
16. **Intermediate nursing care.** Provides health-related services (skilled nursing care and social services) to residents with a variety of physical conditions or functional disabilities. These residents do not require the care provided by a hospital or skilled nursing facility, but do need supervision and support services.
17. **Acute long-term care.** Provides specialized acute hospital care to medically complex patients who are critically ill, have multisystem complications and/or failure, and require hospitalization averaging 25 days, in a facility offering specialized treatment programs and therapeutic intervention on a 24-hour/7 day a week basis.
18. **Other long-term care.** Provision of long-term care other than skilled nursing care or intermediate care for those who do not require daily medical or nursing services, but may requires some assistance in the activities of daily living. This can include residential care, elderly care, or sheltered care facilities for developmentally disabled.
19. **Other care.** (specify) Any type of care other than those listed above.
    The sum of the beds reported in Section C 1-19 should equal what you have reported in Section D(1b) for beds set up and staffed.
20. **Adult day care program.** Program providing supervision, medical and psychological care, and social activities for older adults who live at home or in another family setting, but cannot be alone or prefer to be with others during the day. May include intake assessment, health monitoring, occupational therapy, personal care, noon meal, and transportation services.

20. **Airborne infection isolation room.** A single-occupancy room for patient care where environmental factors are controlled in an effort to minimize the transmission of those infectious agents, usually spread person to person by droplet nuclei associated with coughing and inhalation. Such rooms typically have specific ventilation requirements for controlled ventilation, air pressure and filtration.

22. **Alcoholism-drug abuse or dependency outpatient services.** Organized hospital services that provide medical care and/or rehabilitative treatment services to outpatients for whom the primary diagnosis is alcoholism or other chemical dependency.

23. **Alzheimer center.** Facility that offers care to persons with Alzheimer's disease and their families through an integrated program of clinical services, research, and education.

24. **Ambulance services.** Provision of ambulance service to the ill and injured who require medical attention on a scheduled and unscheduled basis.

25. **Ambulatory surgery center.** Facility that provides care to patients requiring surgery that are admitted and discharged on the same day. Ambulatory surgery centers are distinct from same day surgical units within the hospital outpatient departments for purposes of Medicare payment.

26. **Arthritis treatment center.** Specifically equipped and staffed center for the diagnosis and treatment of arthritis and other joint disorders.

27. **Assisted living.** A special combination of housing, supportive services, personalized assistance and health care designed to respond to the individual needs of those who need help in activities of daily living and instrumental activities of daily living. Supportive services are available, 24 hours a day, to meet scheduled and unscheduled needs, in a way that promotes maximum independence and dignity for each resident and encourages the involvement of a resident's family, neighbor and friends.

28. **Auxiliary.** A volunteer community organization formed to assist the hospital in carrying out its purpose and to serve as a link between the institution and the community.

29. **Bariatric/weight control services.** The medical practice of weight reduction.

30. **Birthing room/LDR room/LDRP room.** A single-room type of maternity care with a more homelike setting for families than the traditional three-room unit (labor/delivery/recovery) with a separate postpartum area. A birthing room combines labor and delivery in one room. An LDR room accommodates three stages in the birthing process--labor, delivery, and recovery. An LDRP room accommodates all four stages of the birth process--labor, delivery, recovery, and postpartum.

31. **Blood donor center.** A facility that performs, or is responsible for the collection, processing, testing or distribution of blood and components.

32. **Breast cancer screening/mammograms.** Mammography screening - The use of breast x-ray to detect unsuspected breast cancer in asymptomatic women. Diagnostic mammography - The x-ray imaging of breast tissue in symptomatic women who are considered to have a substantial likelihood of having breast cancer already.

33. **Cardiology and cardiac surgery services.** Services which include the diagnosis and treatment of diseases and disorders involving the heart and circulatory system.

    a-b. Cardiology services. An organized clinical service offering diagnostic and interventional procedures to manage the full range of heart conditions.

    c-d. Diagnostic catheterization. (also called coronary angiography or coronary arteriography) is used to assist in diagnosing complex heart conditions. Cardiac angiography involves the insertion of a tiny catheter into the artery in the groin then carefully threading the catheter up into the aorta where the coronary arteries originate. Once the catheter is in place, a dye is injected which allows the cardiologist to see the size, shape, and distribution of the coronary arteries. These images are used to diagnose heart disease and to determine, among other things, whether or not surgery is indicated.

    e-f. Interventional cardiac catheterization. Nonsurgical procedure that utilizes the same basic principles as diagnostic catheterization and then uses advanced techniques to improve the heart's function. It can be a less-invasive alternative to heart surgery.

    g-h. Cardiac surgery. Includes minimally invasive procedures that include surgery done with only a small incision or no incision at all, such as through a laparoscope or an endoscope and more invasive major surgical procedures that include open chest and open heart surgery.

    i-j. Cardiac electrophysiology. Evaluation and management of patients with complex rhythm or conduction abnormalities, including diagnostic testing, treatment of arrhythmias by catheter ablation or drug therapy, and pacemaker/defibrillator implantation and follow-up.

    k. Cardiac rehabilitation. A medically supervised program to help heart patients recover quickly and improve their overall physical and mental functioning. The goal is to reduce risk of another cardiac event or to keep an already present heart condition from getting worse. Cardiac rehabilitation programs include: counseling to patients, an exercise program, helping patients modify risk factors such as smoking and high blood pressure, providing vocational guidance to enable the patient to return to work, supplying information on physical limitations and lending emotional support.

34. **Case management.** A system of assessment, treatment planning, referral and follow-up that ensures the provision of comprehensive and continuous services and the coordination of payment and reimbursement for care.

35. **Chaplaincy/pastoral care services.** A service ministering religious activities and providing pastoral counseling to patients, their families, and staff of a health care organization.

36. **Chemotherapy.** An organized program for the treatment of cancer by the use of drugs or chemicals.

37. **Children's wellness program.** A program that encourages improved health status and a healthful lifestyle of children through health education, exercise, nutrition and health promotion.

38. **Chiropractic services.** An organized clinical service including spinal manipulation or adjustment and related diagnostic and therapeutic services.

39. **Community outreach.** A program that systematically interacts with the community to identify those in need of services, alerting persons and their families to the availability of services, locating needed services, and enabling persons to enter the service delivery system.

40. **Complementary and alternative medicine services.** Organized hospital services or formal arrangements to providers that provide care or treatment not based solely on traditional western allopathic medical teachings as instructed in most U.S. medical schools. Includes any of the following: acupuncture, chiropractic, homeopathy, osteopathy, diet and lifestyle changes, herbal medicine, massage therapy, etc.

41. **Computer assisted orthopedic surgery (CAOS).** Orthopedic surgery using computer technology, enabling three-dimensional graphic models to visualize a patient's anatomy.

42. **Crisis prevention.** Services provided in order to promote physical and mental wellbeing and the early identification of disease and ill health prior to the onset and recognition of symptoms so as to permit early treatment.

43. **Dental Services.** An organized dental service or dentists on staff, not necessarily involving special facilities, providing dental or oral services to inpatients or outpatients.

44. **Emergency services.** Health services that are provided after the onset of a medical condition that manifests itself by symptoms of sufficient severity, including severe pain, that the absence of immediate medical attention could reasonably be expected by a prudent layperson, who possesses an average knowledge of health and medicine, to result in placing the patient's health in serious jeopardy.

    a-b. Emergency department. Hospital facilities for the provision of unscheduled outpatient services to patients whose conditions require immediate care.

    c. Satellite Emergency Department. A facility owned and operated by the hospital but physically separate from the hospital for the provision of unscheduled outpatient services to patients whose conditions require immediate care. A freestanding ED is not physically connected to a hospital, but has all necessary emergency staffing and equipment on-site.

    e. Trauma center (certified). A facility to provide emergency and specialized intensive care to critically ill and injured patients. Level 1: A regional resource trauma center, which is capable of providing total care for every aspect of injury and plays a leadership role in trauma research and education. Level 2: A community trauma center, which is capable of providing trauma care to all but the most severely injured patients who require highly specialized care. Level 3: A rural trauma hospital, which is capable of providing care to a large number of injury victims and can resuscitate and stabilize more severely injured patients so that they can be transported to level 1 or 2 facilities. Please provide an explanation in the supplement section on page 13 if necessary.

45. **Enabling services.** A program that is designed to help the patient access health care services by offering any of the following: transportation services and/or referrals to local social services agencies.

46. **Endoscopic services.**
   a. **Optical colonoscopy.** An examination of the interior of the colon using a long, flexible, lighted tube with a small built-in camera.
   b. **Endoscopic ultrasound.** Specially designed endoscope that incorporates an ultrasound transducer used to obtain detailed images of organs in the chest and abdomen. The endoscope can be passed through the mouth or the anus. When combined with needle biopsy the procedure can assist in diagnosis of disease and staging of cancer.
   c. **Ablation of Barrett's esophagus.** Premalignant condition that can lead to adenocarcinoma of the esophagus. The nonsurgical ablation of premalignant tissue in Barrett's esophagus by the application of thermal energy or light through an endoscope passed from the mouth into the esophagus.
   d. **Esophageal impedance study.** A test in which a catheter is placed through the nose into the esophagus to measure whether gas or liquids are passing from the stomach into the esophagus and causing symptoms.
   e. **Endoscopic retrograde cholangiopancreatography (ERCP).** A procedure in which a catheter is introduced through an endoscope into the bile ducts and pancreatic ducts. Injection of contrast material permits detailed x-ray of these structures. The procedure is used diagnostically as well as therapeutically to relieve obstruction or remove stones.

47. **Enrollment (insurance) assistance services.** A program that provides enrollment assistance for patients who are potentially eligible for public health insurance programs such as Medicaid, State Children's Health Insurance, or local/state indigent care programs. The specific services offered This could include explanation of benefits, assist applicants in completing the application and locating all relevant documents, conduct eligibility interviews, and/or forward applications and documentation to state/local social service or health agency.

48. **Extracorporeal shock wave lithotripter (ESWL).** A medical device used for treating stones in the kidney or urethra. The device disintegrates kidney stones noninvasively through the transmission of acoustic shock waves directed at the stones.

49. **Fertility clinic.** A specialized program set in an infertility center that provides counseling and education as well as advanced reproductive techniques such as: injectable therapy, reproductive surgeries, treatment for endometriosis, male factor infertility, tubal reversals, in vitro fertilization (IVF), donor eggs, and other such services to help patients achieve successful pregnancies.

50. **Fitness center.** Provides exercise, testing, or evaluation programs and fitness activities to the community and hospital employees.

51. **Freestanding outpatient care center.** A facility owned and operated by the hospital, that is physically separate from the hospital and provides various medical treatments and diagnostic services on an outpatient basis only. Laboratory and radiology services are usually available.

52. **Geriatric services.** The branch of medicine dealing with the physiology of aging and the diagnosis and treatment of disease affecting the aged. Services could include: Adult day care; Alzheimer's diagnostic-assessment services; Comprehensive geriatric assessment; Emergency response system; Geriatric acute care unit; and/or Geriatric clinics.

53. **Health fair.** Community health education events that focus on the prevention of disease and promotion of health through such activities as audiovisual exhibits and free diagnostic services.

54. **Community health education.** Education that provides health information to individuals and populations as well as support for personal, family and community health decisions with the objective of improving health status.

55. **Genetic testing/counseling.** A service equipped with adequate laboratory facilities and directed by a qualified physician to advise parents and prospective parents on potential problems in cases of genetic defects. A genetic test is the analysis of human DNA, RNA, chromosomes, proteins, and certain metabolites in order to detect heritable disease-related genotypes, mutations, phenotypes, or karyotypes for clinical purposes. Genetic tests can have diverse purposes, including the diagnosis of genetic diseases in newborns, children, and adults; the identification of future health risks; the prediction of drug responses; and the assessment of risks to future children.

56. **Health screening.** A preliminary procedure such as a test or examination to detect the most characteristic sign or signs of a disorder that may require further investigation.

57. **Health research.** Organized hospital research program in any of the following areas: basic research, clinical research, community health research, and/or research on innovative health care delivery.

58. **Hemodialysis.** Provision of equipment and personnel for the treatment of renal insufficiency on an inpatient or outpatient basis.

59. **HIV-AIDS services.** Could include: HIV-AIDS unit-Special unit or team designated and equipped specifically for diagnosis, treatment, continuing care planning, and counseling services for HIV-AIDS patients and their families. General inpatient care for HIV-AIDS-Inpatient diagnosis and treatment for human immunodeficiency virus and acquired immunodeficiency syndrome patients, but dedicated unit is not available. Specialized outpatient program for HIV-AIDS-Special outpatient program providing diagnostic, treatment, continuing care planning, and counseling for HIV-AIDS patients and their families.

60. **Home health services.** Service providing nursing, therapy, and health-related homemaker or social services in the patient's home.

61. **Hospice.** A program providing palliative care, chiefly medical relief of pain and supportive services, addressing the emotional, social, financial, and legal needs of terminally ill patients and their families. Care can be provided in a variety of settings, both inpatient and at home.

62. **Hospital-based outpatient care center-services.** Organized hospital health care services offered by appointment on an ambulatory basis. Services may include outpatient surgery, examination, diagnosis, and treatment of a variety of medical conditions on a nonemergency basis, and laboratory and other diagnostic testing as ordered by staff or outside physician referral.

63. **Immunization program.** Program that plans, coordinates and conducts immunization services in the community.

64. **Indigent care clinic.** Health care services for uninsured and underinsured persons where care is free of charge or charged on a sliding scale. This would include "free clinics" staffed by volunteer practitioners, but could also be staffed by employees with the sponsoring health care organization subsidizing the cost of service.

65. **Linguistic/translation services.** Services provided by the hospital designed to make health care more accessible to non-English speaking patients and their physicians.

66. **Meals on wheels.** A hospital sponsored program which delivers meals to people, usually the elderly, who are unable to prepare their own meals. Low cost, nutritional meals are delivered to individuals' homes on a regular basis.

67. **Mobile health services.** Vans and other vehicles used for delivery to primary care services.

68. **Neurological services.** Services provided by the hospital dealing with the operative and nonoperative management of disorders of the central, peripheral, and autonomic nervous systems.

69. **Nutrition programs.** Services within a health care facility which are designed to provide inexpensive, nutritionally sound meals to patients.

70. **Occupational health services.** Includes services designed to protect the safety of employees from hazards in the work environment.

71. **Oncology services.** Inpatient and outpatient services for patients with cancer, including comprehensive care, support and guidance in addition to patient education and prevention, chemotherapy, counseling and other treatment methods.

72. **Orthopedic services.** Services provided for the prevention or correction of injuries or disorders of the skeletal system and associated muscles, joints and ligaments.

73. **Outpatient surgery.** Scheduled surgical services provided to patients who do not remain in the hospital overnight. The surgery may be performed in operating suites also used for inpatient surgery, specially designated surgical suites for outpatient surgery, or procedure rooms within an outpatient care facility.

74. **Pain management program.** A recognized clinical service or program providing specialized medical care, drugs or therapies for the management of acute or chronic pain and other distressing symptoms, administered by specially trained physicians and other clinicians, to patients suffering from acute illnesses of diverse causes.

75. **Palliative care program.** An organized program providing specialized medical care, drugs or therapies for the management of acute or chronic pain and/or the control of symptoms administered by specially trained physicians and other clinicians; and supportive care services, such as counseling on advanced directives, spiritual care, and social services, to patients with advanced diseases and their families.

76. **Palliative care inpatient unit.** An inpatient palliative care ward is a physically discreet, inpatient nursing unit where the focus is palliative care. The patient care focus is on symptom relief for complex patients who may be continuing to undergo primary treatment. Care is delivered by palliative medicine specialists.

77. **Patient controlled analgesia (PCA).** Intravenously administered pain medicine under the patient's control. The patient has a button on the end of a cord than can be pushed at will, whenever more pain medicine is desired. This button will only deliver more pain medicine at pre-determined intervals, as programmed by the doctor's order.

78. **Patient education center.** Written goals and objectives for the patient and/or family related to therapeutic regimens, medical procedures, and self-care.

79. **Patient representative services.** Organized hospital services providing personnel through whom patients and staff can seek solutions to institutional problems affecting the delivery of high quality care and services.

80. **Physical rehabilitation services.** Program providing medical, health-related, therapy, social, and/or vocational services to help disabled persons attain or retain their maximum functional capacity.

    a. **Assistive technology center.** A program providing access to specialized hardware and software with adaptations allowing individuals greater independence with mobility, dexterity, or increased communication options.

    b. **Electrodiagnostic services.** Diagnostic testing services for nerve and muscle function including services such as nerve conduction studies and needle electromyography.

    c. **Physical rehabilitation outpatient services.** Outpatient program providing medical, health-related, therapy, social, and/or vocational services to help disabled persons attain or retain their maximum functional capacity.

    d. **Prosthetic and orthotic services.** Services providing comprehensive prosthetic and orthotic evaluation, fitting, and training.

    e. **Robot-assisted walking therapy.** A form of physical therapy that uses a robotic device to assist patients who are relearning how to walk.

    f. **Simulated rehabilitation environment.** Rehabilitation focused on retraining functional skills in a contextually appropriate environment (simulated home and community settings) or in a traditional setting (gymnasium) using motor learning principles.

81. **Primary care department.** A unit or clinic within the hospital that provides primary care services (e.g. general pediatric care, general internal medicine, family practice, gynecology) through hospital-salaried medical and/or nursing staff, focusing on evaluating and diagnosing medical problems and providing medical treatment on an outpatient basis.

82. **Psychiatric services.** Services provided by the hospital that offer immediate initial evaluation and treatment to patients with mental or emotional disorders.

    a. **Psychiatric child-adolescent services.** Provides care to emotionally disturbed children and adolescents, including those admitted for diagnosis and those admitted for treatment.

    b. **Psychiatric consultation-liaison services.** Provides organized psychiatric consultation/liaison services to nonpsychiatric hospital staff and/or departments on psychological aspects of medical care that may be generic or specific to individual patients.

    c. **Psychiatric education services.** Provides psychiatric educational services to community agencies and workers such as schools, police, courts, public health nurses, welfare agencies, clergy, and so forth. The purpose is to expand the mental health knowledge and competence of personnel not working in the mental health field and to promote good mental health through improved understanding, attitudes, and behavioral patterns.

    d. **Psychiatric emergency services.** Services of facilities available on a 24-hour basis to provide immediate unscheduled out-patient care, diagnosis, evaluation, crisis intervention, and assistance to persons suffering acute emotional or mental distress.

    e. **Psychiatric geriatric services.** Provides care to emotionally disturbed elderly patients, including those admitted for diagnosis and those admitted for treatment.

    f. **Psychiatric outpatient services.** Provides medical care, including diagnosis and treatment, of psychiatric outpatients.

    g. **Psychiatric partial hospitalization program.** Organized hospital services of intensive day/evening outpatient services of three hours or more duration, distinguished from other outpatient visits of one hour.

    h. **Psychiatric residential treatment.** Overnight psychiatric care in conjunction with an intensive treatment program in a setting other than a hospital.

83. **Radiology, diagnostic.** The branch of radiology that deals with the utilization of all modalities of radiant energy in medical diagnoses and therapeutic procedures using radiologic guidance. This includes, but is not restricted to, imaging techniques and methodologies utilizing radiation emitted by x-ray tubes, radionuclides, and ultrasonographic devices and the radiofrequency electromagnetic radiation emitted by atoms.

    a. **CT Scanner.** Computed tomographic scanner for head or whole body scans.

    b. **Diagnostic radioisotope facility.** The use of radioactive isotopes (Radiopharmaceuticals) as tracers or indicators to detect an abnormal condition or disease.

    c. **Electron beam computed tomography (EBCT).** A high tech computed tomography scan used to detect coronary artery disease by measuring coronary calcifications. This imaging procedure uses electron beams which are magnetically steered to produce a visual of the coronary artery and the images are produced faster than conventional CT scans.

    d. **Full-field digital mammography (FFDM).** Combines the x-ray generators and tubes used in analog screen-film mammography (SFM) with a detector plate that converts the x-rays into a digital signal.

    e. **Magnetic resonance imaging (MRI).** The use of a uniform magnetic field and radio frequencies to study tissue and structure of the body. This procedure enables the visualization of biochemical activity of the cell in vivo without the use of ionizing radiation, radioisotopic substances or high-frequency sound.

    f. **Intraoperative magnetic resonance imaging.** An integrated surgery system which provides an MRI system in an operating room. The system allows for immediate evaluation of the degree to tumor resection while the patient is undergoing a surgical resection. Intraoperative MRI exists when a MRI (low-field or high-field) is placed in the operating theater and is used during surgical resection without moving the patient from the operating room to the diagnostic imaging suite.

    g. **Magnetoencephalography (MEG).** A noninvasive neurophysiological measurement tool used to study magnetic fields generated by neuronal activity of the brain. MEG provides direct information about the dynamics of evoked and spontaneous neural activity and the location of their sources in the brain. The primary uses of MEG include assisting surgeons in localizing the source of epilepsy, sensory mapping, and the study of brain function. When it is combined with structural imaging, it is known as *magnetic source imaging* (MSI).

    h. **Multi-slice spiral computed tomography (<64+slice CT).** A specialized computed tomography procedure that provides three-dimensional processing and allows narrower and multiple slices with increased spatial resolution and faster scanning times as compared to a regular computed tomography scan.

    i. **Multi-slice spiral computed tomography (64+ slice CT).** Involves the acquisition of volumetric tomographic x-ray absorption data expressed in Hounsfield units using multiple rows of detectors. 64+ systems reconstruct the equivalent of 64 or greater slices to cover the imaged volume.

    j. **Positron emission tomography (PET).** A nuclear medicine imaging technology which uses radioactive (positron emitting) isotopes created in a cyclotron or generator and computers to produce composite pictures of the brain and heart at work. PET scanning produces sectional images depicting metabolic activity or blood flow rather than anatomy.

    k. **Positron emission tomography/CT (PET/CT).** Provides metabolic functional information for the monitoring of chemotherapy, radiotherapy and surgical planning.

    l. **Single photon emission computerized tomography (SPECT).** A nuclear medicine imaging technology that combines existing technology of gamma camera imaging with computed tomographic imaging technology to provide a more precise and clear image.

    m. **Ultrasound.** The use of acoustic waves above the range of 20,000 cycles per second to visualize internal body structures.

84. **Radiology, therapeutic.** The branch of medicine concerned with radioactive substances and using various techniques of visualization, with the diagnosis and treatment of disease using any of the various sources of radiant energy. Services could include: megavoltage radiation therapy; radioactive implants; stereotactic radiosurgery; therapeutic radioisotope facility; X-ray radiation therapy.

    a. **Image-guided radiation therapy (IGRT).** Automated system for image-guided radiation therapy that enables clinicians to obtain high-resolution x-ray images to pinpoint tumor sites, adjust patient positioning when necessary, and complete a treatment, all within the standard treatment time slot, allowing for more effective cancer treatments.

    b. **Intensity-Modulated Radiation Therapy (IMRT).** A type of three-dimensional radiation therapy, which improves the targeting of treatment delivery in a way that is likely to decrease damage to normal tissues and allows varying intensities.

    c. **Proton beam therapy.** A form of radiation therapy which administers proton beams. While producing the same biologic effects as x-ray beams, the energy distribution of protons differs from conventional x-ray beams in that they can be more precisely focused in tissue volumes in a three-dimensional pattern resulting in less surrounding tissue damage than conventional radiation therapy permitting administration of higher doses.

    d. **Shaped beam radiation system.** A precise, non-invasive treatment that involves targeting beams of radiation that mirrors the exact size and shape of a tumor at a specific area of a tumor to shrink or destroy cancerous cells. This procedure delivers a therapeutic dose of radiation that conforms precisely to the shape of the tumor, thus minimizing the risk to nearby tissues.

    e. **Stereotactic radiosurgery.** A radiotherapy modality that delivers a high dosage of radiation to a discrete treatment area in as few as one treatment session. Includes gamma knife, cyberknife, etc.

85. **Retirement housing.** A facility that provides social activities to senior citizens, usually retired persons, who do not require health care but some short-term skilled nursing care may be provided. A retirement center may furnish housing and may also have acute hospital and long-term care facilities, or it may arrange for acute and long-term care through affiliated institutions.

86. **Robotic surgery.** The use of mechanical guidance devices to remotely manipulate surgical instrumentation.

87. **Rural health clinic.** A clinic located in a rural, medically under-served area in the United States that has a separate reimbursement structure from the standard medical office under the Medicare and Medicaid programs.

88. **Sleep center.** Specially equipped and staffed center for the diagnosis and treatment of sleep disorders.

89. **Social work services.** Could include: organized services that are properly directed and sufficiently staffed by qualified individuals who provide assistance and counseling to patients and their families in dealing with social, emotional, and environmental problems associated with illness or disability, often in the context of financial or discharge planning coordination.

90. **Sports medicine.** Provision of diagnostic screening and assessment and clinical and rehabilitation services for the prevention and treatment of sports-related injuries.

91. **Support groups.** A hospital sponsored program that allows a group of individuals with the same or similar problems who meet periodically to share experiences, problems, and solutions in order to support each other.

92. **Swing bed services.** A hospital bed that can be used to provide either acute or long-term care depending on community or patient needs. To be eligible a hospital must have a Medicare provider agreement in place, have fewer than 100 beds, be located in a rural area, do not have a 24 hour nursing service waiver in effect, have not been terminated from the program in the prior two years, and meet various service conditions.

93. **Teen outreach services.** A program focusing on the teenager which encourages an improved health status and a healthful lifestyle including physical, emotional, mental, social, spiritual and economic health through education, exercise, nutrition and health promotion.

94. **Tobacco treatment/cessation program.** Organized hospital services with the purpose of ending tobacco-use habits of patients addicted to tobacco/nicotine.

95. **Transplant services.** The branch of medicine that transfers an organ or tissue from one person to another or from one body part to another to replace a diseased structure or to restore function or to change appearance. Services could include: Bone marrow transplant program; heart, lung, kidney, intestine, or tissue transplant. Please include heart/lung or other multi-transplant surgeries in 'other'.

96. **Transportation to health facilities.** A long-term care support service designed to assist the mobility of the elderly. Some programs offer improved financial access by offering reduced rates and barrier-free buses or vans with ramps and lifts to assist the elderly or handicapped; others offer subsidies for public transport systems or operate mini-bus services exclusively for use by senior citizens.

97. **Urgent care center.** A facility that provides care and treatment for problems that are not life threatening but require attention over the short term.

98. **Virtual colonoscopy.** Noninvasive screening procedure used to visualize, analyze and detect cancerous or potentially cancerous polyps in the colon.

99. **Volunteer services department.** An organized hospital department responsible for coordinating the services of volunteers working within the institution.

100. **Women's health center/services.** An area set aside for coordinated education and treatment services specifically for and promoted to women as provided by this special unit. Services may or may not include obstetrics but include a range of services other than OB.

101. **Wound management services.** Services for patients with chronic wounds and nonhealing wounds often resulting from diabetes, poor circulation, improper seating and immunocompromising conditions. The goals are to progress chronic wounds through stages of healing, reduce and eliminate infections, increase physical function to minimize complications from current wounds and prevent future chronic wounds. Wound management services are provided on an inpatient or outpatient basis, depending on the intensity of service needed.

102a. **Physician arrangements.** An integrated healthcare delivery program implementing physician compensation and incentive systems for managed care services.

    a. **Independent practice association (IPA).** A legal entity that holds managed care contracts. The IPA then contracts with physicians, usually in solo practice, to provide care either on a fee-for-services or capitated basis. The purpose of an IPA is to assist solo physicians in obtaining managed care contracts.

    b. **Group practice without walls.** Hospital sponsors the formation of, or provides capital to physicians to establish, a "quasi" group to share administrative expenses while remaining independent practitioners.

    c. **Open physician-hospital organization (PHO).** A joint venture between the hospital and all members of the medical staff who wish to participate. The PHO can act as a unified agent in managed care contracting, own a managed care plan, own and operate ambulatory care centers or ancillary services projects, or provide administrative services to physician members.

    d. **Closed physician-hospital organization (PHO).** A PHO that restricts physician membership to those practitioners who meet criteria for cost effectiveness and/or high quality.

e. **Management services organization (MSO).** A corporation, owned by the hospital or a physician/hospital joint venture, that provides management services to one or more medical group practices. The MSO purchases the tangible assets of the practices and leases them back as part of a full-service management agreement, under which the MSO employs all non-physician staff and provides all supplies/administrative systems for a fee.

f. **Integrated salary model.** Physicians are salaried by the hospital or another entity of a health system to provide medical services for primary care and specialty care.

g. **Equity model.** Allows established practitioners to become shareholders in a professional corporation in exchange for tangible and intangible assets of their existing practices.

h. **Foundation.** A corporation, organized either as a hospital affiliate or subsidiary, which purchases both the tangible and intangible assets of one or more medical group practices. Physicians remain in a separate corporate entity but sign a professional services agreement with the foundation.

102b. Of all physician arrangements listed in question 102a (a-i), indicate the total number of physicians (count each physician only once) that are engaged in an arrangement with your hospital that allows for joint contracting with payers or shared responsibility for financial risk or clinical performance between the hospital and physician (arrangement may be at the hospital, system or network level). *Joint contracting* does not include contracting between physicians participating in an independent practice.

103. Joint venture. A contractual arrangement between two or more parties forming an unincorporated business. The participants in the arrangement remain independent and separate outside of the ventures purpose.

104a. Accountable Care Organization (ACO) Contract. An ACO contract has two essential elements: (1) accountability for the total costs of care for the population of patients attributed to the primary care physicians in the organization; (2) financial incentives that link the magnitude of bonus payments to performance on quality measures (which could include technical quality, patient experience and/or health outcome measures). This will generally involve a contract where the payer establishes a target budget for one or more years for the total costs of care for the agreed-upon patient population, the payer tracks actual spending and performance on quality; and the provider receives bonus payments that could include a share of savings that are (or are not) contingent on meeting quality targets, with (or without) additional bonuses related to performance on those quality measures.

105. Patient-Centered Medical Home. The medical home concept refers to the provision of comprehensive primary care services that facilitates communication and shared decision-making between the patient, his/her primary care providers, other providers, and the patient's family.

106. Bundling. Bundling is a payment mechanism whereby a provider entity receives a single payment for services provided across one or parts of the care continuum. For example, an entity might receive a single payment for the hospital and physician services provided as part of an inpatient stay or might receive a single payment for the post-acute care services involved in a single episode of care. The entity then has responsibility for compensating each of the individual providers involved in the episode of care.

109. Capitation. An at-risk payment arrangement in which an organization receives a fixed prearranged payment and in turn guarantees to deliver or arrange all medically necessary care required by enrollees in the capitated plan. The fixed amount is specified within contractual agreements between the payor and the involved organization. The fixed payment amount is based on an actuarial assessment of the services required by enrollees and the costs of providing these services, recognizing enrollees' adjustment factors such as age, sex, and family size.

110. Shared risk payments. A payment arrangement in which a hospital and a managed care organization share the risk of adverse claims experience. Methods for sharing risk could include: capitation with partial refunds or supplements if billed hospital charges or costs differ from capitated payments, and service or discharge-based payments with withholds and bonus payouts that depend on expenditure targets.

SECTION D
TOTAL FACILITY BEDS, UTILIZATION, FINANCES, AND STAFFING
Instructions and Definitions

For the purposes of this survey, nursing home type unit/facility provides **long-term care for the elderly or other patients requiring chronic care** in a non-acute setting in any of the following categories: *Skilled nursing care *Intermediate care *Other Long-term Care (*see page 16 definitions)The nursing home type units/facilities are to be owned and operated by the hospital. Only one legal entity may be vested with title to the physical property or operate under the authority of a duly executed lease of the physical property.

1 a. **Total licensed beds** are the total number of beds authorized by the state licensing (certifying agency).

b. Report the number of **beds** regularly available (those **set up and staffed for use**) at the end of the reporting period. Report only operating beds, not constructed bed capacity. Include all bed facilities that are set up and staffed for use by inpatients that have no other bed facilities, such as pediatric bassinets, isolation units, quiet rooms, and reception and observation units assigned to or reserved for them. Exclude newborn bassinets and bed facilities for patients receiving special procedures for a portion of their stay and who have other bed facilities assigned to or reserved for them. Exclude, for example, labor room, post anesthesia, or postoperative recovery room beds, psychiatric holding beds, and beds that are used only as holding facilities for patients prior to their transfer to another hospital.

c. Report the number of normal newborn **bassinets**. Do not include neonatal intensive care or intermediate care bassinets. These should be reported on page 3, C6 and C7.

d. Total **births** should exclude fetal deaths.

e. Include the number of adult and pediatric **admissions** only (exclude births). This figure should include all patients admitted during the reporting period, including neonatal and swing admissions.

f. Report the number of adult and pediatric **days of care** rendered during the entire reporting period. Do not include days of care rendered for normal infants born in the hospital, but do include those for their mothers. Include days of care for infants born in the hospital and transferred into a neonatal care unit. Also include swing bed inpatient days. **Inpatient day** of care (also commonly referred to as a **patient day** or a **census day**, or by some federal hospitals as an **occupied bed day**) is a period of service between the census-taking hours on two successive calendar days, the day of discharge being counted only when the patient was admitted the same day.

g. **Emergency department visits** should reflect the number of visits to the emergency unit. Emergency outpatients can be admitted to the inpatient areas of the hospital, but they are still counted as emergency visits and subsequently as inpatient admissions.

h. An **Outpatient visit** is a visit by a patient who is not lodged in the hospital while receiving medical, dental, or other services. Each appearance of an outpatient in each unit constitutes one visit regardless of the number of diagnostic and/or therapeutic treatments that the patient receives. Total outpatient visits should include all clinic visits, referred visits, observation services, outpatient surgeries (also reported on line D1k), home health service visits, and emergency department visits (also reported on line D1g).
Clinic visits should reflect total number of visits to each specialized medical unit that is responsible for the diagnosis and treatment of patients on an outpatient, nonemergency basis (i.e., alcoholism, dental, gynecology, etc.). Visits to the satellite clinics and primary group practices should be included if revenue is received by the hospital.
Referred visits should reflect total number of outpatient ancillary visits to each specialty unit of the hospital established for providing technical aid used in the diagnosis and treatment of patients. Examples of such units are diagnostic radiology, EKG, pharmacy, etc.
Observation services are those services furnished on a hospital's premises, including use of a bed and periodic monitoring by a hospital's nursing

or other staff, which are reasonable and necessary to evaluate an outpatient's condition or determine the need for a possible admission to the hospital as an inpatient. Observation services usually do not exceed 24 hours. However, there is no hourly limit on the extent to which they may be used.

Home health service visits are visits by home health personnel to a patient's residence.

i. **Inpatient surgical operation.** Count each patient undergoing surgery as one surgical operation regardless of the number of surgical procedures that were performed while the patient was in the operating or procedure room.

j. **Operating room.** A unit/room of a hospital or other health care facility in which surgical procedures requiring anesthesia are performed.

k. **Outpatient surgical operation.** For outpatient surgical operations, please record operations performed on patients who do not remain in the hospital overnight. Include all operations whether performed in the inpatient operating rooms or in procedure rooms located in an outpatient facility. Include an endoscopy only when used as an operative tool and not when used for diagnosis alone. Count each patient undergoing surgery as one surgical operation regardless of the number of surgical procedures that were performed while the patient was in the operating or procedure room.

2a2. Managed Care Medicare Discharges. A discharge day where a Medicare Managed Care Plan is the source of payment.

2b2. Managed Care Medicare Inpatient Days. An inpatient day where a Medicare Managed Care Plan is the source of payment.

2c2. Managed Care Medicaid Discharges. A discharge day where a Medicaid Managed Care Plan is the source of payment.

2d2. Managed Care Medicaid Inpatient Days. An inpatient day where a Medicaid Managed Care Plan is the source of payment.

3a. Net patient revenue. Reported at the estimated net realizable amounts from patients, third-party payors, and others for services rendered, including estimated retroactive adjustments under reimbursement agreements with third-party payors. Retroactive adjustments are accrued on an estimated basis in the period the related services are rendered and adjusted in future periods, as final settlements are determined.

3b. Tax appropriations. A predetermined amount set aside by the government from its taxing authority to support the operation of the hospital.

3c. Other operating revenue. Revenue from services other than health care provided to patients, as well as sales and services to nonpatients. Revenue that arises from the normal day-to-day operations from services other than health care provided to patients. Includes sales and services to nonpatients, and revenue from miscellaneous sources (rental of hospital space, sale of cafeteria meals, gift shop sales). Also include operating gains in this category.

3d. Nonoperating revenue. Includes investment income, extraordinary gains and other nonoperating gains.

3e. Total revenue. Add net patient revenue, tax appropriations, other operating revenue and nonoperating revenue.

3f. Payroll expenses. Include payroll for all personnel including medical and dental residents/interns and trainees.

3g. Employee benefits. Includes social security, group insurance, retirement benefits, workman's compensation, unemployment insurance, etc.

3h. Depreciation expense (for reporting period only) report only the depreciation expense applicable to the reporting period. The amount also Should be included in accumulated depreciation (D7b).

3i. Interest expense. Report interest expense for the reporting period only.

3j. Supply expense. The net cost of all tangible items that are expensed including freight, standard distribution cost, and sales and use tax minus rebates. This would exclude labor, labor-related expenses and services as well as some tangible items that are frequently provided as part of labor costs.

3k.Total expenses. Includes all payroll and non-payroll expenses as well as any nonoperating losses (including extraordinary losses). **Treat bad debt as a deduction from gross patient revenue and not as an expense.**

4a. Total gross inpatient revenue. The hospitals full-established rates(charges) for all services rendered to inpatients.

4b. Total gross outpatient revenue. The hospitals full-established rates(charges) for all services rendered to outpatients.

4c. Total gross patient revenue. Total gross patient revenue (add total gross inpatient revenue and total gross outpatient revenue).

5. **Uncompensated care.** Care for which no payment is expected or no charge is made. It is the sum of bad debt and charity care absorbed by a hospital or other health care organization in providing medical care for patients who are uninsured or are unable to pay.

5a. Bad debt. The provision for actual or expected uncollectibles resulting from the extension of credit. Report as a deduction from revenue.

5b. Financial Assistance (Includes **Charity care).** Financial assistance and charity care refer to health services provided free of charge or at reduced rates to individuals who meet certain financial criteria . For purposes of this survey, charity care is measured on the basis of revenue forgone, at full-established rates.

5d. Medicaid Provider Tax, Fee or Assessment. Dollars paid as a result of a state law that authorizes collecting revenue from specified categories of providers. Federal matching funds may be received for the revenue collected from providers and some or all of the revenues may be returned directly or indirectly back to providers in the form of a Medicaid payment.

6. **REVENUE BY PAYOR**

6a1   Medicare. Should agree with the Medicare utilization reported in questions D2a1-D2b2.

6a1a Fee for service patient revenue. Include traditional Medicare fee-for-service.

6a1c. Total. Medicare revenue (add Medicare fee for service patient revenue and Medicare managed care revenue).

6a2. Medicaid. Should agree with Medicaid utilization reported in questions D2c1-D2d2.

6a2a. Fee for service patient revenue. Do not include Medicaid disproportionate payments(DSH) or Medicaid supplemental payments that are non-Medicaid disproportionate payments (DSH).

6a2c. Medicaid disproportionate share payments. DSH minus associated provider taxes or assessments. Report in 'Net' column only.

6a2d. Medicaid supplemental payments. Not including Medicaid DSH payments (these are supplemental payments the Medicaid program pays the hospital that are NOT Medicaid DSH) and minus associated provider taxes or assessments. Report in 'Net' column only.

7 **a-c. Fixed Assets.** Represent land and physical properties that are consumed or used in the creation of economic activity by the health care entity. The historical or acquisition costs are used in recording fixed assets. Net plant, property, and equipment represent the original costs of these items less accumulated depreciation and amortization.

7d. Gross Square Footage. Include all inpatient, outpatient, office, and support space used for or in support of your health care activities. Exclude exterior, roof, and garage space in the figure.

8. **Capital Expenses.** Expenses used to acquire assets, including buildings, remodeling projects, equipment, or property.

9. **Information Technology.**

   a. **IT Operating expense.** Exclude department depreciation and operating dollars paid against capital leases.

   b. **IT Capital expense.** Include IT capital expense for the current year only. Any capital expense that is carried forward from the previous year should be excluded from this figure. Include IT related capital included in the budget of other departments. (i.e. lab, radiology, etc., if known or can be reasonably estimated.) Include the total value of capital leases to be signed in the current year.

   c. **Number of Employed IT staff (in FTEs).** Number of full-time equivalent (FTE) staff employed in the IT department/organization and on the hospital payroll.

   d. **Total number of outsourced IT staff (in FTEs).** i.e. contracted staff.

   e. **Electronic Health Record.** An electronic health record (EHR) integrates electronically originated and maintained patient-level clinical health information, derived from multiple sources, into one point of access. An EHR replaces the paper medical record as the primary source of patient information.

10. Full-Time Equivalent (FTE) is the total number of hours worked by all employees over the full (12 month) reporting period divided by the normal number of hours worked by a full-time employee for that same time period. For example, if your hospital considers a normal workweek for a full-time employee to be 40 hours, a total of 2,080 would be worked over a full year (52 weeks). If the total number of hours worked by all employees on the payroll is 208,000, then the number of Full-Time Equivalents (FTE) is 100 (employees). The FTE calculation for a specific occupational category such as registered nurses is exactly the same. The calculation for each occupational category should be based on the number of hours worked by staff employed in that specific category.

a-b. Physicians and dentists. Include only those physicians and dentists engaged in clinical practice and on the payroll. Those who hold administrative positions should be reported in "All other personnel."

d. Other trainees. A trainee is a person who has not completed the necessary requirements for certification or met the qualifications required for full salary under a related occupational category. Exclude medical and dental residents/interns who should be reported on line 10c.

e. Registered nurses. Nurses who have graduated from approved schools of nursing and who are currently registered by the state. They are responsible for the nature and quality of all nursing care that patients receive. Do not include any registered nurses more appropriately reported in other occupational categories, such as facility administrators, and therefore listed under "All other personnel."

f. Licensed practical (vocational) nurses. Nurses who have graduated from an approved school of practical (vocational) nursing who work under the supervision of registered nurses and/or physicians.

g. Nursing assistive personnel. Certified nursing assistant or equivalent unlicensed staff assigned to patient care units and reporting to nursing.

h. Radiology Technicians. Technical positions in imaging fields, including, but not limited to, radiology, sonography, nuclear medicine, radiation therapy, CT, MRI.

i. Laboratory professional/technical. Professional and technical positions in all areas of the laboratory, including, but not limited to, histology, phlebotomy, microbiology, pathology, chemistry, etc.

j. Pharmacists, licensed. Persons licensed within the state who are concerned with the preparation and distribution of medicinal products.

k. Pharmacy technicians. Persons who assist the pharmacist with selected activities, including medication profile reviews for drug incompatibilities, typing labels and prescription packaging, handling of purchase records and inventory control.

l. Respiratory Therapists. An allied health professional who specializes in scientific knowledge and theory of clinical problems of respiratory care. Duties include the collection and evaluation of patient data to determine and appropriate care plan, selection and assembly of equipment, conduction of therapeutic procedures, and modification of prescribed plans to achieve one or more specific objectives.

m. All other personnel. This should include all other personnel not already accounted for in other categories.

n. Total facility personnel. This line is to include the total facility personnel - hospital plus nursing home type unit/facility personnel (for those hospitals that own and operate a nursing home type unit/facility).

o-p. Nursing home type unit/facility personnel. These lines should be filled out only by hospitals that own and operate a nursing home type unit/facility, where only one legal entity is vested with title to the physical property or operates under the authority of a duly executed lease of the physical property. If nursing home type unit/facility personnel are reported on the total facility personnel line, but cannot be broken out, please write "cannot break out" on this line.

11. Privileged Physicians. Report the total number of physicians (by type) on the medical staff with privileges except those with courtesy, honorary and provisional privileges. Do not include residents or interns.

Employed by your hospital. Physicians that are either direct hospital employees or employees of a hospital subsidiary corporation. Physicians that are employed for non-clinical services (administrative services, medical director services, etc.) should be excluded.

Individual contract. An independent physician under a formal contract to provide services at your hospital including at outpatient facilities, clinics and offices. Physicians that are contracted only for non-clinical services (administrative services, medical director services, etc.) should be excluded.

Group contract. A physician that is part of a group (group practice, faculty practice plan or medical foundation) under a formal contract to provide services at your hospital including at inpatient and outpatient facilities, clinics and offices. Physicians that are contracted only for non-clinical services (administrative services, medical director services, etc.) should be excluded.

Not employed or under contract. Other physicians with privileges that have no employment or contractual relationship with the hospital to provide services.

The sum of the physicians reported in 11a-11f should equal the total number of privileged physicians in the hospital.

a. Primary care. A physician that provides primary care services including general practice, general internal medicine, family practice, general pediatrics, obstetrics/gynecology and geriatrics.

b. Emergency medicine. Physicians who provide care in the emergency department.

c. Hospitalist. Physician whose primary professional focus is the care of hospitalized medical patients (through clinical, education, administrative and research activity).

d. Intensivist. A physician with special training to work with critically ill patients. Intensivists generally provided medical-surgical, cardiac, neonatal, pediatric and other types of intensive care.

e. Radiologist/pathologist/anesthesiologist. Radiologist. A physician who has specialized training in imaging, including but not limited to radiology, sonography, nuclear medicine, radiation therapy, CT, MRI. **Pathologist.** A physician who examines samples of body tissues for diagnostic purposes. **Anesthesiologist.** A physician who specializes in administering medications or other agents that prevent or relieve pain, especially during surgery.

f. Other specialist. Other physicians not included in the above categories that specialize in a specific type of medical care.

14. Advanced Practice Registered Nurses. Registered nurses with advanced didactic and clinical education, knowledge, skills, and scope of practice. Includes: **Physician assistant.** A healthcare professional licensed to practice medicine with supervision of a licensed physician. **Nurse practitioner.** A registered nurse with at least a master's degree in nursing and advanced education in primary care, capable of independent practice in a variety of settings. **Clinical nurse specialist (CNS).** A registered nurse who, through a formal graduate degree (masters or doctorate) CNS education program, is prepared as CNS with expertise in a specialty area of nursing practice. CNSs are clinical experts in the diagnosis and treatment of illness, and the delivery of evidence-based nursing interventions.

14c. Primary care. Medical services including general practice, general internal medicine, family practice, general pediatrics, obstetrics/gynecology.

Emergency department care. The provision of unscheduled outpatient services to patients whose conditions require immediate care in the emergency department setting.

Other specialty care. A clinician that provides specialized medical care beyond the scope of primary care.

Patient education. Goals and objectives for the patient and/or family related to therapeutic regimens, medical procedures and self-care.

Case management. A system of assessment, treatment planning, referral and follow-up that ensures the provision of comprehensive and continuous services and the coordination of payment and reimbursement for care.

Other. Any type of care other than those listed above.

15. Foreign-educated nurses. Individuals who are foreign born and received basic nursing education in a foreign country. In general many of these nurses come to the US on employment-based visas which allow them to obtain a green card.

2c. Diversity plan. A set of goals and objectives that are linked to the organization's strategic plan to promote the elimination of disparities and identify strategies to ensure the ethnic and racial composition of the workforce better reflects the composition of the communities being served.

3a. Satellite facility(ies). Services are available at a facility geographically remote from the hospital campus.

3b. Group Purchasing Organization. An organization whose primary function is to negotiate contracts for the purpose of purchasing for members of the group or has a central supply site for its members.

3c. Distributor. An entity that typically does not manufacture most of its own products but purchases and re-sells these products. Such a business usually maintains an inventory of products for sales to hospitals and physician offices and others.